Lecture Notes in Computer Science   7509

Commenced Publication in 1973
Founding and Former Series Editors:
Gerhard Goos, Juris Hartmanis, and Jan van Leeuwen

Pew-Thian Yap   Tianming Liu
Dinggang Shen   Carl-Fredrik Westin
Li Shen (Eds.)

Multimodal Brain Image Analysis

Second International Workshop, MBIA 2012
Held in Conjunction with MICCAI 2012
Nice, France, October 1-5, 2012
Proceedings

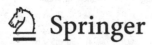 Springer

Volume Editors

Pew-Thian Yap
Dinggang Shen
The University of North Carolina at Chapel Hill, School of Medicine
Department of Radiology and Biomedical Reserach Imaging Center
130 Mason Farm Road, Chapel Hill, NC 27599, USA
E-mail: {ptyap, dgshen}@med.unc.edu

Tianming Liu
The University of Georgia
Department of Computer Science and Bioimaging Research Center
Boyd GSRC 422, Athens, GA 30602, USA
E-mail: tliu@cs.uga.edu

Carl-Fredrik Westin
Harvard Medical School, Brigham and Women's Hospital
Department of Radiology
1249 Boylston Street, Boston, MA 02215, USA
E-mail: westin@bwh.harvard.edu

Li Shen
Indiana University, School of Medicine
Department of Radiology and Imaging Sciences
950 W Walnut Street, R2 E124, Indianapolis, IN 46202, USA
E-mail: shenli@iupui.edu

ISSN 0302-9743   e-ISSN 1611-3349
ISBN 978-3-642-33529-7   e-ISBN 978-3-642-33530-3
DOI 10.1007/978-3-642-33530-3
Springer Heidelberg Dordrecht London New York

Library of Congress Control Number: 2012947117

CR Subject Classification (1998): I.4, I.5, H.3, I.3.5-8, I.2.10, J.3

LNCS Sublibrary: SL 6 – Image Processing, Computer Vision, Pattern Recognition,
and Graphics

Typesetting: Camera-ready by author, data conversion by Scientific Publishing Services, Chennai, India

Printed on acid-free paper

Springer is part of Springer Science+Business Media (www.springer.com)

Preface

The 2nd international workshop on Multimodal Brain Image Analysis (MBIA) was held on October 1, 2012 in conjunction with the 15th international conference on Medical Image Computing and Computer Assisted Intervention (MICCAI) at the Nice Acropolis Convention Center, Nice, France, with the objective of moving forward the state of the art in analysis methodologies, algorithms, software systems, validation approaches, benchmark datasets, neuroscience, and clinical applications.

Brain imaging technologies such as structural MRI, diffusion MRI, perfusion MRI, functional MRI, EEG, MEG, PET, SPECT, and CT are playing increasingly important roles in unraveling brain structural and functional patterns that give unprecedented insights into how the brain orchestrates an immense web of intricate functions. It is widely held that these imaging modalities provide distinctive yet complementary information that is critical to the understanding of the working dynamics of the brain. However, effective processing, fusion, analysis, and visualization of images from multiple sources are significantly more challenging, owing to the variation in imaging resolutions, spatial-temporal dynamics, and the fundamental biophysical mechanisms that determine the characteristics of the images. The MBIA workshop is a forum dedicated to the exchange of ideas, data, and software among researchers, with the goal of fostering the development of innovative technologies that will propel hypothesis testing and data-driven discovery in brain science.

This year the workshop received 23 submissions (including 7 invited papers). Based on the scores and recommendations provided by the Program Committee, which consists of 25 notable experts in the field, 19 papers were selected for poster presentations. Out of these 14 were selected for podium presentation.

We are enormously grateful to the authors for their high-quality submissions, the Program Committee for evaluating the papers, the presenters for their excellent presentations, and all who supported MBIA 2012 by attending the meeting.

July 2012

Pew-Thian Yap
Tianming Liu
Dinggang Shen
Carl-Fredrik Westin
Li Shen

Organization

Program Committee

John Ashburner	University College London, UK
Christian Barillot	IRISA Rennes, France
Vince Calhoun	University of New Mexico, USA
Gary Christensen	University of Iowa, USA
Moo K. Chung	University of Wisconsin-Madison, USA
Rachid Deriche	INRIA, France
James Gee	University of Pennsylvania, USA
Xiujuan Geng	UNC Chapel Hill, USA
Dewen Hu	National University of Defense Technology, China
Xiaoping Hu	Emory University, USA
Heng Huang	University of Texas, Arlington, USA
Tianzi Jiang	Chinese Academy of Science, China
David Kennedy	University of Massachusetts Medical School, USA
Xiaofeng Liu	GE Global Research, USA
Jerry Prince	Johns Hopkins University, USA
Daniel Rueckert	Imperial College London, UK
Feng Shi	UNC Chapel Hill, USA
Yalin Wang	Arizona State University, USA
Yongmei Wang	University of Illinois at Urbana-Champaign, USA
Simon Warfield	Harvard Medical School and Boston Children's Hospital, USA
Chong-Yaw Wee	UNC Chapel Hill, USA
Thomas Yeo	Duke-NUS Graduate Medical School, Singapore
Daoqiang Zhang	Nanjing University of Aeronautics and Astronautics, China
Gary Zhang	University College London, UK
Dajiang Zhu	University of Georgia, USA

Table of Contents

Multimodal Neuroimaging Predictors for Cognitive Performance Using Structured Sparse Learning

Jingwen Yan[1,2], Shannon L. Risacher[1], Sungeun Kim[1], Jacqueline C. Simon[1,3], Taiyong Li[1,4], Jing Wan[1,5], Hua Wang[6], Heng Huang[6,*], Andrew J. Saykin[1,*], and Li Shen[1,2,5,*], for the Alzheimer's Disease Neuroimaging Initiative[**]

[1] Radiology and Imaging Sciences, Indiana University School of Medicine, IN, USA
[2] School of Informatics, Indiana University Indianapolis, IN, USA
[3] Biomedical Engineering and Mathematics, Rose-Hulman Inst. of Tech., IN, USA
[4] Economic Info. Eng., Southwestern Univ. of Finance & Economics, Chengdu, China
[5] Computer and Information Science, Purdue University Indianapolis, IN, USA
[6] Computer Science and Engineering, University of Texas at Arlington, TX, USA

Abstract. Regression models have been widely studied to investigate whether multimodal neuroimaging measures can be used as effective biomarkers for predicting cognitive outcomes in the study of Alzheimer's Disease (AD). Most existing models overlook the interrelated structures either within neuroimaging measures or between cognitive outcomes, and thus may have limited power to yield optimal solutions. To address this issue, we propose to incorporate an $\ell_{2,1}$ norm and/or a group $\ell_{2,1}$ norm ($G_{2,1}$ norm) in the regression models. Using ADNI-1 and ADNI-GO/2 data, we apply these models to examining the ability of structural MRI and AV-45 PET scans for predicting cognitive measures including ADAS and RAVLT scores. We focus our analyses on the participants with mild cognitive impairment (MCI), a prodromal stage of AD, in order to identify useful patterns for early detection. Compared with traditional linear and ridge regression methods, these new models not only demonstrate superior and more stable predictive performances, but also identify a small set of imaging markers that are biologically meaningful.

1 Introduction

Alzheimer's disease (AD) is a neurodegenerative disorder characterized by gradual loss of brain function, especially the memory and cognitive capabilities.

[*] Correspondence to Li Shen (shenli@iupui.edu), Heng Huang (heng@uta.edu), or Andrew J. Saykin (asaykin@iupui.edu).
[**] Data used in preparation of this article were obtained from the Alzheimer's Disease Neuroimaging Initiative (ADNI) database (adni.loni.ucla.edu). As such, the investigators within the ADNI contributed to the design and implementation of ADNI and/or provided data but did not participate in analysis or writing of this report. A complete listing of ADNI investigators can be found at: http://adni.loni.ucla.edu/wp-content/uploads/how_to_apply/ADNI_Acknowledgement_List.pdf

P.-T. Yap et al. (Eds.): MBIA 2012, LNCS 7509, pp. 1–17, 2012.
© Springer-Verlag Berlin Heidelberg 2012

Multimodal neuroimaging has been studied as a potential biomarker for early detection of AD, since brain characteristics relevant to memory and cognitive decline may be captured by magnetic resonance imaging (MRI) morphometry [5,7] and positron emission tomography (PET) metabolism [8,11]. Regression models have been used to study whether these neuroimaging measures can help predict clinical scores and track AD progression [14,17,18,20,21,25,26].

Early studies focused on predicting selected cognitive scores one at a time using statistical learning approaches such as stepwise regression [17] and relevance vector regression [14]. Recent studies employed advanced multi-task learning strategies, aiming for performance enhancement via joint prediction of multiple scores simultaneously. While $\ell_{2,1}$-norm [20,21,25,26] was commonly used to select features that could predict all or most clinical scores, a sparse Bayesian method [18] was proposed to explicitly estimate the covariance structure among multiple outcome measures and demonstrated improved prediction rates.

The studies mentioned above all analyzed the neuroimaging, biomarker and cognitive data from the Alzheimer's Disease Neuroimaging Initiative (ADNI) database [22,23]. The MRI, FDG-PET, and cerebrospinal fluid (CSF) biomarker data from the ADNI-1 phase were used either individually (e.g., MRI [14,17,18, 20,21], FDG-PET [17]) or jointly (e.g., MRI and FDG-PET [26]; MRI, FDG-PET and CSF [25]) to predict selected cognitive scores from neuropsychological tests such as Mini-Mental State Examination (MMSE) [14,18,20,25,26], Alzheimer's Disease Assessment Scale-Cognitive subtest (ADAS-Cog) [14,25,26], Rey Auditory Verbal Learning Test (RAVLT) [14,17,18,20,21], and Trail-making test (TRAILS) [18,20].

Although some of the above methods considered the correlation among cognitive measures, none modeled the interrelated structure within the predictor variables. To address this issue, we propose to employ a new structured sparse learning model called G-SMuRFS (Group-Sparse Multi-task Regression and Feature Selection) [19] for multivariate regression of cognitive scores on neuroimaging data. Motivated by Lasso [16] and group Lasso [24], G-SMuRFS was proposed by us in an imaging genetic application [19], where an $\ell_{2,1}$-norm was used to bundle all the outcome imaging measures together and a group $\ell_{2,1}$-norm ($G_{2,1}$-norm) was used to model the block structure within genetic predictors.

In this study, we demonstrate the effectiveness of structured sparse learning models (including $\ell_{2,1}$-norm and $G_{2,1}$-norm) by applying them to analyze the new data collected at the ADNI-GO and ADNI-2 phases. In particular, we concentrate on the participants with mild cognitive impairment (MCI, thought to be a prodromal stage of AD), including the newly enrolled cohort called early MCI (EMCI) and the cohort of amnestic MCI (now referred to as late MCI, or LMCI). In addition to the MRI data, we evaluate the predictive power of the new AV45-PET data (for amyloid plaque imaging) available for all the ADNI-GO/2 participants, as well as examine whether combining MRI and AV45-PET can help improve the prediction performance. For comparison purpose, we also conduct the same analyses on the MRI data of the ADNI-1 MCI cohort.

Table 1. Participant characteristics

| Category | ADNI-1 | ADNI-GO/2 | |
	LMCI	EMCI	LMCI
Number	388	181	57
Gender(M/F)	250/138	105/76	32/25
Handness(R/L)	353/35	160/21	50/7
Baseline Age(mean±std)	74.8±7.4	70.6±7.4	72.6±7.7
Education(mean±std)	15.7±3.0	16.0±2.6	16.8±2.4

2   Materials and Methods

2.1   Imaging and Cognition Data

All the data used in this study are obtained from the Alzheimer's Disease Neu-roimaging Initiative (ADNI) database (adni.loni.ucla.edu). One goal of ADNI has been to test whether serial MRI, PET, other biological markers, and clinical and neuropsychological assessment can be combined to measure the progression of MCI and early AD. For up-to-date information, see www.adni-info.org.

In this study, we first focus on analyzing the MRI and AV45-PET data ob-tained at the ADNI-GO and ADNI-2 phases, and then conduct a similar analysis on the ADNI-1 MRI data for performance comparison. All the participants with a baseline diagnosis of MCI (EMCI or LMCI) are included in the study, including 388 from ADNI-1 and 238 from ADNI-GO/2 (Table 1). Corrected 3T structural MRI scans [6], pre-processed AV-45 PET scans [9], and clinical and psychometric performance data are downloaded from the ADNI website (adni.loni.ucla.edu).

Structural MRI scans are processed with voxel-based morphometry (VBM) in SPM8 [1], as previously described [13]. Briefly, scans are aligned to a T1-weighted template image, segmented into gray matter (GM), white matter (WM) and cerebrospinal fluid (CSF) maps, normalized to MNI space, and smoothed with an 8mm FWHM kernal. All scans are also processed using automated segmentation and parcellation using Freesurfer version 5.1 [2–4]. Using the regression weights derived from the healthy control participants, VBM measures are pre-adjusted for removing the effects of the baseline age, gender, education, and handedness, and FreeSurfer measures are pre-adjusted for removing the effects of the baseline age, gender, education, handedness, and intracranial volume (ICV).

AV-45 PET scans are pre-processed using techniques identical to the previ-ously described techniques for processing of ADNI PiB PET scans [9]. Stan-dardized uptake value ratio (SUVR) AV-45 PET images are created by intensity normalizing to a mean cerebellar GM region of interest (ROI). Downloaded scans are co-registered to the structural MRI scan from the corresponding visit and normalized to MNI space using SPM8, as described previously [15]. Mean AV-45 measures are calculated for seven ROIs, including frontal lobe, parietal lobe, temporal lobe, occipital lobe, anterior cingulate, poster cingulate, and precuneus.

To sum up, we have 90 VBM measures (Table 2), 95 Freesurfer measures (Table 2) and seven AV45 measures (Figure 7). Using these imaging measures as

Table 2. MRI data: 95 Freesurfer measures and 90 VBM measures

Regional Group	FreeSurfer Volume (29 in total)
Subcortical (temporal)	AmygVol, HippVol
Subcortical (striatum/basal ganglia)	AccumVol, CaudVol, PallVol, PutamVol
Subcortical (thalamus)	ThalVol
Cerebellum	CerebellCtx, CerebellWM
Ventricles	InfLatVent, LatVent, CSF*
Corpus Collosum (WM)	CC_Ant*, CC_Cent*, CC_Post*, CC_MidPost*, CC_MidAnt*
Brainstem	BrainStem*
	*Seven measures are unilateral.

Regional Group	FreeSurfer Thickness (66 in total)
Frontal Lobe	CaudMidFrontal, FrontalPole, LatOrbFrontal, MedOrbFrontal, ParsOper, ParsOrb, ParsTriang, RostMidFrontal, SupFrontal
Cingulate	CaudAntCing, IsthmCing, PostCing, RostAntCing
Parietal Lobe	InfParietal, Precuneus, SupParietal, Supramarg
Temporal Lobe	BanksSTS, EntCtx, Fusiform, InfTemporal, Lingual, MidTemporal, Parahipp, SupTemporal, TemporalPole, TransvTemporal
Occipital Lobe	Cuneus, LatOccipital, Pericalc
Sensory-Motor Cortex	Paracentral, Postcentral, Precentral

Regional Group	VBM GM Density (90 in total)
Subcortical (temporal)	Amygdala, Hippocampus
Subcortical (striatum/basal ganglia)	Caudate, Pallidum, Putamen
Subcortical (thalamus)	Thalamus
Frontal Lobe	InfFrontal_Oper, InfOrbFrontal, MidFrontal, InfFrontal_Triang, MedOrbFrontal, Rectus, MedSupFrontal, MidOrbFrontal, SupFrontal, SupOrbFrontal, Rolandic_Oper, SuppMotorArea
Cingulate	AntCingulate, MidCingulate, PostCingulate
Parietal Lobe	Angular, InfParietal, SupParietal, Precuneus, Supramarg
Temporal Lobe (cortical)	Fusiform, Heschl, Lingual, Olfactory, Parahipp, InfTemporal, MidTemporal, MidTempPole, SupTempPole, SupTemporal
Occiptal Lobe	Calcarine, Cuneus, InfOccipital, MidOccipital, SupOccipital
Insula	Insula
Sensory-Motor Cortex	Paracentral, Postcentral, Precentral

predictor variables, we perform regression analyses using the methods described below for predicting two types of cognitive scores: (1) Alzheimer's Disease Assessment Scale-Cognitive test (ADAS), where the response variable is the ADAS total score; (2) Rey Auditory Verbal Learning Test (RAVLT), where the response variables include RAVLT total score (TOTAL), 30 minute delayed recall total score (T30), and 30 minute delayed recognition total score (RECOG).

2.2 Structured Sparse Regression Methods

Throughout this section, we write matrices as boldface uppercase letters and vectors as boldface lowercase letters. Given a matrix $\mathbf{M} = (m_{ij})$, its i-th row and j-th column are denoted as $\mathbf{m}^i$ and $\mathbf{m}_j$ respectively. The Frobenius norm and $\ell_{2,1}$-norm (also called as $\ell_{1,2}$-norm) of a matrix are defined as $||\mathbf{M}||_F = \sqrt{\sum_i ||\mathbf{m}^i||_2^2}$ and $||\mathbf{M}||_{2,1} = \sum_i \sqrt{\sum_j m_{ij}^2} = \sum_i ||\mathbf{m}^i||_2$, respectively.

We focus on multi-task learning paradigm, where imaging measures are used to predict one or more cognitive outcomes. Let $\{\mathbf{x}_1, \cdots, \mathbf{x}_n\} \subseteq \Re^d$ be imaging measures and $\{\mathbf{y}_1, \cdots, \mathbf{y}_n\} \subseteq \Re^c$ cognitive outcomes, where n is the number of samples, d is the number of predictors (feature dimensionality) and c is the number of response variables (tasks). Let $\mathbf{X} = [\mathbf{x}_1, \ldots, \mathbf{x}_n]$ and $\mathbf{Y} = [\mathbf{y}_1, \ldots, \mathbf{y}_n]$.

Linear Regression and Ridge Regression. The linear regression (LR) is a basic least square approach designed to solve:

$$\min_{\mathbf{W}} ||\mathbf{W}^T\mathbf{X} - \mathbf{Y}||_F^2, \tag{1}$$

where the entry w_{ij} of weight matrix $\mathbf{W}$ measures the relative importance of the i-th predictor in predicting the j-th response. To avoid over-fitting and increase numerical stability, ridge regression (RR) is proposed to solve:

$$\min_{\mathbf{W}} ||\mathbf{W}^T\mathbf{X} - \mathbf{Y}||_F^2 + \gamma||\mathbf{W}||_F^2, \tag{2}$$

where $\gamma > 0$ is a tradeoff parameter. The RR model has a few limitations. Given its non-sparse weight matrix $\mathbf{W}$, this model is not designed for identifying important biomarkers via feature selection. Second, the tasks in the RR model are decoupled and each of them can be learned separately. As a result, the information of underlying interacting relationships between cognitive outcomes are ignored. To address these issues, the $\ell_{2,1}$ norm method is proposed as follows.

The $\ell_{2,1}$ Norm Method. Motivated by using the ℓ_1 norm (Lasso, [16]) to impose sparsity on relevant features, the $\ell_{2,1}$ norm [12] is proposed to solve:

$$\min_{\mathbf{W}} ||\mathbf{W}^T\mathbf{X} - \mathbf{Y}||_F^2 + \gamma||\mathbf{W}||_{2,1}. \tag{3}$$

This approach couples multiple tasks together, with ℓ_2 norm within tasks and ℓ_1 norm within features. While the ℓ_2 norm enforces the selection of similar

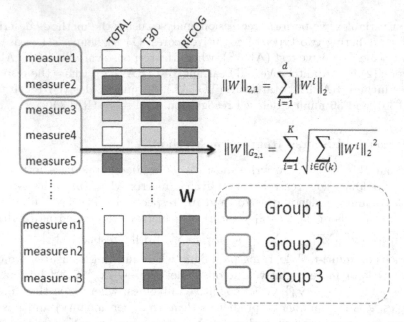

Fig. 1. Illustration of the G-SMuRFS method. The $\ell_{2,1}$-norm regularization ($\|\mathbf{W}\|_{2,1}$) is used to select imaging features that are associated with all or most cognitive outcomes. The group $\ell_{2,1}$-norm regularization ($\|\mathbf{W}\|_{G_{2,1}}$) is used to select imaging feature sets based on the pre-defined grouping structure.

features across tasks, the ℓ_1 norm helps achieve the final sparsity. Objective function Eq. (3) can be solved in many different ways [10,12,21]. Here we use the simplest one proposed in [21], which applied an iterative optimization procedure. By setting the derivative with respect to $\mathbf{W}$ to zero, $\mathbf{W}$ can be solved as:

$$\mathbf{W} = (\mathbf{XX}^T + \gamma\mathbf{D})^{-1}\mathbf{XY}^T, \tag{4}$$

where $\mathbf{D}$ is a diagonal matrix with the i-th diagonal element as $\frac{1}{2\|\mathbf{w}^i\|_2}$. For further optimization information, please refer to [21].

G-SMuRFS. In each of the above models, the rows of $\mathbf{W}$ are equally treated, which implies that the underlying structures among predictors are overlooked. However, in some cases, predictors can be partitioned into non-overlapping groups so that those within each group are highly correlated to each other. For example, in voxel-based analysis, voxels can be grouped based on brain regions. Thus, the predictors within each group are more homogeneous and should be considered together for predicting the response variables. To solve this issue, we have proposed a novel Group-Sparse Multi-task Regression and Feature Selection (G-SMuRFS) method [19] to exploit the interrelated structures within and between the predictor and response variables (Fig. 1). Our approach is to add a new group $\ell_{2,1}$-norm term ($\|\mathbf{W}\|_{G_{2,1}}$) to the $\ell_{2,1}$ norm model (Eq. (3)) as follows:

$$\min_{\mathbf{W}} ||\mathbf{W}^T\mathbf{X} - \mathbf{Y}||_F^2 + \gamma_1||\mathbf{W}||_{G_{2,1}} + \gamma_2||\mathbf{W}||_{2,1} \,, \qquad (5)$$

where $||\cdot||_{G_{2,1}}$ is our proposed *group $\ell_{2,1}$-norm ($G_{2,1}$-norm)* of a matrix with respect to a partition $\Pi \equiv \{\pi_k\}_{k=1}^K$ and defined as:

$$||\mathbf{W}||_{G_{2,1}} = \sum_{k=1}^K \sqrt{\sum_{i\in\pi_k}\sum_{j=1}^c w_{ij}^2} = \sum_{k=1}^K ||\mathbf{W}^k||_F \,.$$

In Eq. (5), the first term measures the regression loss. The second term couples all the regression coefficients of a group of features over all the c tasks together, which incorporates the grouping information on features. Finally, the third term penalizes all c regression coefficient of each individual feature as whole to select features across multiple learning tasks. We call Eq. (5) as Group-Sparse Multi-task Regression and Feature Selection (G-SMuRFS) method.

Solution of the objective function Eq. (5) can be obtained through an iterative optimization procedure, as shown in Eq. (6).

$$\mathbf{W} = (\mathbf{XX}^T + \gamma_1\mathbf{D} + \gamma_2\tilde{\mathbf{D}})^{-1}\mathbf{XY}^T, \qquad (6)$$

where $\mathbf{D}$ is a block diagonal matrix with the k-th diagonal block as $\frac{1}{2||\mathbf{W}^k||_F}\mathbf{I}_k$, $\mathbf{I}_k$ is an identity matrix with size of m_k, m_k is the total feature numbers included in group k, $\tilde{\mathbf{D}}$ is a diagonal matrix with the i-th diagonal element as $\frac{1}{2||\mathbf{w}^i||_2}$. Detailed optimization procedure and algorithm can be found in [19].

3   Results and Discussion

3.1   Experimental Setting

In our regression analyses, we have three sets of predictor variables: (1) 90 VBM GM density measures, (2) 95 FreeSurfer (FS in short) volume and thickness measures, and (3) seven AV45-PET (AV45 in short) measures; and have two sets of response variables: (1) ADAS, and (2) RAVLT scores including TOTAL, T30 and RECOG. We compare five regression methods: (1) Linear, (2) Ridge, (3) $\ell_{2,1}$ norm, and (4-5) G-SMuRFS with two different grouping strategies. The grouping strategies for G-SMuRFS are only applied to VBM and FS measures, including (1) *regional grouping* based on Table 2, and (2) *symmetric grouping* by coupling the left and right sides of the same structure together.

To provide an unbiased estimate of prediction performance of each method tested in the experiments, we employ five-fold cross-validation; and the partition schemes are consistent across all the methods tested in each comparison. Correlation coefficients between predicted scores and actual scores of all the test samples were used to compare the prediction performances across different methods. To test whether different imaging modalities can provide complementary information, we perform four sets of analyses using (1) FS alone, (2) VBM alone, (3) AV45 alone, and (4) ALL (i.e., combined FS, VBM and AV45).

3.2 Prediction Performance

As mentioned earlier, we calculate the correlation coefficient between the actual and predicted cognitive scores of the testing samples in each cross-validation trial, and use that to obtain an unbiased estimate of the prediction performance of each regression analysis. Fig. 2 shows performance comparison among two sparse methods (G-SMuRFS and $\ell_{2,1}$ norm) and two traditional methods (Linear and Ridge). Using AV45 to predict ADAS and RAVLT scores, all four methods perform similarly. Given only seven AV45 measures available, it is possible that the sparse methods do not play to their full potential. In all the other cases, G-SMuRFS and $\ell_{2,1}$ norm demonstrate a generally better performance than Ridge, and a much better one than Linear. G-SMuRFS performs similarly to $\ell_{2,1}$ norm in some cases and does slightly better in others. As to the two group strategies used in G-SMuRFS, they perform very similarly in most cases; and in a few cases the symmetric grouping works slightly better than regional grouping.

Shown in Fig. 3 is the performance comparison between each individual set (AV45, VBM, or FS) and the combined set (ALL = AV45 + VBM + FS), using G-SMuRFS as the regression model. For each comparison, a p value is calculated from paired t test between two sets of cross-validation correlation coefficients, to show whether the performance difference is significant. ALL performs significantly better (1) than AV45 on predicting all the tested scores, (2) than VBM on predicting ADAS, TOTAL and RECOG, and (3) than FS on predicting ADAS. For predicting RAVLT scores, ALL performs similarly to FS.

Shown in Fig. 4 is the performance comparison of running G-SMuRFS with symmetric and regional grouping strategies on the VBM and FS data of the ADNI-1 and ADNI-GO/2 cohorts. AV45 is not compared because it is not available in ADNI-1. G-SMuRFS performs significantly better on ADNI-GO/2 than on ADNI-1 in the following cases: (1) using VBM to predict T30 and RECOG, and (2) using FS to predict all three RAVLT scores. Note that the ADNI-1 MCI cohort contains only LMCI participants and ADNI-GO/2 has both EMCI and LMCI participants. As a result, ADNI-GO/2 data spans a wider range of imaging and cognitive measurement values, which may have a potential to result in a stronger correlation.

Our best prediction performance is comparable with prior results applied to the ADNI-1 data. However, we do observe that some prior studies [14,17,18,25, 26] have reported higher correlation coefficients. There are a couple of possible reasons. First, our study is focused on MCI only. Most prior studies analyze multiple groups including AD, MCI and healthy controls (HC). So the ranges of their cognitive scores and imaging measures are wider, making it easier to yield stronger correlations. Second, some studies calculate the correlation coefficients by pooling together all the test samples across cross-validation trials, which tends to yield a more optimistic estimate.

3.3 Biomarker Identification

Both G-SMuRFS and $\ell_{2,1}$ norm are sparse models that are able to identify a compact set of relevant imaging biomarkers and to explain the underlying brain

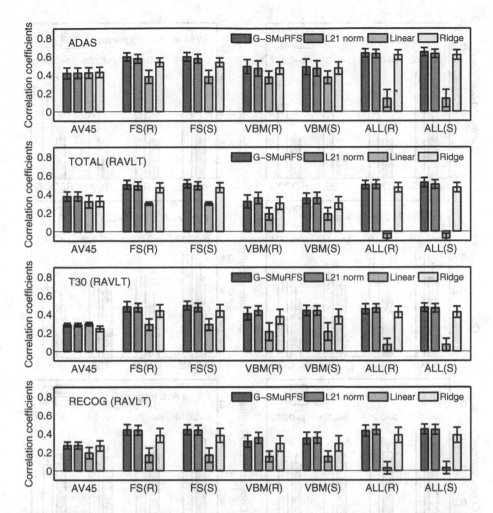

Fig. 2. Performance comparison between four methods: two sparse ones (G-SMuRFS and $\ell_{2,1}$ norm) and two traditional ones (Linear and Ridge). The prediction performances are measured by correlation coefficients; and the mean of five correlation coefficients obtained from cross-validation trials, coupled with the standard error shown as the error bar, is plotted for each experiment. Each panel shows the prediction performance for each cognitive score using different methods and different predictor sets. Note that all three RAVLT scores are predicted jointly. Labels on the X axes indicate the predictor data sets. Regional and symmetric grouping strategies used in G-SMuRFS are respectively denoted by "(R)" and "(S)" and attached to the predictor data sets. In the case of AV45, G-SMuRFS is equivalent to $\ell_{2,1}$ norm, since no grouping is applied.

structural changes related to cognitive status. Shown in Fig. 5 are the maps of regression weights for predicting RAVLT scores using the FS measures. Average regression weights of 5-fold cross-validation trials are plotted for G-SMuRFS(S) (symmetric grouping), G-SMuRFS(R) (regional grouping), $\ell_{2,1}$ norm, Linear,

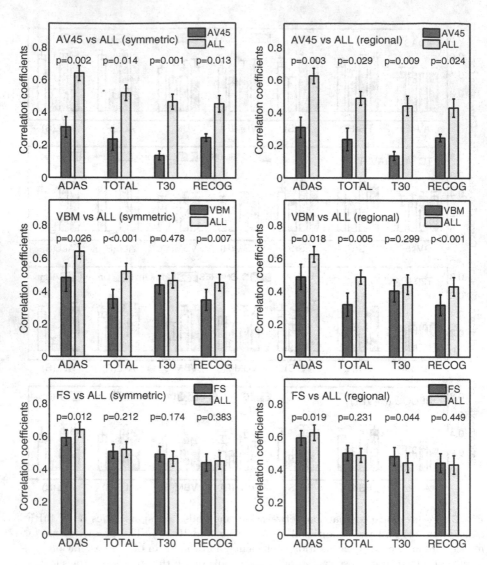

Fig. 3. Performance comparison between each individual set and combined data as the predictors: AV45 vs ALL (1st row), VBM vs ALL (2nd row), and FS vs ALL (3rd row). The left column shows G-SMuRFS results using symmetric grouping strategy; and the right column shows G-SMuRFS results using regional grouping strategy. The prediction performances are measured by correlation coefficients; and the mean of five correlation coefficients obtained from cross-validation trials, coupled with the standard error shown as the error bar, is plotted for each experiment. The p value is calculated from paired t test between two sets of cross-validation correlation coefficients.

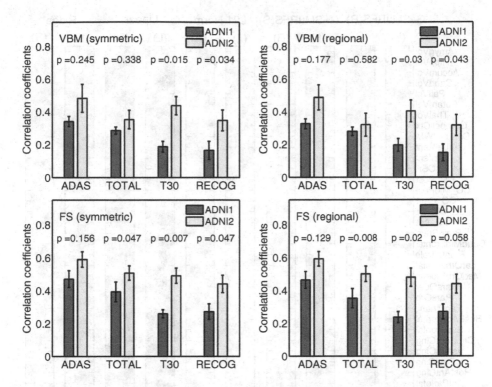

Fig. 4. Performance comparison of running G-SMuRFS with symmetric (left column) and regional (right column) grouping strategies on the VBM (top row) and FS (bottom row) data of the ADNI-1 and ADNI-GO/2 cohorts. AV45 is not compared because it is not available in ADNI-1. The prediction performances are measured by correlation coefficients; and the mean of five correlation coefficients obtained from cross-validation trials, coupled with the standard error shown as the error bar, is plotted for each experiment. The p value is calculated from paired t test between two sets of cross-validation correlation coefficients.

and Ridge. Each row corresponds to an FS measure and each column to a cognitive score. The FS measures are ordered according to the regional grouping structure shown in Table 2. Blue indicates negative correlation, while red indicates positive correlation. The bigger the magnitude of a coefficient is, the more important its imaging measure is in predicting the corresponding cognitive score. Clearly, G-SMuRFS and $\ell_{2,1}$ norm yield more sparse patterns than Linear and Ridge, making the results easier to interpret. The identified patterns match our expectation based on the prior knowledge. RAVLT examines verbal learning memory; and thus the identified regions include hippocampus, fusiform, and middle temporal gyri, which are all relevant to learning and memory.

In addition, the grouping strategies used in G-SMuRFS do seem to work in terms of structuring the identified patterns. For example, in Fig. 5, regional grouping method yields a cluster of cortical measures in the temporal lobe, and

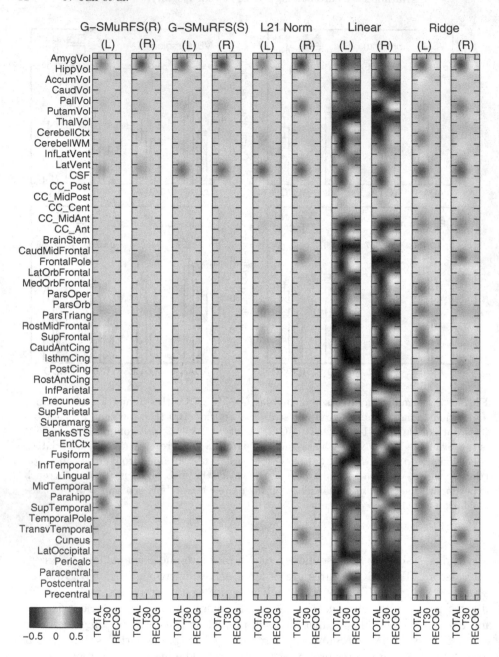

Fig. 5. Heat maps of regression weights for predicting RAVLT scores using FS measures. Average regression weights of 5-fold cross-validation trials are plotted for G-SMuRFS(S) (symmetric grouping), G-SMuRFS(R) (regional grouping), $\ell_{2,1}$ norm, Linear, and Ridge. Each row corresponds to an FS measure and each column to a cognitive score. Each method has two panels, corresponding to measures from the left (L) and right (R) hemispheres. Blue indicates negative correlation, while red indicates positive correlation.

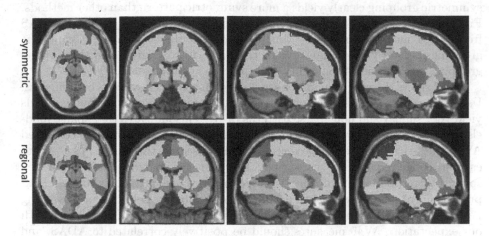

Fig. 6. Brain maps of regression weights for predicting ADAS from VBM measures using G-SMuRFS with symmetric (top panel) and regional (bottom panel) grouping strategies. The color scale is the same as the one used in Fig. 5.

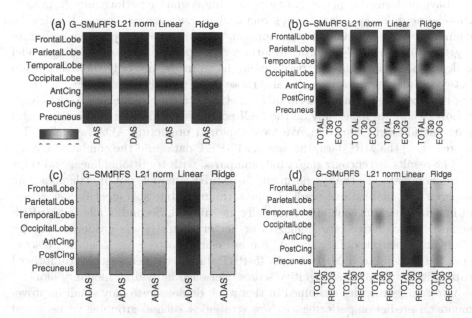

Fig. 7. Heat maps of regression weights for predicting cognitive scores using (a-b) AV45 measures only and (c-d) ALL measures (only AV45 shown here). The first two panels in each of (c-d) show the AV45 part of the results of G-SMuRFS using two grouping strategies. Blue indicates negative correlation, while red indicates positive correlation.

symmetric grouping clearly yields a more symmetric pattern than other methods. Fig. 6 shows the regression weights mapped on the brain while predicting ADAS from VBM measures using G-SMuRFS. We also observe that the symmetric grouping method yields a more symmetric pattern (top panel) and the regional grouping method yields some clustering patterns (bottom panel).

Fig. 7 shows the weight maps for seven AV45 measures in various experiments. Using these seven measures alone to predict cognitive scores, all four methods yield very similar and non-sparse patterns (a-b). This indicates that sparse models may not be necessary for low dimensional learning tasks. If we use combined AV45 and MRI measures for predicting cognitive scores, the weight maps of Linear and Ridge remain non-sparse (c-d). However, the sparse models yield much sparser patterns: only precuneus is selected in terms of contributing to the ADAS prediction (c), and only precuneus and occipital lobe are selected for predicting RAVLT scores (d). The directionality of these correlations is in accordance with our expectation: AV45 measures should be positively correlated to ADAS, and negatively correlated to RAVLT scores.

4   Conclusions

We have performed experiments for predicting cognitive performance from multimodal neuroimaging data using structured sparse learning models. Besides the commonly used $\ell_{2,1}$ norm for encouraging sparsity, we propose to incorporate a group $\ell_{2,1}$ norm ($G_{2,1}$ norm) to form a new sparse multitask learning model called G-SMuRFS. This strategy enables us to model not only the relationship between outcome measures, but also those among predictor variables. We have applied both $\ell_{2,1}$ norm and G-SMuRFS methods to analyze the new ADNI-GO/2 cohort, where we focus only on the MCI participants in order to identify useful patterns for early detection. We have explored predicting ADAS and RAVLT scores using the MRI data, the new AV45-PET data, and the combined data.

The results are encouraging. First, compared with traditional linear and ridge regression methods, the $\ell_{2,1}$ norm and G-SMuRFS models not only demonstrate superior and more stable predictive performances, but also identify a small set of imaging markers that are biologically meaningful. Second, while G-SMuRFS achieves a predictive rate similar to or better than $\ell_{2,1}$, its grouping strategy offers additional flexibility to yield a user-desired pattern for biomarker discovery. Third, combined MRI and AV45-PET data have demonstrated improved capability for predicting cognitive scores over each individual modality alone.

Grouping strategies examined in this work demonstrate only small improvements on prediction performance. New strategies, such as grouping voxels based on brain regions, warrant further investigation. Another possible future direction is to expand these models to handle longitudinal data [26], or to conduct joint classification and regression [20, 25] for simultaneous estimation of both disease and cognitive statuses, since these existing studies [20, 25, 26] have demonstrated that improved performance can potentially be achieved.

Acknowledgement. This research was supported by NSF IIS-1117335, NIH UL1 RR025761, U01 AG024904, NIA RC2 AG036535, NIA R01 AG19771, and NIA P30 AG10133-18S1 at IU; and by NSF CCF-0830780, CCF-0917274, DMS-0915228, and IIS-1117965 at UTA.

Data collection and sharing for this project was funded by the Alzheimer's Disease Neuroimaging Initiative (ADNI) (National Institutes of Health Grant U01 AG024904). ADNI is funded by the National Institute on Aging, the National Institute of Biomedical Imaging and Bioengineering, and through generous contributions from the following: Abbott; Alzheimers Association; Alzheimers Drug Discovery Foundation; Amorfix Life Sciences Ltd.; AstraZeneca; Bayer Health-Care; BioClinica, Inc.; Biogen Idec Inc.; Bristol-Myers Squibb Company; Eisai Inc.; Elan Pharmaceuticals Inc.; Eli Lilly and Company; F. Hoffmann-La Roche Ltd and its affiliated company Genentech, Inc.; GE Healthcare; Innogenetics, N.V.; IXICO Ltd.; Janssen Alzheimer Immunotherapy Research & Development, LLC.; Johnson & Johnson Pharmaceutical Research & Development LLC.; Medpace, Inc.; Merck & Co., Inc.; Meso Scale Diagnostics, LLC.; Novartis Pharmaceuticals Corporation; Pfizer Inc.; Servier; Synarc Inc.; and Takeda Pharmaceutical Company. The Canadian Institutes of Health Research is providing funds to support ADNI clinical sites in Canada. Private sector contributions are facilitated by the Foundation for the National Institutes of Health (www.fnih.org). The grantee organization is the Northern California Institute for Research and Education, and the study is coordinated by the Alzheimer's Disease Cooperative Study at the University of California, San Diego. ADNI data are disseminated by the Laboratory for Neuro Imaging at the University of California, Los Angeles. This research was also supported by NIH grants P30 AG010129 and K01 AG030514.

References

1. Ashburner, J., Friston, K.J.: Voxel-based morphometry–the methods. Neuroimage 11(6), 805–821 (2000)
2. Dale, A.M., Fischl, B., Sereno, M.I.: Cortical surface-based analysis. i. segmentation and surface reconstruction. Neuroimage 99(2), 179–194 (1999)
3. Fischl, B., Salat, D.H., Busa, E., Albert, M., Dieterich, M., Haselgrove, C., van der Kouwe, A., Killiany, R., Kennedy, D., Klaveness, S., Montillo, A., Makris, N., Rosen, B., Dale, A.M.: Whole brain segmentation: automated labeling of neuroanatomical structures in the human brain. Neuron 33(3), 341–355 (2002)
4. Fischl, B., Sereno, M.I., Dale, A.M.: Cortical surface-based analysis. ii: Inflation, flattening, and a surface-based coordinate system. Neuroimage 99(2), 195–207 (1999)
5. Jack Jr., C.R., Bernstein, M.A., Borowski, B.J., Gunter, J.L., Fox, N.C., Thompson, P.M., Schuff, N., Krueger, G., Killiany, R.J., Decarli, C.S., Dale, A.M., Carmichael, O.W., Tosun, D., Weiner, M.W.: Update on the magnetic resonance imaging core of the alzheimer's disease neuroimaging initiative. Alzheimers Dement 6(3), 212–220 (2010)
6. Jack Jr., C.R., Bernstein, M.A., Borowski, B.J., Gunter, J.L., Fox, N.C., Thompson, P.M., Schuff, N., Krueger, G., Killiany, R.J., Decarli, C.S., Dale, A.M.,

Carmichael, O.W., Tosun, D., Weiner, M.W.: Update on the magnetic resonance imaging core of the alzheimer's disease neuroimaging initiative. Alzheimers Dement 6(3), 212–220 (2010)

7. Jack Jr., C.R., Bernstein, M.A., Fox, N.C., Thompson, P., Alexander, G., Harvey, D., Borowski, B., Britson, P.J., L Whitwell, J., Ward, C., Dale, A.M., Felmlee, J.P., Gunter, J.L., Hill, D.L., Killiany, R., Schuff, N., Fox-Bosetti, S., Lin, C., Studholme, C., DeCarli, C.S., Krueger, G., Ward, H.A., Metzger, G.J., Scott, K.T., Mallozzi, R., Blezek, D., Levy, J., Debbins, J.P., Fleisher, A.S., Albert, M., Green, R., Bartzokis, G., Glover, G., Mugler, J., Weiner, M.W.: The alzheimer's disease neuroimaging initiative (adni): Mri methods. J. Magn. Reson. Imaging 27(4), 685–691 (2008)

8. Jagust, W.J., Bandy, D., Chen, K., Foster, N.L., Landau, S.M., Mathis, C.A., Price, J.C., Reiman, E.M., Skovronsky, D., Koeppe, R.A.: The alzheimer's disease neuroimaging initiative positron emission tomography core. Alzheimers Dement 6(3), 221–229 (2010)

9. Jagust, W.J., Bandy, D., Chen, K.W., Foster, N.L., Landau, S.M., Mathis, C.A., Price, J.C., Reiman, E.M., Skovronsky, D., Koeppe, R.A., Initi, A.D.N.: The alzheimer's disease neuroimaging initiative positron emission tomography core. Alzheimers Dementia 6(3), 221–229 (2010)

10. Liu, J., Ji, S., Ye, J.: Multi-task feature learning via efficient l2,1-norm minimization. In: Proceedings of the Twenty-Fifth Conference on Uncertainty in Artificial Intelligence (UAI 2009), pp. 339–348.

11. Nordberg, A., Rinne, J.O., Kadir, A., Langstrom, B.: The use of pet in alzheimer disease. Nat. Rev. Neurol. 6(2), 78–87 (2010)

12. Obozinski, G., Taskar, B., Jordan, M.: Multi-task feature selection. Technical Report, Technical report, Statistics Department, UC Berkeley (2006)

13. Risacher, S.L., Saykin, A.J., West, J.D., Shen, L., Firpi, H.A., McDonald, B.C.: Baseline mri predictors of conversion from mci to probable ad in the adni cohort. Curr. Alzheimer Res. 6(4), 347–361 (2009)

14. Stonnington, C.M., Chu, C., et al.: Predicting clinical scores from magnetic resonance scans in alzheimer's disease. Neuroimage 51(4), 1405–1413 (2010)

15. Swaminathan, S., Shen, L., Risacher, S.L., Yoder, K.K., West, J.D., Kim, S., Nho, K., Foroud, T., Inlow, M., Potkin, S.G., Huentelman, M.J., Craig, D.W., Jagust, W.J., Koeppe, R.A., Mathis, C.A., Jack Jr., C.R., Weiner, M.W., Saykin, A.J.: Amyloid pathway-based candidate gene analysis of [(11)c]pib-pet in the alzheimer's disease neuroimaging initiative (adni) cohort. Brain Imaging Behav. 6(1), 1–15 (2012)

16. Tibshirani, R.: Regression shrinkage and selection via the LASSO. J. Royal. Statist. Soc. B. 58, 267–288 (1996)

17. Walhovd, K.B., Fjell, A.M., Dale, A.M., McEvoy, L.K., Brewer, J., Karow, D.S., Salmon, D.P., Fennema-Notestine, C.: Multi-modal imaging predicts memory performance in normal aging and cognitive decline. Neurobiology of Aging 31(7), 1107–1121 (2010)

18. Wan, J., Zhang, Z., Yan, J., Li, T., Rao, B.D., Fang, S., Kim, S., Risacher, S.L., Saykin, A.J., Shen, L.: Sparse bayesian multi-task learning for predicting cognitive outcomes from neuroimaging measures in alzheimer's disease. In: IEEE Int. Conf. on Computer Vision and Pattern Recognition (accepted, 2012)

19. Wang, H., Nie, F., Huang, H., Kim, S., Nho, K., Risacher, S.L., Saykin, A.J., Shen, L.: Identifying quantitative trait loci via group-sparse multitask regression and feature selection: an imaging genetics study of the adni cohort. Bioinformatics 28(2), 229–237 (2012)

20. Wang, H., Nie, F., Huang, H., Risacher, S., Saykin, A.J., Shen, L.: Identifying AD-sensitive and cognition-relevant imaging biomarkers via joint classification and regression. Med. Image Comput. Comput. Assist. Interv. 14(Pt 3), 115–123 (2011)
21. Wang, H., Nie, F., Huang, H., Risacher, S.L., Ding, C., Saykin, A.J., L, Shen, A.D.N.I.: A new sparse multi-task regression and feature selection method to identify brain imaging predictors for memory performance. In: IEEE Conference on Computer Vision, pp. 557–562 (2011)
22. Weiner, M.W., Aisen, P.S., Jack Jr., C.R., Jagust, W.J., Trojanowski, J.Q., Shaw, L., Saykin, A.J., Morris, J.C., Cairns, N., Beckett, L.A., Toga, A., Green, R., Walter, S., Soares, H., Snyder, P., Siemers, E., Potter, W., Cole, P.E., Schmidt, M.: The alzheimer's disease neuroimaging initiative: progress report and future plans. Alzheimers Dement. 6(3), 202–211, e7 (2010)
23. Weiner, M.W., Veitch, D.P., Aisen, P.S., Beckett, L.A., Cairns, N.J., Green, R.C., Harvey, D., Jack, C.R., Jagust, W., Liu, E., Morris, J.C., Petersen, R.C., Saykin, A.J., Schmidt, M.E., Shaw, L., Siuciak, J.A., Soares, H., Toga, A.W., Trojanowski, J.Q.: The alzheimer's disease neuroimaging initiative: a review of papers published since its inception. Alzheimers Dement. 8(Suppl. 1), S1–S68 (2012)
24. Yuan, M., Lin, Y.: Model selection and estimation in regression with grouped variables. Journal of The Royal Statistical Society Series B 68(1), 49–67 (2006)
25. Zhang, D., Shen, D.: Multi-modalmulti-task learning for joint prediction of multiple regression and classification variables in alzheimers disease. Neuroimage (2011)
26. Zhang, D., Shen, D.: Predicting future clinical changes of mci patients using longitudinal and multimodal biomarkers. PLoS One 7(3), e33182 (2012)

Combining DTI and MRI for the Automated Detection of Alzheimer's Disease Using a Large European Multicenter Dataset

Martin Dyrba[1,15], Michael Ewers[2,3], Martin Wegrzyn[1], Ingo Kilimann[1],
Claudia Plant[4], Annahita Oswald[5], Thomas Meindl[6], Michela Pievani[7],
Arun L.W. Bokde[8,9], Andreas Fellgiebel[10], Massimo Filippi[11],
Harald Hampel[12], Stefan Klöppel[13], Karlheinz Hauenstein[14], Thomas Kirste[15],
Stefan J. Teipel[1,16], and the EDSD Study Group

[1] German Center for Neurodegenerative Diseases (DZNE), Rostock, Germany
[2] Department of Radiology, University of California, San Francisco, USA
[3] Center for Imaging of Neurodegenerative Diseases,
VA Medical Center, San Francisco, USA
[4] Department of Scientific Computing, Florida State University, Tallahassee, USA
[5] Institute for Informatics,
Ludwig-Maximilians-Universität München, Munich, Germany
[6] Institute for Clinical Radiology, Department of MRI,
Ludwig-Maximilians-Universität München, Munich, Germany
[7] LENITEM Laboratory of Epidemiology, Neuroimaging and Telemedicine, IRCCS
Centro San Giovanni di Dio, FBF, Brescia, Italy
[8] Cognitive Systems Group, Discipline of Psychiatry, School of Medicine, Trinity
College Dublin; Dublin, Ireland
[9] Trinity College Institute of Neuroscience (TCIN),
Trinity College Dublin, Dublin, Ireland
[10] Department of Psychiatry, University Medical Center of Mainz, Mainz, Germany
[11] Neuroimaging Research Unit, Institute of Experimental Neurology,
Division of Neuroscience,
Scientific Institute and University Vita-Salute San Raffaele, Milan, Italy
[12] Department of Psychiatry, Goethe University, Frankfurt, Germany
[13] Department of Psychiatry and Psychotherapy, Department of Neurology, Freiburg
Brain Imaging, University Medical Center Freiburg, Freiburg, Germany
[14] Department of Radiology, University of Rostock, Rostock, Germany
[15] Mobile Multimedia Information Systems Group (MMIS),
University of Rostock, Rostock, Germany
[16] Department of Psychiatry, University of Rostock, Rostock, Germany

Abstract. Diffusion tensor imaging (DTI) allows assessing neuronal
fiber tract integrity in vivo to support the diagnosis of Alzheimer's disease (AD). It is an open research question to which extent combinations of different neuroimaging techniques increase the detection of AD.
In this study we examined different methods to combine DTI data and
structural T_1-weighted magnetic resonance imaging (MRI) data. Further,
we applied machine learning techniques for automated detection of AD.
We used a sample of 137 patients with clinically probable AD (MMSE
20.6 ± 5.3) and 143 healthy elderly controls, scanned in nine different

P.-T. Yap et al. (Eds.): MBIA 2012, LNCS 7509, pp. 18–28, 2012.

scanners, obtained from the recently created framework of the European
DTI study on Dementia (EDSD). For diagnostic classification we used
the DTI derived indices fractional anisotropy (FA) and mean diffusivity
(MD) as well as grey matter density (GMD) and white matter density
(WMD) maps from anatomical MRI. We performed voxel-based classification using a Support Vector Machine (SVM) classifier with tenfold
cross validation. We compared the results from each single modality with
those from different approaches to combine the modalities. For our sample, combining modalities did not increase the detection rates of AD. An
accuracy of approximately 89% was reached for GMD data alone and for
multimodal classification when GMD was included. This high accuracy
remained stable across each of the approaches. As our sample consisted
of mildly to moderately affected patients, cortical atrophy may be far
progressed so that the decline in structural network connectivity derived
from DTI may not add additional information relevant for the SVM classification. This may be different for predementia stages of AD. Further
research will focus on multimodal detection of AD in predementia stages
of AD, e.g. in amnestic mild cognitive impairment (aMCI), and on evaluating the classification performance when adding other modalities, e.g.
functional MRI or FDG-PET.

Keywords: Alzheimer's disease, Magnetic Resonance Imaging, Diffusion Tensor Imaging, Support Vector Machine, multimodal analysis, combining classifiers, multicenter study.

1 Introduction

In the recent years, researchers investigated the use of different neuroimaging
techniques as possible biomarkers for the diagnosis of Alzheimer's disease (AD).
Information from structural T_1-weighted magnetic resonance imaging (MRI) can
be used to evaluate the volume and density of cerebral white matter (WM) tissue and gray matter (GM) structures in order to find disease-related atrophy.
Diffusion tensor imaging (DTI) can be used to assess the integrity of cerebral
WM fiber tracts and, hence, can support the diagnosis of AD. From DTI we
can derive scalar indices of anisotropic diffusion, the most widely used being
the fractional anisotropy (FA) and mean diffusivity (MD). Reduced FA or increased MD indicate impaired WM fiber tract integrity [1,2]. Earlier studies
showed superior classification results of MRI measures compared to DTI measures [3] for the detection of AD. In contrast, in predementia stages of AD, such
as amnestic mild cognitive impairment (aMCI), regions of interest analysis of
the hippocampus showed a more accurate separation between MCI and healthy
control (HC) subjects using markers of diffusion anisotropy compared to hippocampus volume [3,4,5]. The question is unresolved to which extent the two
imaging techniques contain complementary information that could be exploited
to improve the performance when these methods are combined. Until today,
only few studies were published that applied machine learning (ML) techniques
to combined neuroimaging datasets for the automated detection of AD. Among

them are [6] who combined DTI data and functional MRI data with N=27 subjects, [7] using structural MRI and fluorodeoxyglucose positron emission tomography (FDG-PET) with N=48 subjects, and [8,9] combining structural MRI, FDG-PET and additionally cerebrospinal fluid (CSF) biomarkers with N=202 and N=233 subjects, respectively. In our previous work [10] we applied ML techniques on a large multicenter dataset with N=280 subjects obtained from the European DTI Study on Dementia (EDSD) to investigate the influence of multi-center acquisition of the DTI data on automatic detection of AD. Based on this work, the present study aims at combining the structural MRI data and DTI data in order to improve the detection accuracy. We examined the following approaches to combine the different modalities: (i) directly merging DTI scans and MRI scans at voxel level, (ii) using a two layer meta classifier in which the predictions of the single modality SVMs were used as input for second classifier, and (iii) a multiple kernel SVM (MK-SVM).

2 Material and Methods

2.1 Data Acquisition

The data were taken from the European DTI Study on Dementia (EDSD), a newly established framework of nine European centers: Amsterdam (Netherlands), Brescia (Italy), Dublin (Ireland), Frankfurt (Germany), Freiburg (Germany), Milano (Italy), Mainz (Germany), Munich (Germany), and Rostock (Germany), with one center including data from two different MRI scanners. Written informed consent was provided by all subjects or their representatives and the study was approved by local ethics committees at each of the participating centers. After strict quality control and preprocessing, 280 DTI and MRI scans derived from nine MRI scanners were retained for the analysis, consisting of scans from 137 patients with clinically probable AD according to NINCDS-ADRCA criteria [11] and 143 healthy elderly control subjects (for details see [12]). All participants were free of any significant neurological, psychiatric or medical condition (except for AD in patients), in particular cerebrovascular apoplexy, vascular dementia, depression, subclinical hypothyroidism as well as substance abuse. Healthy controls were required to have no cognitive complaints and scored within one standard deviation of the age and education adjusted norm in all subtests of the Consortium to Establish a Registry of Alzheimer's Disease (CERAD) cognitive battery [13]. Patients were significantly older and had less years of education than the controls (Table 1). Gender was not different between groups. As expected, MMSE scores [14] were significantly lower in AD patients compared to controls, with the patients ranging in the mild to moderate stages of dementia [14]. The number of subjects per scanner ranged between 13 and 46 with a median of 29.

2.2 Data Preprocessing

Preprocessing of DTI data was performed using the diffusion toolbox of FSL (Version 4.1, FMRIB, Oxford, UK) [15]. FSL preprocessing included

Table 1. Demographic data and MMSE of the subjects

	AD	controls
No. of subjects (women)	137 (79)	143 (72)
Age (SD) in years *	72.5 (8.3)	69.2 (5.9)
MMSE (SD) *	20.6 (5.3)	28.8 (1.1)
Years of education (SD) *	10.2 (3.3)	13.1 (3.8)

*Highly significant difference between groups, $p < 0.001$

(i) corrections for eddy currents and head motion, (ii) skull stripping, and (iii) fitting of the data to the diffusion tensor model to compute maps of fractional anisotropy (FA) and mean diffusivity (MD). Deformation-based analysis of MPRAGE data and of the FA and MD maps was performed using SPM8 (Wellcome Trust Centre for Neuroimaging, London, UK) implemented in Matlab 7 (Mathworks, Natwick). The images in native space were manually aligned to set the anterior commissure as the origin of coordinate system. Then FA and MD maps were affinely aligned to the corresponding MPRAGE scans. For spatial normalization, the VBM8 toolbox (Version 414) [16] implemented in SPM8 was used to create a customized DARTEL template. We created the template out of N=54 images by randomly selecting six scans (three AD patients and three healthy controls) from each of the nine scanners. The resulting template was used for high-dimensional DARTEL normalization of the MPRAGE scans as implemented in VBM8. Images were segmented into GM and WM and transformed to MNI space applying modulation for non-linear components only. The Deformation fields derived from this step were applied to the spatially coregistered FA and MD maps, without modulation. To exclude all voxels outside the WM of the FA and MD maps, we used a binary WM mask based on the average WM image derived from the random sample of N=54 normalized images described above. Additionally, we created a corresponding binary GM mask following the same procedure. The GM and WM segments as well as the masked FA and MD maps in MNI space were smoothed using an 8mm full width at half maximum (FWHM) isotropic Gaussian kernel. After smoothing, all scans were again masked with the WM or GM mask, respectively, to restrict the subsequent analysis to be performed based on the voxels within the corresponding areas, only. Without additional masking after smoothing our subsequent analysis detected group differences in areas outside the respective tissues, e.g. in the ventricles. These artifacts were caused by imperfect smoothing at the segment or tissue borders. As this study is based on our preceding work [10], we omitted any correction steps to remove variance introduced by confounding factors, such as age, gender or the acquisition scanner.

2.3 Classification Methods

For classification we pooled all 280 scans from the different centers and divided them into the four modalities: GM density (GMD), WM density (WMD), WM FA and WM MD which we processed separately. For learning and classification we used the WEKA machine learning toolkit (Version 3.6.6) [17] and the Lib-SVM toolbox (Version 3.12) [18]. The learning and classification process involves three steps: (i) feature selection, (ii) learning and classification, and (iii) evaluation. To estimate the performance of our methods objectively, we used the tenfold cross validation technique. Therefore, all scans from the 280 subjects were randomized and stratified by the diagnosis into ten folds using WEKA. Additionally, we repeated this procedure ten times to avoid our results being biased due to randomization artifacts.

Feature Selection. After image segmentation and masking, WM and GM tissue maps included approximately 250 thousand voxels. To reduce the computation time and memory space needed for data processing the number of features was further reduced using Plant's approach [19]: Voxels that do not contribute any information to the separation of the data were excluded using the entropy-based information gain (IG) criterion [20] and a rather liberal threshold of $min_{IG} = 0.05$.

Learning and Classification. For classification we used a multivariate Support Vector Machine (SVM) [21] with a radial basis function (RBF) kernel. SVM performed highly accurately in former neuroimaging studies [6,7,8,19] For the SVM we needed to define two parameters including the complexity or cost constant C and the radial basis function kernel width ($\gamma > 0$). The parameter $C > 0$ determines the trade-off between margin maximization and training error minimization for the soft margin SVM. To estimate suitable values for C and γ we used a grid search in the range of $C = 2^{-3}, 2^{-2}, ..., 2^{8}$ and $\gamma = 2^{-14}, 2^{-13}, ..., 2^{-1}$ which we performed for each modality separately. Each of the input features was rescaled to range between zero and one before applying the SVM algorithm. Due to high computational costs of SVM parameter estimation we used a two-step approach: First, we computed the accuracy of the SVM classifier for the whole range of parameters with only two arbitrarily selected folds. Then, we selected a smaller area for the parameter range in which we repeated the parameter estimation process for all of the other folds. For the parameter estimation we performed an internal fourfold cross-validation for the training data. Thus, we ensured that the test data were not used for parameter selection. The parameters which gave the best average results for all repetitions were applied for the final classification and validation process.

Combining Data. The simplest approach for combining modalities is to directly merge the scans at voxel level. That means that the feature vector for each subject x_i was constructed by concatenating the voxel intensity values for each modality: $x_i = [voxel_j^{(FA)}, ..., voxel_k^{(MD)}, ..., voxel_l^{(WMD)}, ..., voxel_m^{(GMD)}]$. This approach was also used in [7] and in [9] (only for comparison). In order to compare the influence of each modality, we determined the classification performance using different combinations of modalities. SVM parameter estimation was performed for each combination separately.

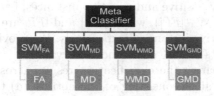

Fig. 1. Structure of the meta classifier

Combining Classifiers. In this approach we used a two layer meta classifier as illustrated in Fig. 1. The predictions of each single modality SVM were used as input for a second classifier. We used the optimal parameters determined earlier for each single modality SVM in the lower layer. Additionally, we repeated evaluating the classification performance using the distance from the separation hyperplane as output of the lower layer SVMs and input of the meta classifier for comparison. As meta classifier we arbitrarily selected a subset of WEKA's [17] classifiers with the goal to cover different methods and types of decision functions: (i) majority voting, (ii) the J48 decision tree – WEKA's implementation of the C4.5 decision tree, (iii) a linear SVM, (iv) a multilayer perceptron, (v) logistic regression, and (vi) a Naïve Bayes classifier. The majority voting meta classifier was also used in [8] (only for comparison).

Multiple Kernel SVM. The multiple kernel learning SVM (MKL-SVM) or multiple kernel SVM (MK-SVM) was first introduced by [22]. This method allows using different types of kernels or datasets concurrently in one single SVM instance. The additionally introduced parameters β_m define the weight for each modality m. The kernel k used for classification (often referred to as 'mixed kernel') is constructed by summing the kernels for each single modality and weighting them as specified: $k(\boldsymbol{x}_i, \boldsymbol{x}_j) = \sum_{m=1}^{M} \beta_m \phi(\boldsymbol{x}_i^{(m)})^T \phi(\boldsymbol{x}_j^{(m)})$ (see [6,8,9] for details). Using this method to compute the final kernel and by predefining the β_m parameters, traditional SVM solvers can be used with multiple kernels. In our case, we used LibSVM [18] and the optimal γ parameters determined earlier for each single modality. For C and the β_m parameters we performed a grid search as described above. Due to the large dimension of the search space, we restricted each β_m to be in the range of $0.5, 0.75, ..., 1.5$. For comparison, we additionally examined the results when arbitrarily setting the β_m parameters such that they reflect the proportion of accuracy obtained for each single modality. The MK-SVM approach was also used in [6], [8] and [9] as main method.

Evaluation. As results we report the mean accuracy, sensitivity and specificity. The accuracy was defined as $acc = (|TP| + |TN|)/n$ where $|TP|$ is the number of true positives, $|TN|$ is the number of true negatives and n is the total number of subjects. Following a common convention, we defined correctly classified patients with AD as true positives. The sensitivity and the specificity measure the ability of a classifier to identify positive and negative instances, i.e. $sen = |TP|/(|TP| + |FN|)$, $spec = |TN|/(|TN| + |FP|)$, where $|FN|$ and $|FP|$ are the number of false negative and false positive instances, respectively. We provide the 2.5 and 97.5 percentiles of our results as 95% confidence interval.

For pairwisely comparing the classification results across the modalities we compiled contingency tables consisting of the entries: (a) the number subjects that were classified correctly by both classifiers N_{11}, (b) the number of subjects classified correctly by the first classifier N_{10}, (c) the number of subjects classified correctly by the second classifier N_{01}, and (d) the number of subjects misclassified by both classifiers N_{00}. From N_{10} and N_{01} we can derive the proportion of subjects classified correctly by one of both classifiers. In case that one of these is relatively small, it is unlikely that the corresponding modality will contribute additional information that would be useful for the group separation of AD and HC.

3   Results

The classification results of the single modalities were obtained in our previous work [10]. They are displayed in the upper four rows of Table 3. The pairwise comparisons of the single modality classifier results are given in Table 2. The results of the combined data sets are shown in the lower part of Table 3. The accuracies for the non-GMD group differed significantly from the GMD group ($p < 0.05$, two-tailed paired t-test). Table 4 and Table 5 report the results obtained by stacking of different classifiers based on the SVM classification labels and the distance from the separation hyperplane, respectively. Except from the accuracy obtained from the J48 classifier (Table 5), no accuracies differed significantly from each other. In Table 6 the results of the multiple kernel SVM are given.

Table 2. Mean contingency table entries obtained from the single modality SVM classification results

First modality	Second modality	N_{11}	N_{10}	N_{01}	N_{00}
FA	GMD	215	10	34	20
MD	GMD	221	12	29	18
WMD	GMD	220	12	30	18
FA	MD	205	20	29	26
FA	WMD	200	25	32	32
MD	WMD	210	24	22	25

Table 3. SVM classification results using the single modalities and the combined data

FA	MD	WMD	GMD	Accuracy	Sensitivity	Specificity	γ	C
×				80.3% [66.0,94.7]	78.8% [57.1,96.6]	81.9% [64.3,100.0]	2^{-10}	4
	×			83.3% [69.1,96.4]	79.6% [57.1,100.0]	86.9% [71.4,100.0]	2^{-12}	32
		×		82.7% [67.9,96.4]	77.9% [55.4,92.9]	87.4% [71.4,100.0]	2^{-14}	8
			×	89.3% [78.6,100.0]	87.4% [69.2,100.0]	91.2% [72.3,100.0]	2^{-12}	4
×	×			83.2% [82.1,96.4]	82.9% [84.6,100.0]	83.5% [65.4,100.0]	2^{-12}	32
×	×	×		83.3% [71.4,96.4]	82.8% [60.5,100.0]	83.6% [62.8,100.0]	2^{-13}	8
		×	×	89.0% [75.0,98.4]	88.7% [71.4,100.0]	89.2% [70.3,100.0]	2^{-14}	4
×			×	89.2% [78.6,98.4]	89.1% [71.4,100.0]	89.1% [71.4,100.0]	2^{-13}	2
	×		×	88.7% [78.6,100.0]	88.6% [71.4,100.0]	88.7% [71.4,100.0]	2^{-13}	4
×	×		×	89.1% [76.7,96.6]	89.2% [71.4,100.0]	88.8% [70.3,100.0]	2^{-14}	4
×	×	×	×	88.8% [78.6,96.4]	88.6% [71.4,100.0]	88.8% [66.6,100.0]	2^{-16}	4

Table 4. Classification results using the prediction labels from optimized SVMs as input for the given classifiers

Classifier	Accuracy	Sensitivity	Specificity
Voting	86.0% [75.0,96.4]	77.9% [57.1,92.9]	93.8% [80.0,100.0]
J48 Decision Tree	82.9% [69.1,96.4]	86.8% [71.4,100.0]	78.9% [57.1,100.0]
Linear SVM	86.4% [71.4,96.4]	91.7% [72.3,100.0]	80.9% [61.5,100.0]
Multilayer Perceptron	88.5% [76.3,100.0]	88.8% [71.4,100.0]	88.1% [71.4,100.0]
Logistic Regression	87.8% [76.3,98.3]	89.3% [71.4,100.0]	86.2% [64.3,100.0]
Naïve Bayes	87.5% [89.3,98.3]	89.8% [71.4,100.0]	85.0% [64.3,100.0]

Table 5. Classification results using the distance from the separation hyperplane of optimized SVMs as input for the given classifiers

Classifier	Accuracy	Sensitivity	Specificity
J48 Decision Tree	56.2% [48.2,66.2]	100.0% [100.0,100.0]	12.4% [0.0,29.7]
Linear SVM	88.7% [78.6,100.0]	88.4% [68.9,100.0]	88.8% [70.3,100.0]
Multilayer Perceptron	88.1% [76.7,98.4]	87.0% [70.3,100.0]	89.0% [70.3,100.0]
Logistic Regression	87.9% [75.0,98.4]	87.7% [70.3,100.0]	88.0% [69.2,100.0]
Naïve Bayes	86.7% [75.4,98.3]	86.8% [71.4,100.0]	86.7% [64.3,100.0]

Table 6. Classification results obtained by the multiple kernel SVM using the given parameters

Classifier	Accuracy	Sensitivity	Specificity	β_{FA}	β_{MD}	β_{WMD}	β_{GMD}	C
MK-SVM*	88.6%[78.6,100.0]	85.9%[66.7,100.0]	91.2%[75.8,100.0]	0.5	0.5	1.5	1.5	2
MK-SVM**	88.1%[75.4,98.4]	85.6%[65.4,100.0]	90.6%[71.4,100.0]	0.5	0.75	0.75	1.5	4

*Optimal parameters determined by grid search. **Arbitrarily set parameters reflecting the proportion of accuracy obtained for each single modality.

4   Discussion

Our diagnostic classification results of approximately 89% accuracy for GMD data are already relatively high and compare favorably with previous studies. But such a high accuracy also lowers the chance for further increase when using multimodal data. For the contingency tables with GMD data, the entries of $N_{10} \leq 12$ (see Table 2) indicate that an increase of at maximum $12/280 \approx 4\%$ is possible if all those subjects were additionally classified correctly. We received the same accuracies using the single modality GMD data as for the combined datasets when containing GMD and the meta classifier approach. In contrast to the results reported in [6], [8], and [9], we could not improve the classification performance using MK-SVM. This may be due to our sample which consisted of mildly to moderately affected patients. There, cortical atrophy may be far progressed such that the decline in structural network connectivity derived from DTI may not add additional information relevant for the SVM classification. This may be different for predementia stages of AD, e.g. in aMCI. Currently, we could not evaluate the performance of our approaches in the prediction of AD dementia. Future work of the EDSD will extend the database to include subjects with aMCI in order to investigate this topic.

Previous studies [6,8,9] reported superior detection rates of AD using multimodal data compared to single modality analysis. They included data from structural neuroimaging techniques, such as MRI and DTI, as well as functional neuroimaging data, e.g. functional MRI and FDG-PET. These and our results together suggest that combined structural/functional datasets are more likely to benefit from multimodal analysis for the detection of AD than using multimodal structural data only, e.g. DTI and MRI. More research is needed to investigate if this hypothesis is true and if it also applies for the detection of AD in predementia stages of AD.

The results obtained by the J48 decision tree using the distance from the SVM separation hyperplane (Table 5) are most likely an artifact of overfitting.

4.1   Limitations

We did not remove variance introduced by confounding factors such as age, gender or acquisition center, so that our results might be biased due to (i) higher variability of the data caused by multicenter acquisition and (ii) atrophy effects caused by age. Nevertheless, the missing differences between the multimodal data analysis and the single modality results should remain persistent when applying data correction methods.

5   Conclusion

In this study we evaluated different approaches (i) to combine the neuroimaging modalities MRI and DTI and (ii) to combine different classifiers. With our sample of mildly to moderately affected patients, combining modalities did not increase the detection rates of AD. Further research will focus on (i) multimodal detection of AD in predementia stages of AD, e.g. in aMCI, and (ii) evaluating the classification performance when adding other modalities, e.g. functional MRI or FDG-PET.

Acknowledgement. We want to thank the members of the EDSD for their support. The work of Claudia Plant was supported by the Alexander von Humboldt-Foundation.

References

1. Concha, L., Gross, D.W., Wheatley, B.M., Beaulieu, C.: Diffusion tensor imaging of time-dependent axonal and myelin degradation after corpus callosotomy in epilepsy patients. NeuroImage 32(3), 1090–1099 (2006)
2. Takagi, T., Nakamura, M., Yamada, M., Hikishima, K., Momoshima, S., Fujiyoshi, K., Shibata, S., Okano, H.J., Toyama, Y., Okano, H.: Visualization of peripheral nerve degeneration and regeneration: Monitoring with diffusion tensor tractography. NeuroImage 44(3), 884–892 (2009)
3. Clerx, L., Visser, P.J., Verhey, F., Aalten, P.: New MRI Markers for Alzheimer's Disease: A Meta-Analysis of Diffusion Tensor Imaging and a Comparison with Medial Temporal Lobe Measurements. Journal of Alzheimer's Disease 29(2), 405–429 (2012)
4. Müller, M.J., Greverus, D., Weibrich, C., Dellani, P.R., Scheurich, A., Stoeter, P., Fellgiebel, A.: Diagnostic utility of hippocampal size and mean diffusivity in amnestic MCI. Neurobiology of Aging 28(3), 398–403 (2007)
5. Scola, E., Bozzali, M., Agosta, F., Magnani, G., Franceschi, M., Sormani, M.P., Cercignani, M., Pagani, E., Falautano, M., Filippi, M., Falini, A.: A diffusion tensor MRI study of patients with MCI and AD with a 2-year clinical follow-up. Journal of Neurology, Neurosurgery & Psychiatry 81(7), 798–805 (2010)
6. Wee, C.-Y., Yap, P.-T., Zhang, D., Denny, K., Browndyke, J.N., Potter, G.G., Welsh-Bohmer, K.A., Wang, L., Shen, D.: Identification of MCI individuals using structural and functional connectivity networks. NeuroImage 59(3), 2045–2056 (2012)
7. Dukart, J., Mueller, K., Horstmann, A., Barthel, H., Möller, H.E., Villringer, A., Sabri, O., Schroeter, M.L.: Combined evaluation of FDG-PET and MRI improves detection and differentiation of dementia. PLoS ONE 6(3), e18111 (2011)
8. Zhang, D., Wang, Y., Zhou, L., Yuan, H., Shen, D.: Multimodal classification of Alzheimer's disease and mild cognitive impairment. NeuroImage 55(3), 856–867 (2011)
9. Hinrichs, C., Singh, V., Xu, G., Johnson, S.C.: Predictive markers for AD in a multi-modality framework: an analysis of MCI progression in the ADNI population. NeuroImage 55(2), 574–589 (2011)
10. Dyrba, M., Ewers, M., Wegrzyn, M., Kilimann, I., Plant, C., Oswald, A., Meindl, T., Pievani, M., Bokde, A.L., Fellgiebel, A., Filippi, M., Hampel, H.J., Klöppel, S., Hauenstein, K., Kirste, T., Teipel, S.J.: Automated detection of structural changes in Alzheimer's disease using multicenter DTI (submitted)

11. McKhann, G., Drachman, D., Folstein, M., Katzman, R., Price, D., Stadlan, E.M.: Clinical diagnosis of Alzheimer's disease: report of the NINCDS-ADRDA Work Group under the auspices of Department of Health and Human Services Task Force on Alzheimer's Disease. Neurology 34(7), 939–944 (1984)
12. Teipel, S.J., Wegrzyn, M., Meindl, T., Frisoni, G., Bokde, A.L.W., Fellgiebel, A., Filippi, M., Hampel, H., Klöppel, S., Hauenstein, K., Ewers, M., and the EDSD study group: Anatomical MRI and DTI in the diagnosis of Alzheimer's disease: a European Multicenter Study. Journal of Alzheimer's Disease (in press)
13. Morris, J.C., Heyman, A., Mohs, R.C., Hughes, J.P., van Belle, G., Fillenbaum, G., Mellits, E.D., Clark, C.: The Consortium to Establish a Registry for Alzheimer's Disease (CERAD). Part I. Clinical and neuropsychological assessment of Alzheimer's disease. Neurology 39(9), 1159–1165 (1989)
14. Folstein, M.F., Folstein, S.E., McHugh, P.R.: Mini-mental state. Journal of Psychiatric Research 12(3), 189–198 (1975)
15. Smith, S.M., Jenkinson, M., Woolrich, M.W., Beckmann, C.F., Behrens, T.E.J., Johansen-Berg, H., Bannister, P.R., Luca, M.d., Drobnjak, I., Flitney, D.E., Niazy, R.K., Saunders, J., Vickers, J., Zhang, Y., Stefano, N.d., Brady, J.M., Matthews, P.M.: Advances in functional and structural MR image analysis and implementation as FSL. NeuroImage 23(0)(Suppl. 1), S208–S219 (2004)
16. Gaser, C., Volz, H.-P., Kiebel, S., Riehemann, S., Sauer, H.: Detecting Structural Changes in Whole Brain Based on Nonlinear Deformations—Application to Schizophrenia Research. NeuroImage 10(2), 107–113 (1999)
17. Witten, I.H., Frank, E.: Data Mining: Practical Machine Learning Tools and Techniques, 2nd edn. The Morgan Kaufmann Series in Data Management Systems. Morgan Kaufmann Publishers, San Francisco and CA (2005)
18. Chang, C.-C., Lin, C.-J.: LIBSVM: A library for support vector machines. ACM Transactions on Intelligent Systems and Technology 2(3), 27:1–27:27 (2011)
19. Plant, C., Teipel, S.J., Oswald, A., Böhm, C., Meindl, T., Mourão-Miranda, J., Bokde, A.W., Hampel, H., Ewers, M.: Automated detection of brain atrophy patterns based on MRI for the prediction of Alzheimer's disease. NeuroImage 50(1), 162–174 (2010)
20. Hall, M.A., Holmes, G.: Benchmarking Attribute Selection Techniques for Discrete Class Data Mining. IEEE Transactions On Knowledge And Data Engineering 15, 1437–1447 (2003)
21. Cortes, C., Vapnik, V.: Support-vector networks. Machine Learning 20, 273–297 (1995)
22. Sonnenburg, S., Rätsch, G., Schäfer, C., Schölkopf, B.: Large Scale Multiple Kernel Learning. Journal of Machine Learning Research 7, 1531–1565 (2006)

Genetics of Path Lengths in Brain Connectivity Networks: HARDI-Based Maps in 457 Adults

Neda Jahanshad[1], Gautam Prasad[1], Arthur W. Toga[1],
Katie L. McMahon[2], Greig I. de Zubicaray[3], Nicholas G. Martin[4],
Margaret J. Wright[4], and Paul M. Thompson[1]

[1] Imaging Genetics Center - Laboratory of Neuro Imaging,
Department of Neurology, UCLA School of Medicine, Los Angeles, CA
[2] University of Queensland, Centre for Advanced Imaging, Brisbane, Australia
[3] University of Queensland, School of Psychology, Brisbane, Australia
[4] Queensland Institute of Medical Research, Brisbane, Australia

Abstract. Brain connectivity analyses are increasingly popular for investigating organization. Many connectivity measures including path lengths are generally defined as the number of nodes traversed to connect a node in a graph to the others. Despite its name, path length is purely topological, and does not take into account the physical length of the connections. The distance of the trajectory may also be highly relevant, but is typically overlooked in connectivity analyses. Here we combined genotyping, anatomical MRI and HARDI to understand how our genes influence the cortical connections, using whole-brain tractography. We defined a new measure, based on Dijkstra's algorithm, to compute path lengths for tracts connecting pairs of cortical regions. We compiled these measures into matrices where elements represent the physical distance traveled along tracts. We then analyzed a large cohort of healthy twins and show that our path length measure is reliable, heritable, and influenced even in young adults by the Alzheimer's risk gene, *CLU*.

Keywords: Structural connectivity, neuroimaging genetics, Dijkstra's algorithm, HARDI tractography, path length.

1 Introduction

Understanding the structural and functional connectivity of the brain's neural networks is critical for determining pathways and mechanisms underlying behavior and brain disease. Diffusion tensor imaging, and its mathematical extensions such as HARDI or q-space imaging, have been used to study anatomical connectivity in development [1] and in disorders such as Alzheimer's disease [2]. Such studies shed light on how connections and pathways are disrupted or altered in various diseases.

Analyses of neural network connectivity are increasingly popular, with a rapid rise in the use of methods to map functional and structural networks in the living brain. With diffusion imaging and tractography, physical connections from one region of the brain to another can be tracked. By tracking pairwise connections between a set of N

P.-T. Yap et al. (Eds.): MBIA 2012, LNCS 7509, pp. 29–40, 2012.

regions of interest on the cortex, we can summarize properties of these connections in a matrix. Graphs can be created, in which the nodes represent cortical regions, and edges represent the connections between them. Standard graph theory measures can often be used to summarize global properties of the network. For example, the 'characteristic path length' measures the average number of nodes that must be traversed to connect any one node in the graph to all the others. Despite its name, this average path length depends only on the network topology and not on how it is embedded in space: it ignores the length of any physical connection between the nodes (such as axons in the brain). When used for brain network analysis, the physical distance between cortical regions may also be relevant, as (among other factors) it may affect how vulnerable the connection is to lesions such as stroke, tumors, trauma, or degenerative processes.

In this work, we use tractography based on both high angular resolution diffusion imaging (HARDI) and co-registered standard anatomical MRI to map fibers in the brain connecting various cortical regions. We created maps of the proportions of fibers that interconnect various cortical regions within and across hemispheres and calculate an optimal path between cortical regions based on the fiber counts. By computing these connection matrices in a large cohort of 457 healthy adult twins, we were able to apply quantitative genetic analysis to discover how strongly our genetic make-up affects the lengths of paths connecting different cortical regions. In addition, regardless of the statistical analysis, the measures representing the length of the trajectory of fibers from one cortical region to another could also be used to weight an overall, topological measure of characteristic path length and determine the average length of fiber trajectory. We note that in network analyses, the metric embedding and spatial configuration of the brain's network nodes is typically overlooked, but that same information may be of interest in trying to discover factors that affect the brain's wiring efficiency.

Combining diffusion imaging with genetic analysis is also fruitful, and very recently several common genetic variants have been discovered that affect the integrity of the brain's white matter [3-6]. In general, genetic studies begin by estimating the overall degree of genetic influence on brain measures, as a helpful precursor to candidate gene studies or genome-wide scans (GWAS) to identify factors that may influence white matter fiber connectivity [7]. Any genetically influenced connections or network properties could be prioritized as endophenotypes in the quest to discover specific genetic variants involved in the formation, insufficiency, and degeneration of these pathways. Twin studies have long been used to determine the degree of genetic influence over human traits. Monozygotic twins (MZ) share all their genes while dizygotic twins (DZ) share, on average, half. Here we used Falconer's heritability statistic (h^2) to study how strongly DTI measures are influence by our genetic make-up. Falconer's heritability estimate is a simple measure that examines differences in intra-class correlations between the two kinds of twins, identical (MZ) and fraternal (DZ). If MZ twins are more highly correlated than DZ twins, we can infer that the trait is affected to some extent by genetic influences, and the proportion of variance due to genetics can also be estimated.

In this study, we use ODF-based tractography on state-of-the-art 4-Tesla HARDI images from 457 young adult subjects to define the first geometric measure of white matter path length underlying cortical connectivity. The resulting measure is heritable, and a topological analysis of the matrix reveals a genetic association to the Alzheimer's risk gene, CLU.

2   Methods

2.1   Image Acquisition and Subject Information

Whole-brain 3D anatomical MRI and HARDI scans were acquired from 457 genotyped subjects with a high magnetic field (4T) Bruker Medspec MRI scanner. T1-weighted images were acquired with an inversion recovery rapid gradient echo sequence. Acquisition parameters were: TI/TR/TE= 700/1500/3.35 ms; flip angle=8 degrees; slice thickness = 0.9mm, with a 256x256 acquisition matrix. Diffusion-weighted images (DWI) were acquired using single-shot echo planar imaging with a twice-refocused spin echo sequence to reduce eddy-current induced distortions. Imaging parameters were: 23 cm FOV, TR/TE 6090/91.7 ms, with a 128x128 acquisition matrix. Each 3D volume consisted of 55 2-mm thick axial slices with no gap and 1.79x1.79 mm^2 in-plane resolution. 105 images were acquired per subject: 11 with no diffusion sensitization (i.e., b_0 images) and 94 DWI (b=1159 s/mm^2) with gradient directions evenly distributed on the hemisphere. Scan time was 14.2 minutes. In total, images from 457 right-handed young adults (mean age: 23.4 years, s.d. 2.0) were included, comprising 124 MZ (62 pairs) and 94 same-sex DZ twins (47 pairs), other subjects included different sex DZ twins, and siblings. Originally 545 scans were analyzed, but after rigorous quality control (removing images with artifacts or poor segmentation), 457 genotyped individuals remained.

2.2   Cortical Extraction and HARDI Tractography

Non-brain regions were automatically removed from each T1-weighted MRI scan, and from a T2-weighted image from the DWI set using the FSL tool "BET" (http://fsl.fmrib.ox.ac.uk/fsl/). A trained neuroanatomical expert manually edited the T1-weighted scans to further refine the brain extraction. All T1-weighted images were linearly aligned using FSL (with 9 DOF) to a common space with 1mm isotropic voxels and a 220x220x220 voxel matrix. DWI were corrected for eddy current distortions using the FSL tools (http://fsl.fmrib.ox.ac.uk/fsl/). For each subject, the 11 images with no diffusion sensitization were averaged, linearly aligned and resampled to a downsampled version of their T1 image (110x110x110, 2x2x2mm). b_0 maps were elastically registered to the T1 scan to compensate for susceptibility artifacts.

The transformation matrix from the linear alignment of the mean b_0 image to the T1-weighted volume was applied to each of the 94 gradient directions to properly re-orient the orientation distribution functions (ODFs). We performed HARDI specific tractography as performed in [8] on the linearly aligned sets of DWI volumes.

Elastic deformations obtained from the EPI distortion correction, mapping the average b_0 image to the T1-weighted image, were then applied to the tract's 3D coordinates for accurate alignment of the anatomy. Each subject's dataset contained 5000-10,000 useable fibers (3D curves) in total.

34 cortical labels per hemisphere, as listed in the Desikan-Killiany atlas [9], were automatically extracted from all aligned T1-weighted structural MRI scans using FreeSurfer (http://surfer.nmr.mgh.harvard.edu/) [10]. Labels were numbered 1-35, with no label segmented for region 4. The resulting T1-weighted images and cortical models were aligned to the original T1 input image space and down-sampled using nearest neighbor interpolation (to avoid intermixing of labels) to the space of the DWIs. To ensure tracts would intersect labeled cortical regions, labels were dilated with an isotropic box kernel of width 5 voxels.

2.3   Calculating the Connectivity Matrix and Fiber Density Maps

For each subject, a full 68×68 structural connectivity matrix was created. Each element described the proportion of the total number of detected fibers in the brain connecting each of the labels; diagonal elements of this matrix describe the total number of fibers passing through a certain cortical region of interest. In what follows, we will use the term *fibers* to designate the 3D streamlines or curves that result from whole brain tractography, even though strictly speaking only *post mortem* validation would reveal whether they correspond to true axonal pathways in the brain. If more than 5% of subjects had no detected fibers connecting the regions denoted by a matrix element, then the connection was considered invalid, or insufficiently consistent in its incidence in the population, and was not included in the analysis. For each connection across two nodes that was considered valid across the full healthy population (200 different connections from the full matrix were present in 95% of the population), a fiber density image was created. This image consists of a voxelwise mapping of the fibers intersecting the two regions, where a count of fibers crossing each voxel was made.

2.4   Path Length Calculations

Level sets and fast marching methods have been previously described to map structural brain connectivity by following the principal directional of diffusion anisotropy in DTI scans [11, 12]; even maps of connectivity defined in this way have been shown to be genetically influenced [13]. However, here, instead of the using the tensor information to propagate the flow of fibers, we use a map of fiber density, or counts of fibers at each voxel as a result of tractography, to map a path between one cortical region to another by following the trajectory of high fiber counts through discrete voxels. We note that this path may correspond, to some extent, with the path of information flow between cortical regions, as impulses are propagated along the axons recovered by tractography. We used Dijkstra's algorithm [14] to trace the path of highest density. Dijkstra's algorithm is a graph search method to find the shortest discrete path from a source node to every other node while minimizing the weight of the edges; it has been previously applied for tractography [15]. Here we focus not on following specific voxelwise paths in which fibers follow for tractography, but focus on the density of fibers at each voxel, following the path of highest density. In essence, this can help trace the most likely path of information flow from one cortical region to another.

All voxels in each person's 3D fiber density map were then considered as nodes in a graph; and each node in the graph is considered to be connected to 26 nodes (3D neighboring voxels) by undirected edges. Note that now we are considering adjacency in the 3D image, not the 2D matrix of cortical connections. Each edge was weighted inversely by the sum of the fiber densities at each of the two voxels on the edge, and the weight was inversely proportional to the Euclidean distance from the center of one voxel to the other. As the edge weights correspond to edge *costs* for our shortest path detection method, a connection between a pair of voxels that each had a high fiber density was assigned to a lower weight, or lower cost. Suppose voxels i and j are voxelwise neighbors with integer fiber counts (densities) di and dj respectively. Then we defined the edge weight as $W_{i,j} = \dfrac{1}{d_i + d_j}$. As most voxels in the density image are not immediate neighbors of each other (the region is generally a elongated path several voxels wide), the path graph can be represented by a sparse matrix. Dijkstra's algorithm would then follow the path of minimal edge weights, or maximal density connections.

To find the shortest path through the graph from one cortical connection to another, Dijkstra's algorithm requires the graph to have specified start and end nodes. A single point was selected at each region to serve as path start and end points to map the trajectory of the path from one cortical region to another.

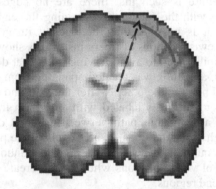

Fig. 1. To select the representative point for each ROI, the spherical coordinates of all label voxels were calculated from the 3D center of the image (yellow circle). The median radial distance was calculated from all points along the cortical label (red curve). Also if two points were only different in their radius (blue solid line and thick black dashed line), then their angular components were only counted once to not over influence the mean. Subsequently, the geometric mean of all these points, back in the Cartesian image space, was calculated as the representative point for the cortical region.

A single representative point was calculated from each of the cortical regions of interest from the parcellated T1 image, and it was defined so as to avoid excessive influence of cortical folding patterns and depth on the position of the selected representative point. The representative point was selected based on all voxels from the entire segmented label (before label dilation). Voxel coordinates were transformed to spherical coordinates (r, radius, θ polar angle, and φ azimuthal angle) from the stereotaxic image center. The median radial distance from the center point was chosen to represent the depth along the surface. Only unique pairs of angles were retained to prevent over representation of inner and outer cortical points with the same angular projection. A 2D illustration of this is shown in **Fig 1.** Retained points were then converted back to the Cartesian space and the corresponding geometric mean was used as the center point. These points then served as the corresponding end points for each ROI. They were defined in such a way as to be less influenced by cortical folding patterns than the centroid of the regions.

Mapping the path from ROI-1 to ROI-2 would not necessarily follow the same path as that from ROI-2 to ROI-1. To ensure symmetry, we select the point with the highest fiber density in the pathway connecting the two regions of interest as the starting point. To make sure that the fibers in the pathway were in fact only those that intersected 2 ROIs, a fiber density map was created for each of 200 pairs of connections, by filtering the tractography output files. The point of maximal fiber density in only those fibers was chosen as the *start point*. If more than one point had the equivalent maximal density, the point with the minimal Euclidean distance from the midpoint of the two ROI endpoints was chosen as the start.

The algorithm will be incapable of finding an accurate connection between the two nodes if the graph structure is such that there are no edges from the subgraph containing the start node with the subgraph containing the end node. As the fibers discretized into voxels, it is possible that the density image would not show a continuous path, but piecewise sections of fibers instead, as shown in 2D in **Figure 1**. To account for this possibility, and to avoid having tracts that do not start and end in different cortical regions, a 3D box was created spanning from the start point in one cortical region to the end point in the other. After the start and end points have been computed, this box is then artificially labeled with a uniform fractional fiber density count (0.5) to allow for a continuous path between different cortical regions to be connected, albeit at a high cost. Additionally, all voxels of the path were dilated (and given the small density count). This helps to ensure a continuous path such that the algorithm can find a set of voxel locations where it can create a representative path connecting the start and end regions.

Once the optimal path has been calculated based on the weights, the length of the path is computed by summing the distances from the center of the neighboring voxel points along the path, starting from the start point, following the path, and ending at the end point in the other cortical region. Alternative approaches might use tensor-derived measures such as FA as weights for each voxel visited along the path, or other scalar diffusion measures to describe the properties of the path.

Once all the path lengths have been calculated from all valid cortical connections to the next, an *observed path length* connectivity matrix can be computed. Instead of using each element to represent the proportion of fibers in the brain that run between the regions, the physical length of fibers connecting the regions is approximated.

Dijkstra's   algorithm   was   implemented   in   Matlab   using
http://www.mathworks.com/matlabcentral/fileexchange/10922-matlabbgl   the
'matlab_bgl' toolbox.

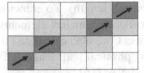

Fig. 2. Discretization of a fiber into a set of voxels in the image (here in 2D, but the 3D case is tackled in the paper) may leave a piecewise path (*dark blue*) rather than a connected one. Voxels are dilated (*light blue*) to ensure a connected path exists.

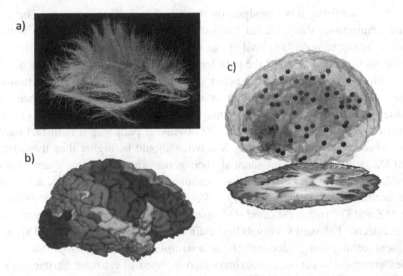

Fig. 3. A) Full brain tractography is performed using HARDI based tractography on high field, high resolution images; B) Automatic cortical parcellation in Freesurfer [10] is simultaneously conducted on the T1-weighted high field scans. Once DWI and T1 scans are registered together to account for susceptibility artifacts, tracts are filtered to include only those going through pairs of cortical regions to create 200 filtered fiber density images, one for each valid pair of connections. C) Fibers that remain going through the left rostral anterior cingulate and left medial orbital frontal cortices are shown in yellow for a single subject. Representative points for each cortical region are extracted; points shown in black across brain surface, points of interest show in red; the highest density point is selected from the filtered fiber density file (shown as a green sphere). To ensure symmetry, the point of highest density is traced to each one of the red endpoints of interest based Dijkstra's algorithm following the highest density path. The resulting path is shown in blue. This represents only one element in the 68x68 path length connectivity matrix as all combinations of connections are calculated in the same way.

2.5   Overall Physical Path Length

In this study, brain network matrices were created by calculating a true path length between individual cortical regions. We used a single point determined from each of the segmented regions of interest, on the cortical surface, as an end point in a path. The distance along this path is calculated. The common topological measure *characteristic path length* (CPL) is an average measure (across the whole network) of the minimum number of edges necessary to travel from one node to another in the network (i.e., average minimum path length). To coincide with this common measure generally calculated using networks with matrix elements based on cortical activation correlations or proportions of fibers, we also calculated this overall path length index, using a weighting based on our 'physical path length'. This was performed using the Brain Connectivity Toolbox in Matlab [16].

2.6   Heritability of Path Length Analysis

In this study, we focused our analysis on the set of 'valid' connections. These at the detected connections that proceed from one brain region to another in almost all individuals in our sample. One goal of our work is to determine genetic influences on the brain, so we tested whether the path length connecting cortical regions across the corpus callosum is heritable. In genetics, the 'heritability' is the proportion of the observed variance in a measure that is attributable to genetic differences across individuals. To assess heritability, we use the fact that our large sample consists of both monozygotic (MZ) and dizygotic (DZ) twins. If path length is in fact heritable, then the observed correlations among MZ twins should be higher than those between pairs of DZ twins, as MZ twins share all their genes while DZ twins share on average only half. If genes had no effect on the measures, then the correlations should not be any higher for MZ than DZ twins [17]. We computed intra-class correlations (ICC) within MZ and DZ twins, rMZ and rDZ respectively, to compute a simple measure of genetic effects: Falconer's heritability estimate, $h^2 = 2(rMZ-rDZ)$ [18] at each subsequent connection (Falconer's h^2 is a simple but widely-used statistic; more complex structural equation models may also be used to estimate heritability). Here the ICC was calculated as

$$ICC = \frac{MSB - MSE}{MSB + MSE}, MSB = 2\sum_{i=1}^{N}\frac{(\mu_i - \tilde{\mu})^2}{N-1}, MSE = \sum_{i=1}^{N}\frac{\sigma_i}{N}, \sigma_i = (N1_i - \mu_i)^2 + (N2_i - \mu_i)^2, \mu_i = \frac{N1_i + N2_i}{2}$$

where MSB corresponds to the mean square error between pairs; MSE is the mean squared error across the full set of pairs. N refers to the total number of pairs, while $N1_i$ and $N2_i$ represent each individual within pair i.

Reproducibility and reliability of the connections were assessed by examining the ICC for 12 unrelated subjects scanned twice with the exact same protocol, approximately 3 months apart. Tractography and cortical surface extractions were performed for both time points. For the reproducibility analysis, only unrelated subjects were analyzed because the inclusion of related subjects (e.g., MZ twins) could bias the estimate of reliability by reducing the MSE relative to what would be obtained by independent sampling of the young adult population.

2.7   Genetic Association of Overall Path Length

In this analysis, we found that our topological measure was quite heritable (see *Results*). To further delve into the possible genetic basis for the heritability, we also assessed effects of a candidate gene that was previously found to influence fractional anisotropy on DTI. The *CLU* single nucleotide polymorphism, at rs11136000, is a very commonly carried variant in the genome that is consistently associated with Alzheimer's disease in vast samples of tens of thousands of subjects [19] in recent work, it has also been shown to alter brain structure in healthy adults without AD [20]. The number of risk alleles a person carries (0,1 or 2) at the rs11136000 locus was regressed against the overall 'characteristic' path length measure, as weighted by the approximate distance traveled as calculated above. As our subjects were related, we used a statistical mixed model, including a kinship matrix, to test associations [21]. We also covaried for the effects of age, sex, and brain size, which can clearly affect our measured lengths.

3   Results

Our path length matrices showed moderate levels of heritability (in 228 twins) and reliability (in 12 unrelated individuals scanned twice with a three month interval with both sMRI and HARDI), with reliability comparable to that observed for fiber count matrices in [22].

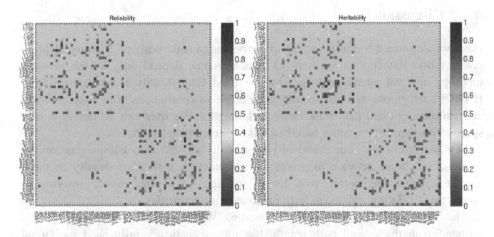

Fig. 4. (A) Connectivity map of the path length estimates for reliability and (B) the heritability. Certain connections, including the connection of the right insula with the right inferior temporal lobe show both high levels of heritability (~0.6) as well as high reliability as measured in 12 individuals (~0.6).

The standard topological measure, *characteristic path length*, was calculated (1) using matrices weighted by the distance between cortical regions as defined in this paper, and also (2) with the more standard "fiber count measure" where matrix elements represent the proportion of traced fibers connecting one region to another [23]. We find the heritability (as measured by Falconer's h^2) of our new more accurately termed characteristic path length measure was 0.76, while for the more traditional measure, it was 0.08. This is promising for genetic studies; even though a high heritability – meaning strong genetic control – is not a guarantee that SNP effects will be large, it is certainly true that SNP effects are unlikely to be found at all for measures whose heritability is very low. For that reason alone, this new measure becomes a strong candidate for very large scale genetic association studies, such as those conducted by the ENIGMA consortium [7].

Such high heritability suggests the value of conducting a search for specific genetic influences on these pathways. We reserve an unguided search of the genome for future analysis, and use a candidate gene to show the potential of our measure here. As the *CLU* SNP has been previously shown to be associated with differences in white matter microstructure in healthy adults, here we tested whether it also was related to the global length of fiber paths traveled around the brain, based on the connection distances defined in this paper. We found that in fact a person's *CLU* genotype was indeed associated with our global path length measure. Each additional copy of the AD-risk *CLU*-C allele was associated with a 0.9 voxel (1.8mm) increase in characteristic path length ($p=0.003$). This can perhaps reveal more mechanistic detail on the effect of the gene, perhaps even suggesting a less efficient brain network in people who carry the adverse variant of this risk gene.

4   Discussion

Here we developed a novel method to probe the genetic basis of anatomical brain connectivity. Rather than use network measures that depend only on the network topology and not on the path lengths, we used fiber density maps derived from HARDI tractography as a way to weight the edges or connections from voxel to voxel and estimate optimal path trajectories and lengths. We used this to define a new symmetric connectivity matrix based on this observed path length.

Our analysis of this large cohort of young adults allowed us to estimate heritability of structural brain network measures. In conjunction with fiber density at these elements across the matrix, path length matrices may offer robust analyses of connections, offering additional detail on connection properties.

This work suggests several follow up studies. While we examined specific genetic influences on the overall path length, the most genetically influenced individual connections may also be promising targets to prioritize in the search for genes influencing brain integrity and risk for psychiatric disease. Connections under strong genetic control may serve as powerful endophenotypes to search for specific genetic variants influencing the human brain.

Acknowledgments. This study was supported by the National Institute of Child Health and Human Development (R01 HD050735), and the National Health and Medical Research Council (NHMRC 486682), Australia. Genotyping was supported by NHMRC (389875). Additional support for algorithm development was provided by NIH R01 grants EB008432, EB008281, and EB007813. GP is additionally supported by the UCLA I2-IDRE Research Informatics and Computational Data Development Grant. GZ is supported by an ARC Future Fellowship (FT0991634).

References

1. Hagmann, P., et al.: White matter maturation reshapes structural connectivity in the late developing human brain. Proc. Natl. Acad. Sci. U S A 107(44), 19067–19072 (2010)
2. Zhou, Y., et al.: Abnormal connectivity in the posterior cingulate and hippocampus in early Alzheimer's disease and mild cognitive impairment. Alzheimers Dement 4(4), 265–270 (2008)
3. Brown, J.A., et al.: Brain network local interconnectivity loss in aging *APOE-4* allele carriers. Proc. Natl. Acad. Sci. U S A 108(51), 20760–20765 (2011)
4. Dennis, E.L., et al.: Altered structural brain connectivity in healthy carriers of the autism risk gene, CNTNAP2. Brain Connect 1(6), 447–459 (2011)
5. Lopez, L.M., et al.: A genome-wide search for genetic influences and biological pathways related to the brain's white matter integrity. Neurobiol Aging (in Press. 2012)
6. Jahanshad, N., et al.: Brain structure in healthy adults is related to serum transferring and the H63D polymorphism in the *HFE* gene. Proc. Natl. Acad. Sci. U S A 109(14), E851–E859 (2012)
7. Kochunov, P., et al.: Genome-wide association of full brain white matter integrity – from the ENIGMA DTI working group. Organization of Human Brain Mapping, Beijing, China (2012)
8. Aganj, I., et al.: A Hough transform global probabilistic approach to multiple-subject diffusion MRI tractography. Med. Image Anal. 15(4), 414–425 (2011)
9. Desikan, R.S., et al.: An automated labeling system for subdividing the human cerebral cortex on MRI scans into gyral based regions of interest. Neuroimage 31(3), 968–980 (2006)
10. Fischl, B., et al.: Automatically parcellating the human cerebral cortex. Cereb. Cortex 14(1), 11–22 (2004)
11. Parker, G.J., Wheeler-Kingshott, C.A., Barker, G.J.: Estimating distributed anatomical connectivity using fast marching methods and diffusion tensor imaging. IEEE Trans. Med. Imaging 21(5), 505–512 (2002)
12. Prados, E., et al.: Control Theory and Fast Marching Techniques for Brain Connectivity Mapping. In: 2006 IEEE Computer Society Conference on Computer Vision and Pattern Recognition (2006)
13. Patel, V., et al.: Scalar connectivity measures from fast-marching tractography reveal heritability of white matter architecture. In: ISBI, pp. 1109–1112. IEEE, Rotterdam (2010)
14. Dijkstra, E.W.: A note on two problems in connexion with graphs. Numerische Mathematik 1(1), 269–271 (1959)
15. Zalesky, A.: DT-MRI fiber tracking: a shortest paths approach. IEEE Trans. Med. Imaging 27(10), 1458–1471 (2008)
16. Rubinov, M., Sporns, O.: Complex network measures of brain connectivity: uses and interpretations. Neuroimage 52(3), 1059–1069 (2010)

17. Thompson, P.M., et al.: Genetic influences on brain structure. Nat. Neurosci. 4(12), 1253–1258 (2001)
18. Veale, A.M.O.: Introduction to Quantitative Genetics - Falconer, D.S. The Royal Statistical Society Series C-Applied Statistics 9(3), 202–203 (1960)
19. Harold, D., et al.: Genome-wide association study identifies variants at *CLU* and *PICALM* associated with Alzheimer's disease. Nat. Genet. 41(10), 1088–1093 (2009)
20. Braskie, M.N., et al.: Common Alzheimer's Disease Risk Variant Within the *CLU* Gene Affects White Matter Microstructure in Young Adults. J. Neurosci. 31(18), 6764–6770 (2011)
21. Kang, H.M., et al.: Efficient control of population structure in model organism association mapping. Genetics 178(3), 1709–1723 (2008)
22. Dennis, E.L., et al.: Test-retest reliability of graph theory measures of structural brain connectivity. In: Medical Image Computing and Computer Assisted Intervention, Nice, France. LNCS (in press, 2012)
23. Jahanshad, N., et al.: Sex differences in the Human Connectome: 4-Tesla high angular resolution diffusion tensor imaging (HARDI) tractography in 234 young adult twins. In: ISBI, pp. 939–943. IEEE, Chicago (2011)

Connectivity Network Breakdown Predicts Imminent Volumetric Atrophy in Early Mild Cognitive Impairment

Talia M. Nir[1,*], Neda Jahanshad[1,*], Arthur W. Toga[1], Clifford R. Jack[2], Michael W. Weiner[3], and Paul M. Thompson[1], and the Alzheimer's Disease Neuroimaging Initiative (ADNI)

[1] Center for Imaging Genetics, Laboratory of Neuro Imaging, UCLA School of Medicine, Los Angeles, CA, USA
[2] Department of Radiology, Mayo Clinic and Foundation, Rochester, MN, USA
[3] Department of Radiology and Biomedical Imaging, UCSF School of Medicine, San Francisco, CA, USA

Abstract. Alzheimer's disease (AD) is characterized both by cortical atrophy and disrupted connectivity, resulting in abnormal interactions between neural systems. Diffusion weighted imaging (DWI) and graph theory can be used to evaluate major brain networks, and detect signs of abnormal breakdown in network connectivity. In a longitudinal study using both DWI and standard MRI, we assessed baseline white matter connectivity patterns in 24 early mild cognitive impairment (eMCI) subjects (mean age: 74.5 +/- 8.3 yrs). Using both standard MRI-based cortical parcellations and whole-brain tractography, we computed baseline connectivity maps from which we calculated global "small-world" architecture measures. We evaluated whether these network measures predicted future volumetric brain atrophy in eMCI subjects, who are at risk for developing AD, as determined by 3D Jacobian "expansion factor maps" between baseline and 6-month follow-up scans. This study suggests that DWI-based network measures may be a novel predictor of AD progression.

Keywords: Graph theory, brain networks, white matter, DTI, tractography, ADNI, TBM, small worldness, connectivity.

1 Introduction

Alzheimer's disease (AD), the most common form of dementia, is characterized by memory loss in its early stages, followed by a progressive decline in other cognitive domains. The Alzheimer's Disease Neuroimaging Initiative (ADNI) is one of several major efforts worldwide to identify sensitive biomarkers that may help track or predict brain tissue loss due to AD progression, and identify those most likely to decline.

AD is marked by pervasive grey matter atrophy, but the brain's white matter (WM) pathways also progressively decline. MRI-based image analysis methods have been used to track structural atrophy of the brain, but diffusion tensor imaging (DTI) is

---

* Corresponding author.

P.-T. Yap et al. (Eds.): MBIA 2012, LNCS 7509, pp. 41–50, 2012.

sensitive to microscopic WM injury not always detectable with standard anatomical MRI. DTI may be used to track the highly anisotropic diffusion of water along axons, revealing microstructural WM fiber bundles connecting cortical and subcortical regions. In both AD and mild cognitive impairment (MCI), cognitive impairment is associated with deterioration in these connecting fiber bundles, including the corpus callosum, cingulum, superior longitudinal fasciculus (SLF), and the inferior fronto-occipital fasciculus (IFO) [1-2].

In this study, we combined DTI with longitudinally acquired standard anatomical MRI (across a 6-month interval) to measure the integrity and connectivity of white matter tracts, and assess whether variations in the degree and extent of connections may be a useful predictor of future brain decline. We created 68x68 structural connectivity matrices based on baseline structural cortical parcellations and whole-brain tractography. We then used graph theory to describe general properties of the anatomical networks and characterize global connectivity patterns. In these graphs, *nodes* designate brain regions, which are thought of as being connected by *edges* representing WM fibers.

"Small-world" networks are marked by low characteristic path length (CPL) and high mean clustering coefficient (MCC), so they are both integrated and segregated. Small-world properties have been regarded as typical properties of many kinds of communication networks, and are found in social networks, efficient biological networks, and even in healthy mammalian brain networks [3]. Networks with a small-world organization can have both functional segregation and specialization of modules and a 'low wiring cost' that supports easy communication across an entire network. AD patients have abnormal small-world architecture in large-scale structural and functional brain networks, with differences in MCC and CPL that imply less optimal network topology [4-6].

Here, we use global network measures, computed from baseline DTI scans, to predict future volumetric atrophy (dynamic tissue loss) over a follow-up period of 6 months. We assessed 24 ADNI participants with early signs of cognitive impairment (eMCI). Predictors of decline in eMCI are sorely needed, as subjects are only mildly impaired and do not have drastic changes in most of the standard biomarkers of AD; even so, eMCI subjects are the target of many clinical trials that aim to slow disease progression, before brain changes are so pervasive that they are irremediable.

We examined whether small-world architecture measures calculated from baseline connectivity maps were able to predict volumetric brain atrophy after 6 months, as determined by 3D Jacobian "expansion factor maps" of T1-weighted structural scans. We found that global network measures may offer a potentially useful biomarker for predicting atrophy at this critical time before the onset of AD.

2   Methods

2.1   Subject Information and Image Acquisition

Data collection for the ADNI-2 project (the second phase of ADNI) is still in progress. Here we performed an initial analysis of 24 eMCI subjects who, by June

2012, had returned for a 6-month follow-up evaluation (mean age at baseline: 74.5+/-8.3 yrs; 14 men/10 women). We additionally analyzed baseline data from 29 cognitively healthy control subjects (HC) to create a study-specific template (mean age at baseline: 73.4+/-5.2 yrs; 15 men/14 women).

All subjects underwent whole-brain MRI scanning on 3-Tesla GE Medical Systems scanners, on at least one of two occasions (baseline and 6 months). T1-weighted SPGR (spoiled gradient echo) sequences (256x256 matrix; voxel size = 1.2x1.0x1.0 mm^3; TI=400 ms; TR = 6.98 ms; TE = 2.85 ms; flip angle = 11°), and diffusion-weighted images (DWI; 256x256 matrix; voxel size: 2.7x2.7x2.7 mm^3; scan time = 9 min) were collected. 46 separate images were acquired for each DTI scan: 5 T2-weighted images with no diffusion sensitization (b_0 images) and 41 diffusion-weighted images (b=1000 s/mm²).

2.2   Image Preprocessing

Preprocessing of Baseline and 6-Month Follow-up Anatomical Scans. All extra-cerebral tissue was removed from both baseline and 6 month T1-weighted anatomical scans using ROBEX, an automated brain extraction program trained on manually "skull-stripped" MRI data from hundreds of healthy young adults [7]. Anatomical scans subsequently underwent intensity inhomogeneity normalization using the MNI "nu_correct" tool (www.bic.mni.mcgill.ca/software/). To align data from different subjects into the same 3D coordinate space, each anatomical image was linearly aligned to a standard brain template (the Colin27; [8]) using FSL FLIRT [9].

Baseline DWI Preprocessing. For each subject, all raw DWI volumes were aligned to the average b_0 image using the FSL "eddy-correct" tool (www.fmrib.ox.ac.uk/fsl) to correct for head motion and eddy current distortions. Non-brain tissue was removed from the diffusion-weighted images using the Brain Extraction Tool (BET) from FSL [10]. To correct for echo-planar induced (EPI) susceptibility artifacts, which can cause distortions at tissue-fluid interfaces, skull-stripped b_0 images were linearly aligned and then elastically registered to their respective baseline T1-weighted structural scans using an inverse consistent registration algorithm with a mutual information cost function [11]. The resulting 3D deformation fields were then applied to the remaining 41 DWI volumes.

2.3   Fiber Tractography

At each voxel, orientation distribution functions (ODFs) were computed using the normalized and dimensionless ODF estimator, derived for Q-ball imaging (QBI) as in [12]. The angular resolution of the ADNI data somewhat limited to avoid long scan times that may tend to increase patient attrition, but the use of an ODF model makes best use of the available angular resolution. Tractography was performed on the linearly aligned sets of DWI volumes by probabilistically seeding voxels with a prior probability based on the FA value. Curves through a seed point receive a score estimating the probability of the existence, computed from the ODFs. We used a voting process provided by the Hough transform to determine the best fitting curves through each point (**Figure 1a;** [13]). Elastic deformations obtained from the EPI distortion correction, mapping the average b_0 image to the T1-weighted image, were then applied to the tracts' 3D coordinates. Each subject's dataset contained approximately 10,000 non-duplicated fibers (3D curves). We removed any erroneous fibers traced on the edge of the brain due to high intensity noise.

2.4   Automated Cortical ROI Segmentation

Using FreeSurfer (http://surfer.nmr.mgh.harvard.edu/;[14]), 34 cortical labels (**Table 1**) were automatically extracted in each hemisphere from the raw baseline T1-weighted structural MRI scans. The resulting T1-weighted images and were then aligned to the corrected T1 images, and the linear transformation matrix was applied to the cortical parcellations using nearest neighbor interpolation (to avoid intermixing of labels). This placed the cortical labels in the same space as the tractography, calculated from the DWIs that were elastically registered to the corrected T1 space (**Figure 1b**). To ensure tracts would intersect cortical labeled boundaries, labels were dilated with an isotropic box kernel of 5x5x5 voxels (**Figure 1c**).

Table 1. Index of cortical labels extracted from the anatomical MRI scans by FreeSurfer [14]

1	Banks of the superior temporal sulcus	19	*Pars orbitalis*
2	Caudal anterior cingulate	20	*Pars triangularis*
3	Caudal middle frontal	21	Peri-calcarine
4	-N/A-	22	Postcentral
5	Cuneus	23	Posterior cingulate
6	Entorhinal	24	Precentral
7	Fusiform	25	Precuneus
8	Inferior parietal	26	Rostral anterior cingulate
9	Inferior temporal	27	Rostral middle frontal
10	Isthmus of the cingulate	28	Superior frontal
11	Lateral occipital	29	Superior parietal
12	Lateral orbitofrontal	30	Superior temporal
13	Lingual	31	Supra-marginal
14	Medial orbitofrontal	32	Frontal pole
15	Middle temporal	33	Temporal pole
16	Parahippocampal	34	Transverse temporal
17	Paracentral	35	Insula
18	*Pars opercularis*		

2.5   NxN Matrices Representing Structural Connectivity

As in [15], for each subject, a baseline 68x68 (34 right hemisphere ROIs and 34 left) connectivity matrix was created. Each element described the estimated proportion of the total number of fibers, in that subject, connecting each of the labels to each of the other labels (**Figure 1d**).

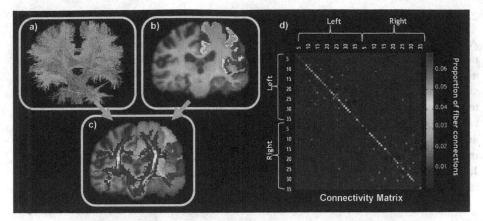

Fig. 1. (a) EPI-corrected whole-brain tractography calculated from the DWI. (b) Anatomical cortical parcellations in one hemisphere are shown, registered to the same subject's DWI space. (c) Red fiber density map overlaid on the dilated labels. (d) Connectivity matrix, in which each colored element represents the proportion of detected fibers connecting each of the colored labels in each hemisphere to each of the other colored labels in (c) – computed as a proportion of the total number of extracted fibers in the brain.

2.6   Network Analysis Based on Graph Theory

We applied the Brain Connectivity Toolbox (https://sites.google.com/a/ brainconnectivity-toolbox.net/bct/Home) to our baseline connectivity matrices generated above, to compute the measures whose values contribute to small world architecture. Characteristic path length (CPL) is an average measure (across the whole network) of the minimum number of edges necessary to travel from one node to another in the network (i.e., average minimum path length). Mean clustering coefficient (MCC) measures how many neighbors of a given node are also connected to each other, relative to the total possible number of connections in the network [16]. The ratio of the MCC in our network to the MCC in a simulated random network is *gamma*. The ratio of CPL in our network to CPL in the same simulated random network is *lambda*. Small-worldness (SW), which measures the balance between network differentiation and network integration, is calculated as a ratio of the MCC and CPL of a network relative to that in a random network with the same number of connections.

$$SW = \frac{MCC\,/\,MCCrand}{CPL\,/\,CPLrand} = \frac{gamma}{lambda} \tag{1}$$

As a *post hoc* analysis, we evaluated two additional global measures of network differentiation and integration, global efficiency (EGLOB) and modularity (MOD). EGLOB is simply the inverse (reciprocal) of CPL. Networks with lower CPL are more efficient than those with greater CPL. MOD is the degree to which a system may be subdivided into smaller networks. The equations to calculate each of these measures can be found in [16].

2.7   Study Specific Template Creation

A study-specific minimal deformation template (MDT) was created using 29 healthy normal (HN) subjects' baseline spatially-aligned corrected anatomical volumes. Using a customized template from subjects in the study (rather than a standard atlas or a single optimally chosen subject) can reduce bias in the registrations. The MDT is the template that deviates least from the anatomy of the subjects, and, in some circumstances, it can improve statistical power [17]. The MDT [18] was generated by creating an initial affine mean template from all 29 subjects, then registering all the aligned individual scans to that mean using elastic registration [11] while regularizing the Jacobians [19]. A new mean was created from the registered scans; this process was iterated several times.

2.8   Tensor Based Morphometry

To quantify 3D patterns of volumetric brain atrophy in eMCI, each subject's 6 month pre-processed T1-weighted scan was elastically registered to its respective corrected baseline T1-weighted scan [11]. A separate 3D Jacobian map (i.e., volumetric expansion factor map) was created for each subject to characterize the local volume differences between their baseline scan and 6 month scan. To ensure the Jacobians had common anatomical coordinates for statistical analysis, each subject's respective 3D deformation field - from the elastic registration of the baseline T1-weighted scan to the MDT - was applied to each Jacobian map.

2.9   Statistics

We ran a voxel-wise multiple linear regression, controlling for sex and age, and a partial F test, using baseline *gamma* and *lambda* as predictors – both jointly and independently – of the longitudinal volumetric changes. In *post hoc* analyses, we further ran a voxel-wise linear regression, controlling for sex and age, to detect any associations between baseline MOD and EGLOB and the Jacobian maps. Computing thousands of association tests at a voxel-wise level can introduce a high false positive error rate in neuroimaging studies, if not corrected. To correct for these errors, we used the searchlight method for false discovery rate correction (FDR) [20]. All statistical maps are thresholded at a corrected p-value to show regression coefficients only in regions that controlled the false discovery rate ($q=0.05$).

3   Results

We found a significant association between the baseline anatomical network measures, *gamma* and *lambda*, used together as predictors in the same regression model, and 3D volumetric changes over the 6-month follow-up interval (**Figure 2a**; corrected $p<0.05$; [20]). When we assessed *gamma* and *lambda* separately, we found no significant association between Jacobian maps and *lambda*, suggesting that the *gamma* measure was driving our findings. *Gamma*, the normalized MCC, was significantly negatively associated with regional volumes in the longitudinal sulcus, the left intra-parietal sulcus, the central sulcus bilaterally, the right superior frontal sulcus, right superior temporal sulcus and the right insular sulcus (**Figure 2b**). This suggests that lower MCC at baseline was associated with increases in CSF expansion, implying an effect driven by tissue loss causing sulci to open up. We also found small positive associations in the posterior *corona radiata* in an area near the precuneus and cingulate gyrus white matter, suggesting higher MCC at baseline corresponds to preservation of volume in these areas.

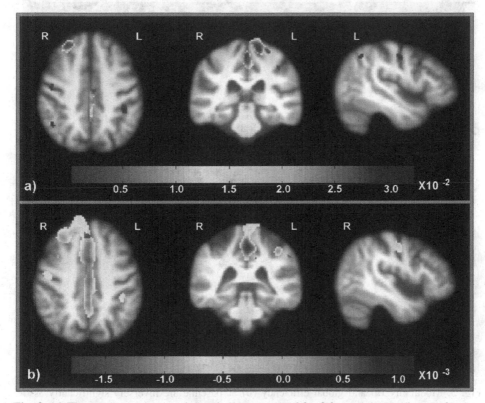

Fig. 2. (a) These *p*-maps show regions where *gamma* and *lambda* are joint predictors of volumetric changes after 6 months (corrected $p<0.05$; [20]) (b) These maps show *Beta*-values (unnormalized slopes of the regression coefficients, in units of percent atrophy over 6 months; per unit of the predictor, *gamma*) within regions where only *gamma* has a significant correlation with volumetric changes (corrected $p<0.05$; [20]). These results suggest that lower *gamma*, the normalized mean clustering coefficient, at baseline is associated with volumetric atrophy after 6 months.

In a *post hoc* analysis, we also found a significant positive association (corrected $p<0.05$; [20]) between MOD and the left supratentorial space between the cerebellum and the occipital lobe, as well as a negative association in the left occipital lobe (**Figure 3a**). This implies that increased modularity at baseline is associated with atrophy in the left occipital lobe after 6 months. Although occipital lobe atrophy is not

always the most prominent change in MCI, the comparatively low cross-subject anatomical variability in this region may have made it easier to pick up consistent associations here. Conversely we found a significant negative association (corrected $p<0.05$;
[20]) between EGLOB and the CSF expansion in the left supratentorial space between
the cerebellum and the occipital lobe, and a positive association in the left occipital
lobe and small parts of the right (**Figure 3b**), implying that lower global efficiency at
baseline is associated with occipital lobe atrophy.

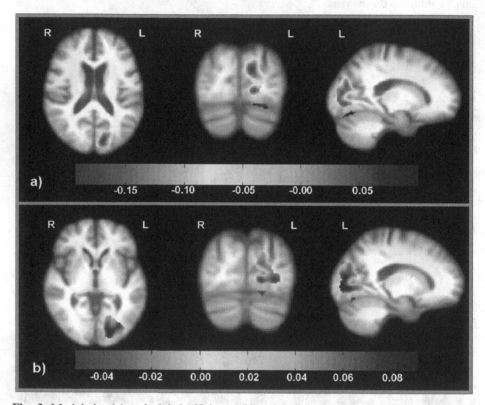

Fig. 3. Modularity (**a**) and global efficiency (**b**) at baseline are inversely significantly associated with 3D patterns of volumetric brain atrophy, implying that increased modularity and
decreased global efficiency are associated with future atrophy in the left occipital lobe. These
maps show *Beta*-values (non-normalized slope of the regression in units of imaging measure
per unit of the network measure, used as a predictor) within regions that show a significant
correlation (corrected $p<0.05$; [20]).

4   Discussion

There is great interest in predicting which subjects with early MCI are likely to decline, as well as in understanding what patterns of organizational decline in the brain
are harbingers of brain tissue loss. Several recent studies have suggested that AD
progression may involve a loss of small world characteristics in the brain's structural

and functional networks [4-6]. This is consistent with theoretical notions that small-world topology may be functionally beneficial and efficient. In this study, we assessed whether abnormalities in small worldness, the balance between network segregation and network integration, at baseline were predictive of volumetric brain decline over a 6-month period. As the small worldness measure (1) may falsely report small world topology in highly segregated, but poorly integrated networks [16], we chose to assess *gamma* and *lambda* as joint predictors instead.

In this study we found an association between baseline small-world global network measures and volumetric changes in T1 structural scans. Moreover, we found that lower mean clustering at baseline is associated with greater atrophy throughout the brain. In a previous study, using DTI based tractography, similar results were found with decreased MCC at baseline associated with decreases in fractional anisotropy (FA) over 6 months [21]. Networks with higher levels of clustering are more densely connected and may indicate a more functionally coherent neural system [22]. Here we found that increased modularity, a measure of segregation and decreased global efficiency, a measure of integration at baseline are associated with atrophy in the left occipital lobe.

It appears that the degree of network integration both globally, EGLOB, and locally within clusters, *gamma,* is an important indication of a more coherent neural system at baseline. Our data suggest that both lower global efficiency, indicating poor integration and high cost of information transfer, and lower *gamma*, a measure of local efficiency within clusters, at baseline, may be predictive of decline. Conversely, increased modularity and segregation at baseline – perhaps a sign of progressive isolation of network hubs - is also predictive of decline. As ADNI is a multisite longitudinal study currently under data collection, we will later investigate which of these subjects eventually develops AD, and if these early aberrations in connectivity can help to predict a patient's conversion to AD, as well as future brain tissue loss. This study offers evidence that DTI-based network measures may be a novel predictor of AD progression.

References

1. Zhang, Y.-Z., et al.: Comparison of diffusion tensor image study in associa-tion fiber tracts among normal, amnestic mild cognitive impairment, and Alzheimer's patients. Neurol. India 59, 168–173 (2011)
2. Liu, Y., et al.: Diffusion tensor imaging and tract-based spatial statistics in Alzheimer's disease and mild cognitive impairment. Neurobiol. Aging 32, 1558–1571 (2011)
3. Hilgetag, C.C., et al.: Anatomical connectivity defines the organization of clusters of cortical areas in the macaque and the cat. Phil. Trans. R. Soc. Lond. 355, 91–110 (2000)
4. He, Y., et al.: Structural insights into aberrant topological patterns of large-scale cortical networks in Alzheimer's disease. J. Neurosci. 28, 4756–4766 (2008)
5. Stam, C.J., et al.: Small-world networks and functional connectivity in Alzheimer's disease. Cereb. Cortex 17, 92–99 (2007)
6. Sanz-Arigita, E.J., et al.: Loss of 'small-world' networks in Alzheimer's disease: graph analysis of FMRI resting-state functional connectivity. PLoS One 5, e13788 (2010)
7. Iglesias, J.E., et al.: Robust brain extraction across datasets and compari-son with publicly available methods. IEEE Trans. on Medical Imaging 30(9), 1617–1634 (2011)

8. Holmes, C.J., et al.: Enhancement of MR images using registration for signal averaging. JCAT 22(2), 324–333 (1998)
9. Jenkinson, M., et al.: Improved optimisation for the robust and accurate linear registration and motion correction of brain images. NeuroImage 17(2), 825–841 (2002)
10. Smith, S.M.: Fast robust automated brain extraction. Hum. Brain Mapp. 17(3), 143–155 (2002)
11. Leow, A.D., et al.: Statistical properties of Jacobian maps and the realiza-tion of unbiased large-deformation nonlinear image registration. IEEE Trans. on Medical Imaging 26(6), 822–832 (2007)
12. Aganj, I., et al.: Reconstruction of the orientation distribution function in single- and mul-tiple-shell q-ball imaging within constant solid angle. Magn. Reson. Med. 64(2), 554–566 (2010)
13. Aganj, I., et al.: A Hough transform global probabilistic approach to mul-tiple-subject dif-fusion MRI tractography. Med. Image Analysis 15, 414–425 (2011)
14. Fischl, B., et al.: Automatically parcellating the human cerebral cortex. Cereb. Cortex 14, 11–22 (2004)
15. Jahanshad, N., et al.: Sex differences in the Human Connectome: 4-Tesla high angular res-olution diffusion tensor imaging (HARDI) tractography in 234 young adult twins. In: ISBI 2011, pp. 939–943 (2011)
16. Rubinov, M., Sporns, O.: Complex network measures of brain connec-tivity: Uses and in-terpretations. NeuroImage 3, 1059–1069 (2010)
17. Leporé, N., Brun, C.A., Pennec, X., Chou, Y.-Y., Lopez, O.L., Aizenstein, H.J., Becker, J.T., Toga, A.W., Thompson, P.M.: Mean Template for Tensor-Based Morphometry Using Deformation Tensors. In: Ayache, N., Ourselin, S., Maeder, A. (eds.) MICCAI 2007, Part II. LNCS, vol. 4792, pp. 826–833. Springer, Heidelberg (2007)
18. Gutman, B., et al.: Creating unbiased minimal deformation templates for brain volume reg-istration. In: OHBM 2010 (2010)
19. Yanovsky, I., et al.: Topology preserving log-unbiased nonlinear image registration: theory and implementation. In: IEEE CVPR 2007, pp. 1–8 (2007)
20. Langers, D.R., et al.: Enhanced signal detection in neuroimaging by means of regional control of the global false discovery rate. NeuroImage 38, 43–56 (2007)
21. Nir, T.M., et al.: Small world network measures predict white matter de-generation in pa-tients with early-stage mild cognitive impairment. In: ISBI 2012 (2012)
22. Bullmore, E., Sporns, O.: Complex brain networks: graph theoretical analysis of structural and functional systems. Nature Rev. Neurosci. 10, 186–198 (2009)

Deconfounding the Effects of Resting State Activity on Task Activation Detection in fMRI

Burak Yoldemir[1], Bernard Ng[2], and Rafeef Abugharbieh[1]

[1] Biomedical Signal and Image Computing Lab, UBC, Canada
[2] Parietal Team, INRIA Saclay, France
{buraky,rafeef}@ece.ubc.ca, bernardyng@gmail.com

Abstract. Inferring brain activation from functional magnetic resonance imaging (fMRI) data is greatly complicated by the presence of strong noise. Recent studies suggest that part of the noise in task fMRI data actually pertains to ongoing resting state (RS) brain activity. Due to the sporadic nature of RS temporal dynamics, pre-specifying temporal regressors to reduce the confounding effects of RS activity on task activation detection is far from trivial. In this paper, we propose a novel approach that exploits the intrinsic task-rest relationships in brain activity for addressing this challenging problem. With an approximate task activation pattern serving as a seed, we first infer areas in the brain that are intrinsically connected to this seed from RS-fMRI data. We then apply principal component analysis to extract the RS component within the task fMRI time courses of the identified intrinsically-connected brain areas. Using the learned RS modulations as confound regressors, we re-estimate the task activation pattern, and repeat this process until convergence. On real data, we show that removal of the estimated RS modulations from task fMRI data significantly improves activation detection. Our results thus provide further support for the presence of continual RS activity superimposed on task fMRI response.

Keywords: activation detection, fMRI, resting state, task-rest interactions.

1 Introduction

Functional magnetic resonance imaging (fMRI) has become a primary means for studying human brain activity. To map brain areas to function, the standard analysis approach models fMRI observations as a combination of expected temporal responses using a general linear model (GLM) [1]. However, the strong noise in fMRI data arising from confounds, such as scanner drifts, motion artifacts, and physiological effects, greatly hampers reliable detection of brain activation. Recent studies have shown that the brain is not idle in the absence of external stimulus [2]. Instead, spontaneous modulations in brain activity, referred to as resting state (RS) activity, are continually present [2]. Moreover, there is evidence indicating that RS activity actually persists during task performance [3]. Thus, part of the noise observed in task fMRI data indeed ascribes to ongoing RS activity. The frequency range at which RS activity resides is typically found to be between 0.01 to 0.1 Hz [2], which overlaps with the

P.-T. Yap et al. (Eds.): MBIA 2012, LNCS 7509, pp. 51–60, 2012.
© Springer-Verlag Berlin Heidelberg 2012

stimulus frequencies employed in most task-based fMRI studies. Thus, standard high pass filtering e.g. at 1/128 Hz, which is the default cutoff frequency in the SPM software, for removing temporal drifts in task fMRI data, would not account for ongoing RS modulations. Also, unlike task-evoked responses, which are time-locked to stimulus, the time at which RS activity peaks and troughs is difficult to predict. Hence, prespecifying temporal regressors to model RS activity is non-trivial.

Albeit its seemingly sporadic temporal dynamics, RS activity is not random [2]. Rather, strong synchrony in RS modulations between specific brain areas has been observed in numerous studies [2]. In fact, many of the detected RS networks exhibit high resemblance to networks seen in task experiments [4]. Further supporting this finding is a recent work [5] that demonstrated enhanced sensitivity in task activation detection by incorporating an RS-connectivity prior. In addition, studies that jointly examined RS-fMRI and diffusion MRI data indicate an anatomical basis for RS activity [6, 7]. In particular, high anatomical connectivity typically predicts high functional connectivity [6, 7]. Thus, the spatial patterns of RS networks would presumably be constrained by the underlying fiber pathways [6, 7]. Taken together, these findings suggest that there is spatial structure in RS activity and that the spatial structure of ongoing RS activity during task would likely remain similar to that during rest [3].

To the best of our knowledge, the only previous work that attempted to tackle this challenging problem of RS activity removal from task fMRI data was by Fox et al. [3]. Specifically, the authors showed that for a right handed motor task, subtracting out fMRI signals in the right somatomotor cortex (RSC) from the left somatomotor cortex (LSC) significantly reduced inter-trial variability in fMRI response. The basis of this approach is twofold. First, the presence of coherent RS activity between the LSC and RSC is well established [8], and is assumed to persist during task performance. Second, right handed motor tasks typically activate only the LSC, thus signals in RSC would largely correspond to RS activity. Subtraction of signals in RSC from LSC would thereby remove the RS components within the task fMRI time courses of the LSC. However, not all tasks evoke only lateralized activation. Thus, simply subtracting signals in one side of the brain from the other side is not always suitable for removing RS modulations from task fMRI data.

In this paper, we propose a novel approach for RS activity removal in more general settings. The key challenge to this problem is that RS activity is internally-driven by the brain, as opposed to being evoked by external stimulus with known timing. It is thus not obvious how the temporal dynamics of RS modulations that occurred during task performance can be determined a priori. Representative time courses reflective of ongoing RS activity must hence be extracted from the task fMRI data itself. Since the brain comprises multiple networks [4], the RS modulations superimposed on the fMRI responses of the task-activated brain areas would be specific to the RS network in which these brain areas belong. Extracting RS activity from task fMRI data would thus require knowing the parts of the brain that are activated and their intrinsically-connected areas, which introduces a circular problem. To deal with this issue, we employ an iterative strategy in which we first apply seed-based analysis [8] with an approximate task activation pattern being the seed to infer the intrinsically-connected brain areas from RS-fMRI data. Assuming the spatial structure of RS networks is sustained during task performance [3], we extract RS modulations from the task fMRI time courses of the identified brain areas and re-estimate the task activation pattern with the learned RS activity as confound regressors. On real fMRI data collected from 19 subjects undergoing a checkerboard-viewing task, we show that repeating this process to remove ongoing RS modulations from task fMRI data significantly improves task activation detection.

2   Proposed RS Activity Removal Approach

Motivated by the recent finding that RS activity contributes to the noise in task fMRI data [3], we propose a novel approach for removing such confounds to improve activation detection. Our approach consists of three steps, as summarized in Fig. 1.

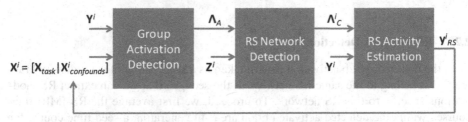

Fig. 1. Depiction of proposed RS activity removal approach. $\mathbf{X}^i = [\mathbf{X}_{task}|\mathbf{X}^i_{confounds}]$ is a regressor matrix, where $\mathbf{X}_{task}$ corresponds to task regressors and $\mathbf{X}^i_{confounds}$ corresponds to confound regressors specific to subject i. $\mathbf{Y}^i$ are the task fMRI time courses of subject i. Λ_A is the set of activated brain areas common across a group of subjects. $\mathbf{Z}^i$ are the RS-fMRI time courses of subject i. Λ^i_C is the set of brain areas estimated to be intrinsically connected to Λ_A for subject i. $\mathbf{y}^i_{RS}$ is the estimated RS activity time course of subject i, which is entered into $\mathbf{X}^i$ as a confound regressor for re-estimating the group activation pattern Λ_A. The three steps: group activation detection, RS network detection, and RS activity estimation, are repeated until Λ_A stabilizes.

In brief, we first approximate the task activation pattern that is common across subjects using standard univariate analysis [1] (Section 2.1). With the detected activation pattern serving as a seed, we infer brain areas that are intrinsically-connected to this seed from RS-fMRI data of each subject [8] (Section 2.2). Assuming that the spatial structure of RS networks remains fixed during task [3], we apply principal component analysis (PCA) to extract the RS component from the task fMRI time courses of the identified intrinsically-connected brain areas (Section 2.3). The estimated RS modulations are then used as confound regressors to re-estimate the task activation pattern of the group, and this process is repeated until the detected activation pattern converges.

2.1   Seed Region Extraction

Our approach begins with the estimation of an approximate task activation pattern (i.e. without accounting for ongoing RS modulations). A standard general linear model (GLM) is first applied to compute the intra-subject activation effects [1]:

$$\mathbf{Y}^i = \mathbf{X}^i\boldsymbol{\beta}^i + \mathbf{E}^i, \tag{1}$$

where $\mathbf{Y}^i$ is an $t\times d$ matrix containing the task fMRI time courses of d brain areas of subject i, $\mathbf{X}^i = [\mathbf{X}_{task}|\mathbf{X}^i_{confounds}]$ is an $t\times p$ matrix with $\mathbf{X}_{task}$ corresponding to task regressors and $\mathbf{X}^i_{confounds}$ corresponding to confound regressors specific to subject i [1], $\boldsymbol{\beta}^i$ is an $p\times d$ activation effect matrix to be estimated, and $\mathbf{E}^i$ is an $t\times d$ residual matrix. Due to the strong noise in task fMRI data, activation patterns estimated at the intra-subject level might be inaccurate [9]. Therefore, we opt to combine information across subjects in generating a group activation map, which is then used as a seed for identifying intrinsically-connected brain areas (Section 2.2). To infer group activation, we apply a max-t permutation test [10] on $\boldsymbol{\beta}^i$ of all subjects, which implicitly accounts for multiple comparisons and provides strong control over false detections. Group activation is declared at a p-value threshold of 0.05. We denote the set of detected brain areas as Λ_A.

2.2   RS Network Detection

With the detected group activation pattern taken as a seed, our goal is to identify brain areas that belong to the same RS network as the seed, so that we can extract RS modulations specific to this RS network. To proceed, we first average the RS-fMRI time courses within the detected activated brain areas in generating a seed time course for each subject. We then apply the standard seed-based analysis [8] to find brain areas intrinsically-connected to this seed for each subject i:

$$\mathbf{Z}^i_{\sim s} = \mathbf{z}^i_s\mathbf{w}^i + \boldsymbol{\Omega}^i, \tag{2}$$

where $\mathbf{Z}^i_{\sim s}$ is an $n\times(d-|\Lambda_A|)$ matrix containing the RS-fMRI time courses of all brain areas except those in Λ_A, $|\Lambda_A|$ is the number of brain areas in Λ_A, $\mathbf{z}^i_s$ is an $n\times 1$ vector containing the seed time course, $\mathbf{w}^i$ is an $1\times(d-|\Lambda_A|)$ vector with each element reflecting the correlation between the seed and each brain area not in Λ_A, and $\boldsymbol{\Omega}^i$ is an $n\times(d-|\Lambda_A|)$ residual matrix. Statistical significance of each element of $\mathbf{w}^i$ is declared at a p-value threshold of 0.05 with false discovery rate (FDR) correction [11] to account for multiple comparisons. FDR correction is used instead of max-t permutation test due to correlations between brain volumes at adjacent time points, which violates the independent sample assumption in max-t permutation test [10]. A max-t permutation test could be applied to identify brain areas that are significantly correlated with the seed at the group level. However, compared to task-based experiments, RS experiments are less prone to motion artifacts, which constitute a major part of fMRI noise. Reliable RS networks could thus potentially be extracted at the intra-subject level. We hence opt to perform intra-subject seed-based analysis to retain subject-specific information. We denote the set of brain areas significantly correlated with the seed as Λ^i_C.

2.3   RS Activity Estimation and Removal

After finding the set of brain areas that is intrinsically-connected to the estimated task activation pattern for each subject i, the next step is to extract the RS components from the task fMRI time courses of these brain areas, which we denote as $\mathbf{Y}^i_C$. To target the specific frequency range at which RS activity resides, we first band-pass filter each column of $\mathbf{Y}^i_C$ at cut-off frequencies of 0.01 and 0.1 Hz. Since the estimated task activation pattern is only an approximation without accounting for the confounding effects of RS activity, some intrinsically-connected brain areas might in fact be activated considering the resemblance between task and RS networks [4]. Thus, $\mathbf{Y}^i_C$ might contain task signals. To remove the task-related response in $\mathbf{Y}^i_C$, we apply PCA through eigendecomposition to separate $\mathbf{Y}^i_C$ into task and non-task components:

$$\mathbf{C}^i = \mathbf{U}^i \mathbf{D}^i \mathbf{U}^{iT}, \tag{3}$$

where $\mathbf{C}^i$ is the $d{\times}d$ covariance matrix of $\mathbf{Y}^i_C$, $\mathbf{U}^i$ is an $d{\times}d$ matrix containing the eigenvectors of $\mathbf{C}^i$, and $\mathbf{D}^i$ is an $d{\times}d$ matrix containing the eigenvalues of $\mathbf{C}^i$ along the diagonal. The columns of $\mathbf{U}^i$ are ordered such that the first column, $\mathbf{U}^i_1$, corresponds to the largest eigenvalue. To identify the task-related components, we compute the correlation between each column of $\mathbf{U}^i$ and the task regressor. Statistical significance in correlation is declared at a p-value threshold of 0.05 with FDR correction. For the data examined in this work (Section 3), the task regressor is found to be most significantly correlated with $\mathbf{U}^i_1$. This high correlation between $\mathbf{U}^i_1$ and the task stimulus, as shown in Fig. 1, signifies a definite need for task response removal from $\mathbf{Y}^i_C$. We remove the task components by reconstructing $\mathbf{Y}^i_C$ with the significantly correlated columns of $\mathbf{U}^i$ discarded. We note that other decomposition techniques, such as independent component analysis (ICA) [12], could be also used. We defer comparisons between various decomposition techniques for future work.

Denoting the reconstructed $\mathbf{Y}^i_C$ as $\mathbf{V}^i_{\sim task}$, we take the mean of $\mathbf{V}^i_{\sim task}$ over brain areas to generate a representative RS activity time course for each subject i, $\mathbf{y}^i_{RS}$,

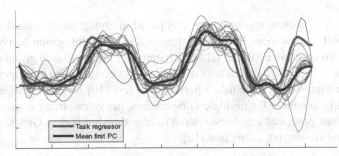

Fig. 2. Dominant principal component (PC) extracted from time courses of intrinsically-connected brain areas. The thick red and blue lines correspond to task regressor and mean dominant PC across subjects. Each thin line corresponds to the dominant PC of a single subject.

which we enter into (1) as a confound regressor to re-estimate the task activation pattern. This process is repeated until the group activation pattern Λ_A stabilizes.

3   Materials

For testing our proposed RS activity removal approach, we used the publicly available Multiband Test-Retest Pilot Dataset, which was released as a part of the 1000 Functional Connectomes Project[1]. Excluding subjects with missing brain volumes, the dataset comprises 19 subjects (14 men, 5 women, mean age 33.1±13.2 years). Each subject performed a passive viewing task in which a checkerboard was displayed on a monitor for 20 s, with 20 s of rest interleaved between stimulus blocks. The total task duration was approximately 2.5 minutes. Task fMRI data were acquired with a TR of 1.4 s and a voxel size of 2 mm (isotropic). RS-fMRI data of 5 minutes duration were also collected with a TR of 2.5 s and a voxel size of 3mm (isotropic).

For each subject's RS-fMRI data, motion correction and spatial normalization were performed using SPM8. The voxel time courses were then bandpass filtered at cutoff frequencies of 0.01 and 0.1 Hz with white matter and cerebrospinal fluid confounds regressed out. In accordance with how the human brain is estimated to comprise ~500 functional regions [13, 14], we functionally divided the brain into 500 parcels as follows. First, we used the Freesurfer atlas to divide the brain into 112 anatomical regions. We then functionally subdivided each anatomical region into N_r parcels, where N_r is chosen based on the number of voxels within each anatomical region relative to the total number of voxels. Parcellation was performed by concatenating RS-fMRI voxel time courses across subjects and applying normalized cut [15] to the correlation matrix computed from the concatenated time courses. RS parcel time courses were then generated by averaging the RS-fMRI voxel time courses within each group parcel. For task fMRI data, similar preprocessing steps were performed, except a highpass filter at 1/128 Hz was used to remove temporal drifts. Task fMRI time courses within each group parcel were averaged to compute task parcel time courses.

4   Results and Discussion

To validate our proposed approach, we compared applying the standard univariate analysis [1] with and without RS activity removal in detecting group activation. We denote these two cases as RSR and GLM, respectively. For increased group activation detection to be a legitimate validation criterion, strong control over false positive rate is critical. For this, we used the max-t permutation test [10] for both RSR and GLM, which implicitly accounts for multiple comparisons, provides strong control on false positive rate, and generates less conservative t-value thresholds than Gaussian random field theory and Bonferroni correction [10].

---

[1] The Multiband Test-Retest Pilot Dataset is available online at:
http://fcon_1000.projects.nitrc.org/indi/pro/eNKI_RS_TRT/
FrontPage.html

Fig. 2 shows the number of detected parcels for different p-value thresholds. For the same specificity, our approach provided higher detection sensitivity than GLM in general. To assess whether the increased detection was statistically significant, we employed a "parcel-label" permutation test. Specifically, for each permutation, we first randomly selected half of the parcels and exchanged the labels (i.e. active or non-active) assigned by RSR and GLM for each p-value threshold. We then computed the difference in the number of detected parcels with and without RS removal, which we denote as N_{diff}. This procedure was repeated 1000 times to generate a null distribution. The original N_{diff} was found to be greater than the 95th percentile of the null distribution for all corrected p-value thresholds within the typical range of [0.01, 0.05]. The detection improvement with RSR compared to GLM was thus statistically significant. We note that improvement in detection was observed even with just one iteration of RSR, and the detected activation pattern stabilized within two iterations, i.e. no more than a couple of parcels changing labels in subsequent iterations.

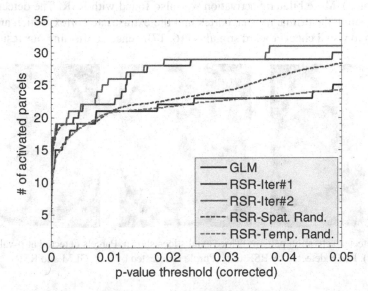

Fig. 3. Activation detection comparison. Number of parcels detected with significant activation vs. p-value thresholds.

To show that there is specific temporal structure in the estimated RS activity time courses that gave rise to the observed detection improvement, we applied RSR on temporally-permuted RS activity time courses 100 times. The average number of detected parcels over the 100 permutations (RSR-Temp. Rand. in Fig. 2) was found to be similar to that of GLM. The difference in detection performance between RSR and RSR-Temp. Rand. was statistically significant based on the parcel-label permutation test with a threshold set at the 95th percentile of the null distribution. Our results thus indicate that there is certain temporal structure in the estimated RS activity time courses that is critical for successful RS activity removal.

Since the brain comprises multiple networks [4], not all parcels would contain the same RS modulations as those superimposed on the underlying task activated brain areas. To illustrate this point, we applied RSR with RS modulations extracted from N_c randomly selected parcels (excluding parcels identified by RSR), where N_c is the number of intrinsically-connected brain areas originally determined with RSR. The average number of detected parcels over 100 random subsets of parcels (RSR-Spat. Rand. in Fig. 2) was found to be similar to that of GLM for p-value thresholds between 0 and 0.02, and modestly better than GLM for p-value thresholds above 0.02. We suspect the increased detection arises from how some parcels might be intrinsically-connected to the task-evoked brain areas, but the estimated correlations were declared not significant due to noise. Such parcels would contain RS modulations common to the task activation pattern, hence the increased activation detection observed. Nevertheless, the increase was not statistically significant based on the parcel-label permutation test with a threshold set at the 95th percentile of the null distribution.

Qualitatively, RSR additionally detected brain areas adjacent to those found by GLM (Fig. 3). More bilateral activation was also found with RSR. The detected brain areas lie within the primary visual cortex and the extrastriate cortex, which are known to pertain to visual checkerboard stimulus [16, 17], hence confirming our results.

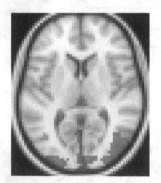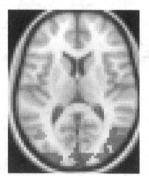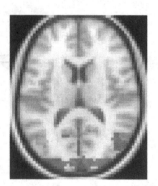

Fig. 4. Detected activation patterns. Three axial slices shown. Parcels detected at p-value < 0.05 (corrected). Red = detected by RSR only. Purple = detected by both GLM and RSR.

5   Conclusions

We proposed a novel approach for the estimation and removal of continual RS activity in task fMRI data. Exploiting how the spatial structure of RS networks are constrained by the underlying fiber pathways hence would remain similar during task performance, our approach first extracts RS modulations from task fMRI time courses within brain areas that are significantly correlated with an approximate task activation pattern at rest. The estimated RS modulations are then entered into a GLM as confound regressors to model the effects of RS activity. Applying our approach on real data resulted in statistically significant improvement in task activation detection. In agreement with the seminal work by Fox et al. [3], our results indicate that RS activity also contributes to the noise seen in task fMRI data, in contrast to the traditional belief that only scanner artifacts, head motions, and physiological confounds contribute to fMRI noise. It is thus important to model RS activity in task fMRI studies.

References

1. Friston, K.J., Holmes, A.P., Worsley, K.J., Poline, J.B., Frith, C.D., Frackowiak, R.S.J.: Statistical Parametric Maps in Functional Imaging: A General Linear Approach. Hum. Brain Mapp. 2, 189–210 (1995)
2. Fox, M.D., Raichle, M.E.: Spontaneous Fluctuations in Brain Activity Observed with Functional Magnetic Resonance Imaging. Nat. Rev. Neurosci. 8, 700–711 (2007)
3. Fox, M.D., Snyder, A.Z., Vincent, J.L., Raichle, M.E.: Intrinsic Fluctuations within Cortical Systems Account for Intertrial Variability in Human Behaviour. Neuron 56, 171–184 (2007)
4. Smith, S.M., Fox, P.T., Miller, K.L., Glahn, D.C., Fox, P.M., Mackay, C.E., Filippini, N., Watkins, K.E., Toro, R., Laird, A.R., Beckmann, C.F.: Correspondence of the Brain's Functional Architecture During Activation and Rest. Proc. Natl. Acad. Sci. 106, 13040–13045 (2009)
5. Ng, B., Abugharbieh, R., Varoquaux, G., Poline, J.B., Thirion, B.: Connectivity-Informed fMRI Activation Detection. In: Fichtinger, G., Martel, A., Peters, T. (eds.) MICCAI 2011, Part II. LNCS, vol. 6892, pp. 285–292. Springer, Heidelberg (2011)
6. Honey, C.J., Thivierge, J.P., Sporns, O.: Can Structure Predict Function in the Human Brain? NeuroImage 52, 766–776 (2010)
7. Damoiseaux, J.S., Greicius, M.D.: Greater than the Sum of its Parts: A Review of Studies Combining Structural Connectivity and Resting-state Functional Connectivity. Brain Struct. Funct. 213, 525–533 (2009)
8. Biswal, B., Yetkin, F.Z., Haughton, V.M., Hyde, J.S.: Functional Connectivity in the Motor Cortex of Resting Human Brain Using Echo-planar MRI. Magn. Reson. Med. 34, 537–541 (1995)
9. Ng, B., Hamarneh, G., Abugharbieh, R.: Modeling Brain Activation in fMRI Using Group MRF. IEEE Trans. Med. Imaging 31, 1113–11123 (2012)
10. Nichols, T., Hayasaka, S.: Controlling the Familywise Error Rate in Functional Neuroimaging: A Comparative Review. Stat. Methods Med. Research 12, 419–446 (2003)
11. Benjamini, Y., Hochberg, Y.: Controlling the False Discovery Rate: A Practical and Powerful Approach to Multiple Testing. J. Royal Stat. Soc. Series B 57, 125–133 (1995)
12. McKeown, M.J., Makeig, S., Brown, G.G., Jung, T.-P., Kindermann, S.S., Bell, A.J., Sejnowski, T.J.: Analysis of fMRI Data by Blind Separation into Independent Spatial Components. Hum. Brain Mapp. 6, 160–188 (1998)
13. Tucholka, A., Thirion, B., Perrot, M., Pinel, P., Mangin, J.-F., Poline, J.-B.: Probabilistic Anatomo-Functional Parcellation of the Cortex: How Many Regions? In: Metaxas, D., Axel, L., Fichtinger, G., Székely, G. (eds.) MICCAI 2008, Part II. LNCS, vol. 5242, pp. 399–406. Springer, Heidelberg (2008)
14. Thyreau, B., Thirion, B., Flandin, G., Poline, J.B.: Anatomo-functional Description of the Brain: A Probabilistic Approach. In: 31st IEEE International Conference on Acoustics, Speech, and Signal Processing, pp. 1109–1112 (2006)

15. Van Den Heuvel, M., Mandl, R., Hulshoff Pol, H.: Normalized Cut Group Clustering of Resting-state fMRI Data. PLoS ONE 3, e2001 (2008)
16. Liu, Z., Zhang, N., Chen, W., He, B.: Mapping the Bilateral Visual Integration by EEG and fMRI. NeuroImage 46, 989–997 (2009)
17. Clare, S.: Magnetic Resonance Imaging of Brain Function. Methods Enzymol. 385, 134–148 (2004)

Hyperbolic Ricci Flow and Its Application in Studying Lateral Ventricle Morphometry

Jie Shi[1], Paul M. Thompson[2], and Yalin Wang[1]

[1] School of Computing, Informatics and Decision Systems Engineering,
Arizona State University, Tempe, AZ 85281, USA
[2] Laboratory of Neuro Imaging, Department of Neurology,
UCLA School of Medicine, Los Angeles, CA 90095, USA
{jie.shi,ylwang}@asu.edu, thompson@loni.ucla.edu

Abstract. Here we propose a novel method to compute surface hyperbolic parameterization for studying brain morphology with the Ricci flow method. Two surfaces are conformally equivalent if there exists a bijective angle-preserving map between them. The Teichmüller space for surfaces with the same topology is a finite-dimensional manifold, where each point represents a conformal equivalence class, and the conformal map is homotopic to the identity map. A shape index can be defined based on Teichmüller space coordinates, and this shape index is intrinsic and invariant under scaling, translation, rotation, general isometric deformation, and conformal deformation. Using the Ricci flow method, we can conformally map a surface with a negative Euler number to the Poincaré disk and the Teichmüller space coordinates can be computed by geodesic lengths under hyperbolic metric. For lateral ventricular surface registration, we further convert the parameterization to the Klein model where a convex polygon is guaranteed for a multiply connected surface. With the Klein model, diffeomorphisms between lateral ventricular surfaces can be computed with some well known surface registration methods. Compared with prior work, the parameterization does not have any singularities and the intrinsic parameterizations help shape indexing and surface registration. Our preliminary experimental results showed its great promise for analyzing anatomical surface morphology.

1 Introduction

Shape analysis is a key research topic in anatomical modeling and statistical comparisons of anatomy. In studies that analyze brain morphology, many shape analysis methods have been proposed, such as spherical harmonic analysis (SPHARM) [1, 2], medial representations (M-reps) [3], and minimum description length approaches [4], etc.; these methods may also be applied to analyze shape changes or abnormalities in subcortical brain structures. Recent work has also taken a population based approach by analyzing surface changes using pointwise displacements of surface meshes, local deformation tensors, or surface expansion factors [5, 6]. Even so, a stable method to compute transformation-invariant shape descriptors and diffeomorphisms between topology complicated surfaces would be highly advantageous in this research field. Here we propose a

P.-T. Yap et al. (Eds.): MBIA 2012, LNCS 7509, pp. 61–76, 2012.
© Springer-Verlag Berlin Heidelberg 2012

novel and intrinsic method to compute hyperbolic conformal parameterization of surfaces with negative Euler numbers with hyperbolic Ricci flow method. We use lateral ventricular morphometry as an example to demonstrate our algorithm in a dataset from our prior research [7, 8].

All oriented surfaces have conformal structures. The conformal structure is, in some respects, more flexible than the Riemannian metric but places more restrictions on the surface morphology than the topological structure. According to Klein's Erlangen program, different geometries study the invariants under different transformation groups. Conformal geometry corresponds to the angle-preserving transformations. If there exists a conformal map between two surfaces, they are conformally equivalent. All surfaces may be classified by the conformal equivalence relation. For surfaces with the same topology, the Teichmüller space is a natural finite-dimensional manifold, where each point represents a conformal equivalence class and the distance between two shapes can be accurately measured. A shape index can be defined based on Teichmüller space coordinates. This shape index is intrinsic and invariant under conformal transformations, rigid motions and scaling. It is simple to compute; no surface registration is needed. It is very general; it can handle all arbitrary topology surfaces with negative Euler numbers.

In this work, only genus-zero surfaces with three boundaries are considered. With the discrete version of the surface Ricci flow method (also called the discrete Ricci flow), we conformally projected the surfaces to the hyperbolic plane and isometrically embedded them in the Poincaré disk. The proposed Teichmüller space coordinates are the lengths of a special set of geodesics under this special hyperbolic metric. Next, we computed the Klein model of the hyperbolic parameterization. The obtained convex polygon provides a stable parameter domain for surface registration. Compared with prior work [8], the new registration method relies on surface intrinsic features and does not have any singularities. It provides a promising way to analyze complex ventricular morphometry using MR images.

We tested our algorithm on cortical and lateral ventricular surfaces extracted from 3D anatomical brain MRI scans. The proposed algorithm can map the profile of differences in surface morphology between healthy controls and subjects with HIV/AIDS. Finally, we applied our algorithm to compare the intrinsic features of two ventricular surfaces with strong shape difference to demonstrate the feasibility of applying the new method for surface registration.

1.1 Related Work

In the computational analysis of brain anatomy, volumetric measures of structures identified on 3D MRI have been used to study group differences in brain structure and also to predict diagnosis [9, 10, 11]. However, early research [12, 13, 14, 15] has demonstrated that surface-based approaches may offer advantages as a method to register brain images. To register brain surfaces, a common approach is to compute a range of intermediate mappings to some canonical parameter space [6, 12, 13, 16, 17, 18]. A flow, computed in the parameter space of the two surfaces, then induces a correspondence field in 3D [19]. This flow can be constrained by anatomical landmark points or curves [20, 21, 22, 23, 24], by subregions of interest [25], by using currents to represent anatomical variation [26, 27], or by metamorphoses [28]. Various ways also exist for optimizing surface registrations [29, 30, 31, 32].

Recent work has also used shape-based features (reviewed in [33]). Many surface based statistics were studied for evaluating disease burden, progression and response to interventions, including m-rep [3], SPHARM [2], principal geodesic analysis [34], random orbit model [35], deformation-based morphometry (DBM) [36, 37], tensor-based morphometry (TBM) [1, 38], Teichmüller shape space [39, 40], Laplace-Beltrami eigen function [41], q-maps [42], and optimal mass transportation [29], etc.

Some work has focused on conformal parameterization of brain surfaces. There are mainly five categories of methods for brain surface study: quasiconformal mapping with circle packing [43], Cauchy-Riemann equation [44, 45, 46], harmonic maps [47], holomorphic differentials [48], and Ricci/Yamabe flow method [49, 50]. Among all these algorithms, only the holomorphic differentials [48, 51], Ricci flow methods [49, 50] and circle packing method [43] work on high genus surfaces while circle packing method can only generate quasi-conformal mapping (see a discussion in [50]).

With the Ricci flow method, Wang et al. [50] solved the Yamabe equation and conformally mapped the cortical surface of the brain to a Euclidean multi-hole punctured disk. Gu et al. applied the surface Ricci flow method to study general 3D shape matching and registration. The hyperbolic Ricci flow has also been applied to study 3D face matching. Recently, Jin et al. [39] and Zeng et al. [52] introduced the Teichmüller shape space to index and compare general surfaces with various topologies, geometries and resolutions.

2 Theoretical Background and Definitions

This section briefly introduces the theoretic background and definitions necessary for the current work.

Conformal Deformation. Suppose S is a surface embedded in $\mathbb{R}^3$ with a Riemannian metric $\mathbf{g}$ induced from the Euclidean metric. Let $u : S \to \mathbb{R}$ be a scalar function on S. It can be verified that $\tilde{\mathbf{g}} = e^{2u}\mathbf{g}$ is also a Riemannian metric on S and angles measured by $\mathbf{g}$ are equal to those measured by $\tilde{\mathbf{g}}$. Thus, $\tilde{\mathbf{g}}$ is called a *conformal deformation* of $\mathbf{g}$.

The Gaussian curvature of the surface will also be changed accordingly and become $\tilde{K} = e^{-2u}(-\Delta_{\mathbf{g}}u + K)$, where $\Delta_{\mathbf{g}}$ is the Laplacian-Beltrami operator under the original metric $\mathbf{g}$. The geodesic curvature will become $\tilde{k}_g = e^{-u}(\partial_{\mathbf{r}}u + k_g)$, where $\mathbf{r}$ is the tangent vector orthogonal to the boundary. According to Gauss-Bonnet theorem, the total curvature is $2\pi\chi(S)$, where $\chi(S)$ is the Euler characteristic number of S.

Uniformization Theorem. [53]. Given a surface S with a Riemannian metric $\mathbf{g}$, there exist an infinite number of metrics conformal to $\mathbf{g}$. The uniformization theorem states that, among all conformal metrics, there exists a unique representative, which induces constant Gaussian curvature everywhere. Moreover, the constant will be one of $\{+1, 0, -1\}$. Therefore, we can embed the universal covering space of any closed surface using its uniformization metric onto one of the three canonical surfaces: the *sphere* $\mathbb{S}^2$ for genus-0 surfaces with positive Euler numbers, the *plane* $\mathbb{E}^2$ for genus-1 surfaces with zero Euler number, and the *hyperbolic space* $\mathbb{H}^2$ for high genus surfaces with negative Euler numbers. Accordingly, we can say that surfaces with positive Euler number admit spherical geometry; surfaces with zero Euler number admit Euclidean geometry; and surfaces with negative Euler number admit hyperbolic geometry.

Poincaré Disk Model. In this work, we specify the background geometry of all surfaces as the hyperbolic space $\mathbb{H}^2$. The hyperbolic space cannot be realized in $\mathbb{R}^3$, thus we use the Poincaré disk to model it. The Poincaré disk is the unit disk $|z| < 1$ in the complex plane with the metric $ds^2 = \frac{4dzd\bar{z}}{(1-z\bar{z})^2}$. The rigid motion in hyperbolic space is the Möbius transformation $z \to e^{i\theta} \frac{z-z_0}{1-\bar{z}_0 z}$, where θ and z_0 are parameters. The geodesics on the Poincaré disk are arcs of Euclidean circles, which intersect the boundary of the the unit circle at right angles.

Hyperbolic Ricci Flow. In this work we use the surface Ricci flow method to conformally project the surfaces to the hyperbolic plane and isometrically embed them in the Poincaré disk. We call this method hyperbolic Ricci flow.

Let S be a smooth surface with a Riemannian metric $\mathbf{g} = (g_{ij})$. The Ricci flow deforms the metric $\mathbf{g}(t)$ according to the Gaussian curvature $K(t)$,

$$\frac{dg_{ij}(t)}{dt} = -2K(t)g_{ij}(t),$$

where t is the time parameter. With $\mathbf{g}(t) = e^{2u(t)}\mathbf{g}(0)$, the Ricci flow can be simplified as

$$\frac{du(t)}{dt} = -2K(t).$$

Fuchsian Transformation. Suppose S is a surface with a negative Euler number and its hyperbolic uniformization metric is $\tilde{\mathbf{g}}$. Then its universal covering space $(\tilde{S}, \tilde{\mathbf{g}})$ can be isometrically embedded in $\mathbb{H}^2$. Any deck transformation of $\tilde{S}$, which is a transformation from one universal covering space to another and keeps projection invariant, is a Möbius transformation and called a *Fuchsian transformation*. Let ϕ be a Fuchsian transformation, let $z \in \mathbb{H}^2$, the *attractor* and *repulser* of ϕ are $\lim_{n\to\infty} \phi^n(z)$ and $\lim_{n\to\infty} \phi^{-n}(z)$, respectively. The *axis* of ϕ is the unique geodesic through its attractor and repulser. The deck transformation group is called the *Fuchsian group* of S.

Fig. 1 (a) and (b) illustrate some basic concepts in hyperbolic geometry. (a) shows a saddle-shape plane which has constant negative Gaussian curvatures. (b) shows Escher's famous prints *Circle Limit III* [54], where the white lines are close to geodesics, i.e. hypercycles, on the Poincaré disk.

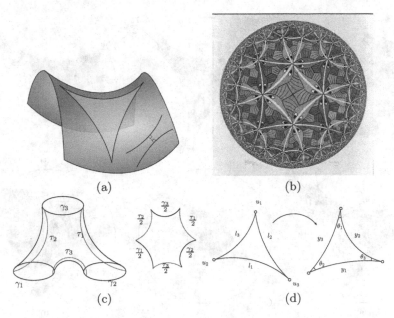

Fig. 1. Some simple illustrations of hyperbolic geometry. (a) a saddle-shape plane with constant negative Gaussian curvatures. (b) Escher's prints Circle Limit III [54]. (c) a pair of hyperbolic pants. (d) conformal transformation between two hyperbolic triangles.

Teichmüller Space. Let $(S_1, \mathbf{g}_1)$ and $(S_2, \mathbf{g}_2)$ be two metric surfaces, and let $f : S_1 \to S_2$ be a differential map between them. If the pull-back metric induced by f satisfies the following condition:

$$\mathbf{g}_1 = e^{2\lambda} f^* \mathbf{g}_2,$$

then we say the map is *conformal*. Two metric surfaces are conformally equivalent, if there exists an invertible conformal map between them. All surfaces may be classified using this conformal equivalence relation.

All conformal equivalence classes of surface with a fixed topology form a finite-dimensional manifold, the so-called Teichmüller space. Teichmüller space is a shape space, where a point represents a class of surfaces, and a curve in Teichmüller space represents a deformation process from one shape to the other. The coordinates of the surface in Teichmüller space can be explicitly computed. The Riemannian metric of The Teichmüller space is also well-defined.

As an example, Fig. 1 (c) shows a genus-zero surface with three boundaries $\partial S = \{\gamma_1, \gamma_2, \gamma_3\}$, which is also called *topological pants*. If the length of boundary γ_i is l_i under the hyperbolic uniformization metric, then (l_1, l_2, l_3) are the Teichmüller coordinates of S in the Teichmüller space of all conformal classes of a pair of pants. Namely, if two surfaces share the same Teichmüller coordinates, they can be conformally mapped to each other. In this work, only surfaces with the pants topology are considered.

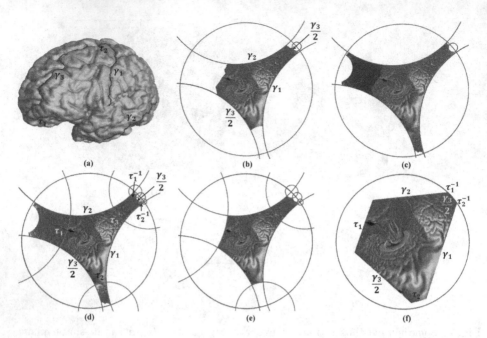

Fig. 2. Illustration of computation of hyperbolic conformal parameterization of a left cortical surface with Ricci flow method.

Klein Model. In additional to Poincaré model, there also exist other models of hyperbolic space. Another commonly used one is the *Klein model* [55]. The Klein model is also the unit disk, where all geodesics are straight Euclidean lines. The obtained convex polygon simplifies the computation and provides a convex domain for further surface registration methods. The conversion from the Poincaré disk to the Klein model is

$$z \rightarrow \frac{2z}{1 + \bar{z}z} \tag{1}$$

The Poincaré model is conformal, whereas the Klein model is not. In our Poincaré model, we compute the shortest lines between two hyperbolic lines. The lines are unique because they are the geodesics on the hyperbolic space. So the converted Klein model is convex and uniquely determined by the intrinsic surface shape. It provides a practical and efficient domain for us to compute diffeomorphisms between topology complicated surfaces.

3   Computational Algorithms

This section details the algorithms for computing the hyperbolic metric, the Teichmüller coordinates and surface diffeomorphisms via the hyperbolic parameterization.

3.1 Computing Hyperbolic Metric of a Surface with the Ricci Flow Method

In practice, most surfaces are approximated by discrete triangular meshes. Let M be a two-dimensional simplicial complex. We denote the set of vertices, edges and faces by V, E, F, respectively. We call the ith vertex v_i; edge $[v_i, v_j]$ runs from v_i to v_j; and the face $[v_i, v_j, v_k]$ has its vertices sorted counter-clockwise. In this work, we assume all faces are hyperbolic triangles. Fig. 1 (d) illustrates the conformal transformation between a pair of hyperbolic triangles and their associated edge lengths l_i, y_i, corner angles θ_i and conformal factor u_i.

A *discrete metric* is a function $l : E \to \mathbb{R}^+$, such that triangle inequality holds on every face, which represents the edge lengths. The *discrete curvature* $K : V \to \mathbb{R}$ is defined as the angle deficit, i.e., 2π minus the surrounding corner angles for an interior vertex, and π minus the surrounding corner angles for a boundary vertex.

Suppose the mesh is embedded in $\mathbb{R}^3$, so it has the induced Euclidean metric. We use l_{ij}^0 to denote the initial induced Euclidean metric on edge $[v_i, v_j]$.

Let $u : V \to \mathbb{R}$ be the *discrete conformal factor*. The discrete conformal metric deformation is defined as

$$\sinh(\frac{y_k}{2}) = e^{u_i} \sinh(\frac{l_k}{2}) e^{u_j}. \tag{2}$$

The *discrete Ricci flow* is defined as

$$\frac{du_i}{dt} = -K_i, \tag{3}$$

where K_i is the curvature at the vertex v_i.

Let $\mathbf{u} = (u_1, u_2, \cdots, u_n)$ be the conformal factor vector, where n is the number of vertices, and $\mathbf{u_0} = (0, 0, \cdots, 0)$. Then the *discrete hyperbolic Yamabe energy* is defined as

$$E(\mathbf{u}) = \int_{\mathbf{u_0}}^{\mathbf{u}} \sum_{i=1}^{n} K_i du_i. \tag{4}$$

The differential 1-form $\omega = \sum_{i=1}^{n} K_i du_i$ is closed. We use c_k to denote $\cosh(y_k)$. By direct computation, it can be shown that on each triangle,

$$\frac{\partial \theta_i}{\partial u_j} = A \frac{c_i + c_j - c_k - 1}{c_k + 1},$$

where

$$A = \frac{1}{\sin(\theta_k) \sinh(y_i) \sinh(y_j)},$$

which is symmetric in i, j, so $\frac{\partial \theta_i}{\partial u_j} = \frac{\partial \theta_j}{\partial u_i}$. It is easy to see that $\frac{\partial K_i}{\partial u_j} = \frac{\partial K_j}{\partial u_i}$, which implies $d\omega = 0$. The discrete hyperbolic Yamabe energy is convex. The unique global minimum corresponds to the hyperbolic metric with zero vertex curvatures.

This requires us to compute the Hessian matrix of the energy. The explicit form is given as follows:

$$\frac{\partial \theta_i}{\partial u_i} = -A \frac{2c_i c_j c_k - c_j^2 - c_k^2 + c_i c_j + c_i c_k - c_j - c_k}{(c_j + 1)(c_k + 1)}$$

The Hessian matrix (h_{ij}) of the hyperbolic Yamabe energy can be computed explicitly. Let $[v_i, v_j]$ be an edge, connecting two faces $[v_i, v_j, v_k]$ and $[v_j, v_i, v_l]$. Then the edge weight is defined as

$$h_{ij} = \frac{\partial \theta_i^{jk}}{\partial u_j} + \frac{\partial \theta_i^{lj}}{\partial u_j}.$$

also for

$$h_{ii} = \sum_{j,k} \frac{\partial \theta_i^{jk}}{\partial u_i},$$

where the summation goes through all faces surrounding v_i, $[v_i, v_j, v_k]$.

The discrete hyperbolic energy can be directly optimized using Newton's method. Because the energy is convex, the optimization process is stable.

Given the mesh M, a conformal factor vector $\mathbf{u}$ is *admissible* if the deformed metric satisfies the triangle inequality on each face. The space of all admissible conformal factors is not convex. In practice, the step length in Newton's method needs to be adjusted. Once the triangle inequality no longer holds on a face, then an edge swap needs to be performed. The target hyperbolic metric computed by the Ricci flow method can be used to isometrically embed the surface in the Poincaré disk.

Fig. 2 (a) and (b) illustrate the hyperbolic Ricci flow method. (a) shows the initial cortical surface with three boundaries $\gamma_1, \gamma_2, \gamma_3$, which were cut along specific anatomical landmarks. The curves τ_1 and τ_2 are the shortest paths connecting γ_2 and γ_3, γ_1 and γ_3, respectively. We cut the surface open along τ_1 and τ_2 to obtain a simply connected surface $\tilde{S}$. By running the hyperbolic Ricci flow, the hyperbolic metric is obtained. With the metric, $\tilde{S}$ can be isometrically embedded onto the Poincaré disk as shown in (b). The boundaries of the original surface, $\gamma_1, \gamma_2, \gamma_3$, map to geodesics.

3.2   Computing the Teichmüller coordinates

In order to compute the Teichmüller coordinates of a surface with the hyperbolic metric obtained with the Ricci flow method in Sec. 3.1, we need to compute the Fuchsian group generators of the surface. As illustrated in Fig. 2, the Möbius transformations ϕ_1 that transforms τ_1 to τ_1^{-1} and ϕ_2 that transforms τ_2 to τ_2^{-1} form the generators of the Fuchsian group of the surface in Fig. 2 (a). In Fig. 2 (c), the embedding of $\tilde{S}$ is transformed by a Fuchsian transformation. Each color represents a copy of $\tilde{S}$. Frame (d) shows the computation of τ_i's, which are the shortest geodesics connecting the geodesic boundaries γ_j and γ_k.

The final result is shown in Fig. 2 (e). The lengths of $\gamma_1, \gamma_2, \gamma_3$ in the hyperbolic space are the Teichmüller coordinates of S.

3.3   Surface Registration with the Klein Model

After we compute the Poincaré model, we can transform the hyperbolic polygon from the Poincaré model to the Klein model with Eqn. 1. The result is shown in Figure 2 (f). The polygon becomes a Euclidean convex polygon. We can apply either constrained harmonic map [8] or surface fluid registration method [56] to compute surface registration. Both methods will generate diffeomorphisms since harmonic maps between convex planar polygons are diffeomorphisms and the surface fluid registration method also guarantees diffeomorphisms. The registered ventricular surfaces may provide a rigorous theoretic foundation to build ventricular atlas with population-based brain imaging approaches [5, 6].

4   Experimental Results

The lateral ventricles - fluid-filled structures deep in the brain - are often enlarged in disease and can provide sensitive measures of disease progression [7, 57, 58, 59]. Ventricular changes reflect atrophy in surrounding structures, and ventricular measures and surface-based maps can provide sensitive assessments of tissue reduction that correlate with cognitive deterioration in illnesses. However, the concave shape, complex branching topology and narrowness of the inferior and posterior horns have made automatic analyses more difficult.

With the hyperbolic Ricci flow method, we proposed two methods to analyze lateral ventricular morphometry: (1) to quantify lateral ventricular surface morphometry with the Teichmüller shape space coordinates; (2) to register lateral ventricular surfaces via the Klein model. In this section, we report our preliminary results on a HIV/AIDS dataset used in our prior research [7, 8].

4.1   Quantifying Lateral Ventricular Surface Morphology with the Teichmüller Shape Space Coordinates

To model the lateral ventricular surface, we automatically locate and introduce three cuts on each ventricle. The cuts are motivated by examining the topology of the lateral ventricles, in which several horns are joined together at the ventricular "atrium" or "trigone". We call this topological model, creating a set of connected surfaces, a *topology optimization* operation. After modeling the topology in this way, a lateral ventricular surface, in each hemisphere, becomes an open boundary surface with 3 boundaries, a topological pant surface.

After the topology optimization, a ventricular surface is topologically equivalent to a topological pant surface. We can then compute its Teichmüller space coordinate. Figure 3 illustrates how to compute Teichmüller space coordinates for a lateral ventricle. In the figure, γ_1, γ_2, and γ_3 are labeled boundaries and τ_1 and τ_2 are the shortest geodesics between boundaries. Figure 3 (d) illustrates the surface with the hyperbolic metric that is isometrically flattened onto the Poincaré disk. When we make the topological change, we make sure each new boundary has the same Euclidean length across different surface. As a result,

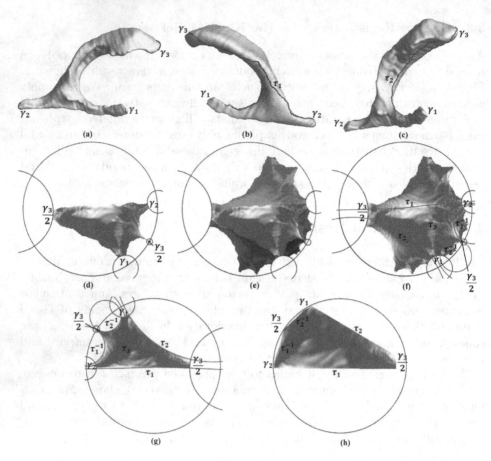

Fig. 3. Illustration of hyperbolic conformal parameterization of a left lateral ventricular surface with Ricci flow method.

the lengths of each boundary under the Poincaré disk metric are valid metrics for studying lateral ventricular surface morphology.

In our experiments [40, 49], we compared ventricular surface models extracted from 3D brain MRI scans of 11 individuals with HIV/AIDS and 8 control subjects [7, 8]. We automatically performed topology optimization on each ventricular surface and computed their lengths in the Poincaré disk by the Ricci flow method. For each pair of ventricular surfaces, we obtained a 6×1 vector, $t = (t_1, t_2, ...t_6)$, which consists of 3 boundary lengths for the left ventricular surface and 3 boundary lengths for right ventricular surface. Given this Teichmüller space coordinate based feature vector, we applied a nearest neighbor classifier based on the Mahalanobis distance, which is

$$d(t) = \sqrt{(t - \mu_{T_c})^T \Sigma_{T_c}^{-1}(t - \mu_{T_c})} + \sqrt{(t - \mu_{T_a})^T \Sigma_{T_a}^{-1}(t - \mu_{T_a})} \quad (5)$$

where μ_{T_c}, μ_{T_a}, Σ_{T_c} and Σ_{T_a} are the feature vector mean and covariance for the two groups, respectively. We classified t based on the sign of the distance of $d(t)$, i.e., the subject that is closer to one group mean is classified into that group. For this data set, we performed a leave-one-out test. Our classifier successfully classified all 19 subjects to the correct group and achieved a 100% accuracy rate.

For comparison, we also tested a nearest neighbor classifier associated with a volume feature vector. For each pair of ventricular surface, we measured their volumes, $v = (v_l, v_r)$. We also used nearest neighbor classifier based on the Mahalanobis distance, which is

$$d(v) = \sqrt{(v - \mu_{V_c})^T \Sigma_{V_c}^{-1}(t - \mu_{V_c})} + \sqrt{(t - \mu_{V_a})^T \Sigma_{V_a}^{-1}(t - \mu_{V_a})} \tag{6}$$

where μ_{V_c}, μ_{V_a}, Σ_{V_c} and Σ_{V_a} are the feature vector mean and covariance for the two groups, respectively. We classified v based on the sign of the distance of $d(v)$, i. e., the subject that is closer to one group mean is classified into that group. In the data set, we performed a leave-one-out test. The classifier based on the simple volume measurement successfully classified only 13 out of 19 subjects to the correct group and achieved a 68.42% accuracy rate.

Studies of ventricular morphology have also used 3D statistical maps to correlate anatomy with clinical measures, but automated ventricular analysis is still difficult because of their highly irregular branching surface shape. The new Teichmüller space shape descriptor requires more validation on other data sets, these experimental results suggest that (1) ventricular surface morphology is altered in HIV/AIDS; (2) volume measures are not sufficient to distinguish HIV patients from controls; and (3) our Teichmüller space feature vector can be used to classify control and patient subjects. Our ongoing work is studying the correlation between the proposed feature vector and clinical measures (e.g., future decline) in an Alzheimer's Disease dataset.

4.2   Registering Lateral Ventricular Surfaces via the Klein Model

Here we report our preliminary study of applying the proposed method for registering lateral ventricular surfaces. Experiments on a pair of lateral ventricular surfaces from two diagnostic groups showed that our method is promising for registration of high-genus surfaces.

Fig. 4 (a) and (d) are the left ventricular surfaces from a healthy control subject and an HIV/AIDS patient, respectively. The boundaries were automatically cut by the topology optimization operation introduced in Sec 4.1. By visual observation, it is obvious that the volume of the lateral ventricular surface of the HIV/AIDS patient is larger than that of the control subject. This characteristic is also represented by the corresponding Poincaré models and Klein models. Furthermore, despite of the shape difference, the Klein disks of the two surface are quite similar, which provides a promising initial condition for further registration with constrained harmonic map [8] or surface fluid registration [56]. One of the most advantageous properties of our method over the method in [8] is that surface conformal parameterization with the new method has no singularities.

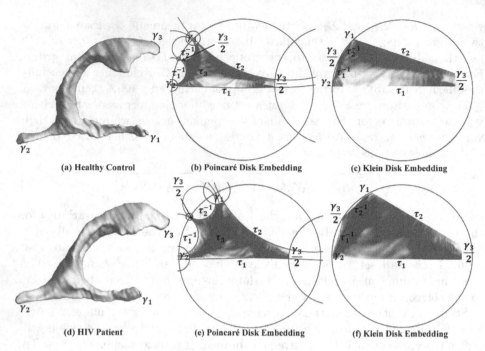

(a) Healthy Control   (b) Poincaré Disk Embedding   (c) Klein Disk Embedding

(d) HIV Patient   (e) Poincaré Disk Embedding   (f) Klein Disk Embedding

Fig. 4. Comparison of two different lateral ventricular surfaces and their hyperbolic parameterizations. The Klein model parameterization provides an intrinsic and stable domain for registration.

All surface information may be used for registration. Intuitively, more usable parameter space in the canonical space is better to match subtle surface features. In our future work, we will apply the proposed pipeline to register high-genus surfaces in big imaging dataset and compare our experimental results with prior methods [8].

5   Discussion and Future Work

In this paper, we propose a stable way to compute hyperbolic conformal parameterization for surfaces with complicated topology structure. Given a topological pant surface, for example, the discrete Ricci flow can be applied to embed it into a Poincaré disk. Its Teichmüller space coordinate is calculated from the lengths of its three boundaries under hyperbolic metric. Further, we may transform the Poincaré disk model to Klein model, where a convex polygon is suitable to generate diffeomorphisms between high genus surfaces. We demonstrated our work in lateral ventricle surfaces for HIV/AIDS research.

Our algorithm is based on solving elliptic partial differential equations, so the computation is stable. The computation is also insensitive to the surface triangular mesh quality so it is robust to the digitization errors in the 3D surface reconstruction. Overall, it provides an intrinsic and stable way to compute surface conformal structure based shape index for further morphometry study. Although our current work focuses on topological pant surfaces, for surfaces with more complicated topologies, their Teichmüller coordinates and Klein model parameterizations can still be computed using the hyperbolic metric. If the surface has Euler number χ, $\chi < 0$, the surface can be decomposed to $-\chi$ number of pants, where the cutting curves are also geodesics under the hyperbolic metric. Furthermore, two pants sharing a common cutting curve can be glued together with a specific twisting angle and it can also be converted to the polygon under the Klein model. The lengths of all cutting geodesics and the twisting angles associated with them form the Teichmüller coordinates of the surface. In the future, we will further explore and validate numerous applications of the hyperbolic Ricci flow method in neuroimaging and shape analysis research.

References

1. Chung, M.K., Dalton, K.M., Davidson, R.J.: Tensor-based cortical surface morphometry via weighted spherical harmonic representation. IEEE Trans. Med. Imaging 27(8), 1143–1151 (2008)
2. Styner, M., Lieberman, J.A., McClure, R.K., Weinberger, D.R., Jones, D.W., Gerig, G.: Morphometric analysis of lateral ventricles in schizophrenia and healthy controls regarding genetic and disease-specific factors. Proc. Natl. Acad. Sci. U. S. A. 102(13), 4872–4877 (2005)
3. Pizer, S.M., Fritsch, D.S., Yushkevich, P.A., Johnson, V.E., Chaney, E.L.: Segmentation, registration, and measurement of shape variation via image object shape. IEEE Trans. Med. Imaging 18(10), 851–865 (1999)
4. Davies, R.H., Twining, C.J., Allen, P.D., Cootes, T.F., Taylor, C.J.: Shape discrimination in the hippocampus using an MDL model. Inf. Process Med. Imaging 18, 38–50 (2003)
5. Miller, M.I., Trouve, A., Younes, L.: On the metrics and euler-lagrange equations of computational anatomy. Annu. Rev. Biomed. Eng. 4, 375–405 (2002)
6. Thompson, P.M., Toga, A.W.: A framework for computational anatomy. Computing and Visualization in Science 5, 1–12 (2002)
7. Thompson, P.M., Dutton, R.A., Hayashi, K.M., Lu, A., Lee, S.E., Lee, J.Y., Lopez, O.L., Aizenstein, H.J., Toga, A.W., Becker, J.T.: 3D mapping of ventricular and corpus callosum abnormalities in HIV/AIDS. NeuroImage 31(1), 12–23 (2006)
8. Wang, Y., Zhang, J., Gutman, B., Chan, T.F., Becker, J.T., Aizenstein, H.J., Lopez, O.L., Tamburo, R.J., Toga, A.W., Thompson, P.M.: Multivariate tensor-based morphometry on surfaces: Application to mapping ventricular abnormalities in HIV/AIDS. NeuroImage 49(3), 2141–2157 (2010)
9. Ashburner, J., Friston, K.: Multimodal image coregistration and partitioning–a unified framework. Neuroimage 6(3), 209–217 (1997)
10. Christensen, G.E., Rabbitt, R.D., Miller, M.I.: Deformable templates using large deformation kinematics. IEEE Trans. Image Process 5(10), 1435–1447 (1996)
11. Shen, D., Davatzikos, C.: HAMMER: hierarchical attribute matching mechanism for elastic registration. IEEE Trans. Med. Imaging 21(11), 1421–1439 (2002)
12. Fischl, B., Sereno, M.I., Dale, A.M.: Cortical surface-based analysis II: Inflation, flattening, and a surface-based coordinate system. NeuroImage 9(2), 195–207 (1999)

13. Thompson, P.M., Hayashi, K.M., Sowell, E.R., Gogtay, N., Giedd, J.N., Rapoport, J.L., de Zubicaray, G.I., Janke, A.L., Rose, S.E., Semple, J., Doddrell, D.M., Wang, Y., van Erp, T.G.M., Cannon, T.D., Toga, A.W.: Mapping cortical change in Alzheimer's disease, brain development, and schizophrenia. NeuroImage 23(suppl. 1), S2–S18 (2004)
14. Thompson, P.M., Toga, A.W.: A surface-based technique for warping 3-dimensional images of the brain. IEEE Trans. Med. Imag. 15(4), 1–16 (1996)
15. Van Essen, D.C., Drury, H.A., Dickson, J., Harwell, J., Hanlon, D., Anderson, C.H.: An integrated software suite for surface-based analyses of cerebral cortex. J. Am. Med. Inform. Assoc. 8(5), 443–459 (2001)
16. Bakircioglu, M., Joshi, S., Miller, M.I.: Landmark matching on brain surfaces via large deformation diffeomorphisms on the sphere. In: Proc. SPIE Medical Imaging, vol. 3661, pp. 710–715 (1999)
17. Leow, A., Yu, C.L., Lee, S.J., Huang, S.C., Nicolson, R., Hayashi, K.M., Protas, H., Toga, A.W., Thompson, P.M.: Brain structural mapping using a novel hybrid implicit/explicit framework based on the level-set method. NeuroImage 24(3), 910–927 (2005)
18. Yeo, B.T., Sabuncu, M.R., Vercauteren, T., Ayache, N., Fischl, B., Golland, P.: Spherical demons: fast diffeomorphic landmark-free surface registration. IEEE Trans. Med. Imaging 29(3), 650–668 (2010)
19. Davatzikos, C., Vaillant, M., Resnick, S.M., Prince, J.L., Letovsky, S., Bryan, R.N.: A computerized approach for morphological analysis of the corpus callosum. J. Comput. Assist. Tomogr. 20(1), 88–97 (1996)
20. Auzias, G., Colliot, O., Glaunes, J.A., Perrot, M., Mangin, J.F., Trouve, A., Baillet, S.: Diffeomorphic brain registration under exhaustive sulcal constraints. IEEE Trans. Med. Imaging 30(6), 1214–1227 (2011)
21. Bookstein, F.L.: Shape and the information in medical images: a decade of the morphometric synthesis. In: Mathematical Methods in Biomedical Image Analysis, Proceedings of the Workshop, pp. 2–12 (June 1996)
22. Joshi, S.H., Cabeen, R.P., Joshi, A.A., Sun, B., Dinov, I., Narr, K.L., Toga, A.W., Woods, R.P.: Diffeomorphic sulcal shape analysis on the cortex. IEEE Trans. Med. Imaging 31(6), 1195–1212 (2012)
23. Pantazis, D., Joshi, A., Jiang, J., Shattuck, D.W., Bernstein, L.E., Damasio, H., Leahy, R.M.: Comparison of landmark-based and automatic methods for cortical surface registration. Neuroimage 49(3), 2479–2493 (2010)
24. Zhong, J., Phua, D.Y., Qiu, A.: Quantitative evaluation of LDDMM, FreeSurfer, and CARET for cortical surface mapping. Neuroimage 52(1), 131–141 (2010)
25. Joshi, S.C., Miller, M.I., Grenander, U.: On the geometry and shape of brain submanifolds. IEEE Trans. Patt. Anal. Mach. Intell. 11, 1317–1343 (1997)
26. Durrleman, S., Pennec, X., Trouve, A., Thompson, P.M., Ayache, N.: Inferring brain variability from diffeomorphic deformations of currents: An integrative approach. Medical Image Analysis 12(5), 626–637 (2008)
27. Vaillant, M., Qiu, A., Glaunes, J., Miller, M.I.: Diffeomorphic metric surface mapping in subregion of the superior temporal gyrus. Neuroimage 34(3), 1149–1159 (2007)
28. Trouvé, A., Younes, L.: Metamorphoses through Lie group action. Found. Comp. Math., 173–198 (2005)
29. Boyer, D.M., Lipman, Y., St Clair, E., Puente, J., Patel, B.A., Funkhouser, T., Jernvall, J., Daubechies, I.: Algorithms to automatically quantify the geometric similarity of anatomical surfaces. Proc. Natl. Acad. Sci. U.S.A. 108, 18221–18226 (2011)

30. Fischl, B., Sereno, M.I., Tootell, R.B., Dale, A.M.: High-resolution intersubject averaging and a coordinate system for the cortical surface. Hum. Brain Mapp. 8(4), 272–284 (1999)
31. Pitiot, A., Delingette, H., Toga, A.W., Thompson, P.M.: Learning object correspondences with the observed transport shape measure. Inf. Process. Med. Imaging 18, 25–37 (2003)
32. Wang, Y., Chiang, M.C., Thompson, P.M.: Mutual information-based 3D surface matching with applications to face recognition and brain mapping. In: Proc. of the Tenth IEEE International Conference on Computer Vision, ICCV 2005, vol. 1, pp. 527–534 (October 2005)
33. Younes, L.: Shapes and Diffeomorphisms. Springer (2010)
34. Fletcher, P.T., Lu, C., Pizer, S.M., Joshi, S.: Principal geodesic analysis for the study of nonlinear statistics of shape. IEEE Trans. Med. Imaging 23(8), 995–1005 (2004)
35. Miller, M.I., Qiu, A.: The emerging discipline of Computational Functional Anatomy. Neuroimage 45(suppl. 1), 16–39 (2009)
36. Ashburner, J., Hutton, C., Frackowiak, R., Johnsrude, I., Price, C., Friston, K.: Identifying global anatomical differences: deformation-based morphometry. Hum. Brain Mapp. 6(5-6), 348–357 (1998)
37. Wang, L., Swank, J.S., Glick, I.E., Gado, M.H., Miller, M.I., Morris, J.C., Csernansky, J.G.: Changes in hippocampal volume and shape across time distinguish dementia of the Alzheimer type from healthy aging. Neuroimage 20(2), 667–682 (2003)
38. Davatzikos, C.: Spatial normalization of 3D brain images using deformable models. J. Comput. Assist. Tomogr. 20(4), 656–665 (1996)
39. Jin, M., Zeng, W., Luo, F., Gu, X.: Computing Teichmüller shape space. IEEE Trans. Vis. Comput. Graphics 15(3), 504–517 (2009)
40. Wang, Y., Dai, W., Gu, X., Chan, T.F., Yau, S.-T., Toga, A.W., Thompson, P.M.: Teichmüller Shape Space Theory and Its Application to Brain Morphometry. In: Yang, G.-Z., Hawkes, D., Rueckert, D., Noble, A., Taylor, C. (eds.) MICCAI 2009, Part II. LNCS, vol. 5762, pp. 133–140. Springer, Heidelberg (2009)
41. Shi, Y., Lai, R., Gill, R., Pelletier, D., Mohr, D., Sicotte, N., Toga, A.W.: Conformal Metric Optimization on Surface (CMOS) for Deformation and Mapping in Laplace-Beltrami Embedding Space. In: Fichtinger, G., Martel, A., Peters, T. (eds.) MICCAI 2011, Part II. LNCS, vol. 6892, pp. 327–334. Springer, Heidelberg (2011)
42. Kurtek, S., Klassen, E., Ding, Z., Jacobson, S.W., Jacobson, J.L., Avison, M.J., Srivastava, A.: Parameterization-invariant shape comparisons of anatomical surfaces. IEEE Trans. Med. Imaging 30(3), 849–858 (2011)
43. Hurdal, M.K., Stephenson, K.: Cortical cartography using the discrete conformal approach of circle packings. NeuroImage 23, S119–S128 (2004)
44. Angenent, S., Haker, S., Tannenbaum, A.R., Kikinis, R.: Conformal Geometry and Brain Flattening. In: Taylor, C., Colchester, A. (eds.) MICCAI 1999. LNCS, vol. 1679, pp. 271–278. Springer, Heidelberg (1999)
45. Ju, L., Hurdal, M.K., Stern, J., Rehm, K., Schaper, K., Rottenberg, D.: Quantitative evaluation of three surface flattening methods. NeuroImage 28(4), 869–880 (2005)
46. Tosun, D., Prince, J.: A geometry-driven optical flow warping for spatial normalization of cortical surfaces. IEEE Trans. Med. Imag. 27(12), 1739–1753 (2008)

47. Gu, X., Wang, Y., Chan, T.F., Thompson, P.M., Yau, S.T.: Genus zero surface conformal mapping and its application to brain surface mapping. IEEE Trans. Med. Imag. 23(8), 949–958 (2004)

48. Wang, Y., Lui, L.M., Gu, X., Hayashi, K.M., Chan, T.F., Toga, A.W., Thompson, P.M., Yau, S.T.: Brain surface conformal parameterization using Riemann surface structure. IEEE Trans. Med. Imag. 26(6), 853–865 (2007)

49. Wang, Y., Dai, W., Gu, X., Chan, T.F., Toga, A.W., Thompson, P.M.: Studying brain morphology using Teichmüller space theory. In: IEEE 12th International Conference on Computer Vision, ICCV 2009, pp. 2365–2372 (September 2009)

50. Wang, Y., Shi, J., Yin, X., Gu, X., Chan, T.F., Yau, S.T., Toga, A.W., Thompson, P.M.: Brain surface conformal parameterization with the Ricci flow. IEEE Trans. Med. Imaging 31(2), 251–264 (2012)

51. Wang, Y., Gu, X., Chan, T.F., Thompson, P.M., Yau, S.T.: Conformal Slit Mapping and Its Applications to Brain Surface Parameterization. In: Metaxas, D., Axel, L., Fichtinger, G., Székely, G. (eds.) MICCAI 2008, Part I. LNCS, vol. 5241, pp. 585–593. Springer, Heidelberg (2008)

52. Zeng, W., Samaras, D., Gu, X.: Ricci flow for 3D shape analysis. IEEE Trans. Patt. Anal. Mach. Intell. 32, 662–677 (2010)

53. Gu, X., Yau, S.T.: Computational Conformal Geometry. International Press (2008)

54. Wikipedia: Hyperbolic geometry — Wikipedia, the free encyclopedia (2012)

55. Luo, F., Gu, X., Dai, J.: Variational Principles for Discrete Surfaces. International Press (2008)

56. Shi, J., Thompson, P.M., Gutman, B., Wang, Y.: Surface fluid registration of conformal representation: application to detect disease effect and genetic influence on hippocampus. Submitted to NeuroImage (2012)

57. Carmichael, O.T., Thompson, P.M., Dutton, R.A., Lu, A., Lee, S.E., Lee, J.Y., Kuller, L.H., Lopez, O.L., Aizenstein, H.J., Meltzer, C.C., Liu, Y., Toga, A.W., Becker, J.T.: Mapping ventricular changes related to dementia and mild cognitive impairment in a large community-based cohort. In: 3rd IEEE International Symposium on Biomedical Imaging: Nano to Macro, pp. 315–318 (April 2006)

58. Ferrarini, L., Palm, W.M., Olofsen, H., van Buchem, M.A., Reiber, J.H., Admiraal-Behloul, F.: Shape differences of the brain ventricles in Alzheimer's disease. NeuroImage 32(3), 1060–1069 (2006)

59. Chou, Y., Leporé, N., de Zubicaray, G.I., Carmichael, O.T., Becker, J.T., Toga, A.W., Thompson, P.M.: Automated ventricular mapping with multi-atlas fluid image alignment reveals genetic effects in Alzheimer's disease. NeuroImage 40(2), 615–630 (2008)

Do We Really Need Robust and Alternative Inference Methods for Brain MRI?

Bennett A. Landman[1,*], Xue Yang[1], and Hakmook Kang[2]

[1] Electrical Engineering, Vanderbilt University, Nasvhille TN, 37235 USA
[2] Biostatistics, Vanderbilt University, Nasvhille TN, 37235 USA
{Bennett.Landman,Xue.Yang,Hakmook.Kang}@vanderbilt.edu

Abstract. Voxel-wise statistical inference lies at the heart of quantitative multi-modal brain imaging. The general linear model with its fixed and mixed effects formulations has been the workhorse of empirical neuroscience for both structural and functional brain assessment. Yet, the validity of estimated p-values hinges upon assumptions of Gaussian distributed errors. Inference approaches based on relaxed distributional assumptions (e.g., non-parametric, robust) have been available in the statistical community for decades. Recently, there has been renewed interest in applying these methods in medical imaging. Despite theoretically attractive behavior, relaxing Gaussian assumptions comes at the practical cost of reduced power (when Gaussian assumptions are met), increased computational complexity, and limited community support. We discuss the challenges of applying robust and alternative statistical methods to medical imaging inference, characterize the conditions under which such approaches are necessary, and present a new quantitative framework to empirically justify selection of inference methods.

Keywords: Robust inference, statistical parametric mapping, neuroimaging.

1 Introduction

Neuroscience and patient care have been transformed by quantitative inference of spatial-temporal brain correlations in normal and patient populations with millimeter resolution and second precision using three-dimensional structural imaging (magnetic resonance imaging – MRI, computed tomography – CT) and functional imaging (positron emission tomography – PET, functional MRI – fMRI) [1]. Classical statistical approaches allow mapping of brain regions associated with planning/execution, response, and default mode behaviors (through task, event, and resting state paradigms, respectively) [2]. While creative and hybrid study designs are broadening the reach of MRI methods to detect subtle brain perturbations with brain state and/or pathology, well-proven techniques for mapping eloquent motor, sensory, and visual areas are now clinically applied to personalize patient care through pre-operative mapping in epilepsy, brain cancers, and implant surgeries. Yet, in the quest to evermore specifically map

---

* Corresponding author.

P.-T. Yap et al. (Eds.): MBIA 2012, LNCS 7509, pp. 77–93, 2012.
© Springer-Verlag Berlin Heidelberg 2012

neural anatomy, cognitive function, and potential pathologies, the resolution limitations of the current generation of clinical MRI scanners are becoming painfully clear. Undersampled imaging (compressed sensing [3]) and ultra-high field (7T [4]) acquisitions promise access to unprecedented spatial-temporal resolution map; yet, the effects of physiological noise (breathing, cardiac, pulsation, flow, etc.), susceptibility artifacts, and hardware induced distortion also increase.

Absolute voxel-wise MRI intensities are rarely used in isolation for inference – rather, the temporal and spatial patterns/correlations of changes over time are of primary interest. Statistical analyses enable *inference* of the probability that observed signals are not observed by chance (i.e., that there exist *significant* associations between the observed signals and model of brain activity). The techniques in wide-spread use are based on classical distributional properties (e.g., Gaussian noise models, auto-regressive temporal correlation, and Gaussian random fields) and have been shown to be appropriate for well-designed studies at traditional field strengths. Violations of statistical assumptions threaten to *invalidate* or (at best) reduce the power of these experiments. Traditional validation guidance involves careful inspection of residuals and evaluation of distributional assumptions [5]. When artifacts are detected, images must be excluded or the analysis approach must be modified. As studies push the limits of resolution and hardware performance, it is uncertain if non-idealities can be controlled or compensated such that their overall impact will be truly negligible.

Modern robust and non-parametric statistical approaches have been pioneered in the statistical community to address precisely these concerns – there were at least 44 panel sessions at the Joint Statistical Meeting (JSM) 2011 discussing aspects of non-parametric and robust inference. With minor adaptations to compensate for the high-dimensionality of image data and study designs, non-parametric techniques have become popular for analysis of small cohorts [6], and the approach has been generalized to include Bayesian [7] and semi-parametric [8] influences. Together, these non- and semi-parametric tests have increased statistical power for studies with small cohorts and have enabled valid inferences with study designs that were previously intractable. Also at JSM, there were 98 (in 2010) and 75 (in 2011) abstracts discussing robust and resilient methods for imaging. However, these efforts have had limited translational impact enabling clinical findings (e.g., [9, 10]), and no abstracts reported using robust fMRI inference at the Organization of Human Brain Mapping 2011 meeting.

In a recent pilot study, we investigated the distributional properties of resting state fMRI (rs-fMRI) at 3T and 7T [11]. The 3T data were well-described by traditional restricted maximum likelihood (ReML) assumptions, while the 7T data exhibited substantial non-Gaussian noise structure and spatial correlations not well-modeled by traditional approaches (as would be expected with data known to be susceptible to artifacts) [12]. The statistics literature is ripe with presentations of "robust/resistant" methods that mimic traditional analyses but are less sensitive to the impacts of outliers and violations of distributional assumptions. For example, a robust empirical Bayesian estimation of longitudinal data is briefly discussed in [13] in a non-imaging context, while temporal artifacts have been previously addressed for 3T fMRI by estimating the covariance matrix of the regression errors [14]. We combined these ideas to extend the traditional ReML approach to use a robust autoregressive model.

When applied to empirical 7T fMRI data, clear differences in statistical parameter maps were observed between inferences based on classical and robust assumptions. Yet, there is a fundamental gap between noting empirical differences in statistical parametric maps and concluding that *improvement* occurred such that one inference method is more appropriate than another (Figure 1).

In 1979, John Tukey, a pioneer in modern statistics, expressed "which robust/resistant methods you use is not important-what is important is that you use some" [15, 16]. Without careful examination of the *possible* impacts of distributional violations, it is difficult (or impossible) to know if violations are impacting data interpretation. Recent advances in statistical image processing software (Table 1) provide reasonable access to robust statistical methods for MRI analyses, but support for these methods is sparse and the challenge of selecting and applying a robust approach given the complexities (variation in possible study design), idiosyncrasies (motion/distortion correction, slice-timing correction, etc.), and high dimensionality (10^4-10^6 voxels per subject per time point) is daunting. There are scores of potential study design choices among the families of robust estimators in the literature — at least 36 packages implement robust estimation in the R Project [17].

Table 1. Comparison of traditional and robust inference tools available for MRI

Traditional	Modern
Fixed Effects [12]	Robust ReML [11, 14]
	Non-parametric ReML [6]
Mixed Effects [18]	Robust Mixed Effects [19]

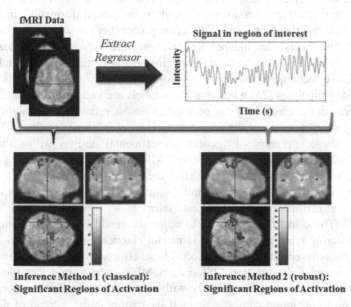

Inference Method 1 (classical):
Significant Regions of Activation

Inference Method 2 (robust):
Significant Regions of Activation

Fig. 1. Quantifying differences between three-dimensional statistical parametric maps produced by different inference methods is challenging, and, to date, has been largely qualitative – i.e., the robust map at right shows less speckle noise

We posit that robust methods have not been widely adapted in medical imaging research because (1) acquisitions at 1.5T and 3T generally result in high quality data and approximately meet parametric distributional assumptions for moderate sized cohorts, (2) robust methods are not routinely accessible and, hence, are not seen as worthwhile as tools for re-validation of the effects of outliers (c.f., Tukey's landmark advice [15, 16]), and, perhaps most importantly, (3) robust methods do not *enable inference* with data for which their classical cousins are suitably adapted. When considering emerging acquisition methods and sequences that push the limits of MRI scanner design, the situation changes:

1. Image reconstruction is technically challenging and plagued by field inhomogeneity and sensitivity to motion, flow, artifacts, etc. [20-22]. Classical distributional assumptions become tenuous and require careful validation and application.
2. Confirmation that results are not corrupted by outliers is critically important, but existing statistical techniques are not easily accessible to the community.
3. Robust methods may provide valid inference in the presence of some imaging artifacts and allow investigators to more fully exploit artifact prone data to reveal new understandings of the human brain.

Paramount to realizing the benefits of these new acquisitions is quantitatively determining when a robust method is more appropriate for a particular empirical dataset than its classical cousins.

Statistical comparison of statistical maps (e.g., t-fields, p-values) can be theoretically challenging given the difficulty in modeling distributional assumptions when the null hypothesis is rejected [23]. Data-driven *prediction* and *reproducibility* metrics enable such quantitative assessments through resampling/information theory [24]. Prediction evaluates the degree (e.g., posterior probability) to which a model can assign correct class labels to an independent test set, while reproducibility measures the similarity (correlation coefficient) of activation maps generated from independent data sets. These techniques can be used to optimize acquisition protocols [25] and post-processing pipelines [26] when true class labels are known. In a related manner, mutual information metrics [18] can be used to assess relative predictability and reproducibility characteristics of the robust and classical inference methods. Yet, generalization of these approaches to generic experimental designs within the general linear model paradigm (i.e., resting state fMRI, structural-functional association studies, etc.) is problematic because true class memberships are unknown.

Herein, we characterize empirical, finite sample performance by quantifying the consistency and resilience of empirical estimators under random data loss (i.e., decimation) [27]. These metrics are simple to compute, readily applied to compare estimators of differing type (robust, non-parametric, classical, etc.), and provide metrics that enable data-driven estimator selection. These efforts build on recent innovations in SIMulation and EXtrapolation [28] (i.e., SIMEX - the notion that the expected value of an estimator diverges smoothly with increasing noise levels, therefore, the mean degree of corruption can be estimated by extrapolating a trend of divergence when synthetic noise is added to *empirical* data) and randomized data subsampling.

The proposed approach does not require acquisition of additional data and is suitable for evaluation on isolated datasets as well as group datasets.

This manuscript is organized as follows. First, we review robust inference in MRI studies. Second, we discuss evaluation of inference methods with simulation. Third, we present calculation of resilience metrics with empirical MRI. Fourth, present a framework for quantitative comparison of inference methods and conclude with an empirical demonstration of the proposed data on rs-fMRI data at 3T and 7T.

This manuscript builds upon (and reanalyzes/reinterprets data from) a previous conference proceeding presenting the theory of decimation resampling [27], our work on robust [29, 30] and alternative [31-33] regression, and empirical studies of distributional assumptions [11, 34].

2   Theory

2.1   Overview

Accounting for temporal correlation, spatio-temporal correlation, and multiple comparisons are fundamental challenges in translating statistical approaches for medical imaging data; these have been addressed from diverse and complementary perspectives. Worsley and Friston accounted for temporal correlations in neuroimaging data in their seminal work [35, 36], which was extended through autoregressive models of order p [37], autoregressive moving averages [38], and wavelet decomposition [39]. Spatio-temporal correlations have been addressed from a spatio-spectral approach in which the hemodynamic response function was allowed to vary voxel to voxel [40]. Katanoda et al. addressed spatial dependency by borrowing information from the six nearest neighboring voxels in three orthogonal directions while working in the Fourier domain [41], while Worsely et al. employed spatial smoothing on the sample autocorrelation [42]. Bowman initially proposed a cluster driven approach [43] to localize brain activity and followed this work with a mixed effects spatio-temporal model with a functionally defined distance metric [44]. A spatio-spectral approach by Ombao et al. employs spatially-varying temporal spectra to characterize underlying spatio-temporal processes [45], while the spatio-spectral mixed effects modeling proposed by Kang et al. accounts for multi-scale spatial correlations and temporal correlation as well [46]. Meanwhile, nonlinear Bayesian hierarchical modeling has been suggested to allowed the hemodynamic response function to be different from voxel to voxel [47]. The Bayesian approach has been generalized to include two-stage hierarchical models [48] and adaptive spatial smoothing [49].

To provide a concrete answer to the title question, "*Do We Really Need Robust and Alternative Inference Methods for Brain MRI?*", we focus on model-based inference with fixed effects and mixed effects models (n.b., random effects are a subset of mixed effects). In particular:

- <u>Fixed Effects Models:</u> $Y = X\beta + \epsilon, \ \epsilon \sim \mathcal{N}(0, \Sigma)$
  - *Ex.:* Single-subject brain activation in response to finger tapping, visual stimulus, or correlation between seed regions. In these models, the effect size is not random – i.e., there is a single true response.

- Mixed Effects Models: $Y = X w + \epsilon,\ w \sim \mathcal{N}(w_{population}, \Sigma_w),\ \epsilon \sim \mathcal{N}(0, \Sigma_\epsilon)$
  - *Ex.:* Between-subject brain activation in response to finger tapping modulated by rate. In this model, each subject has a subject-specific effect size, but the effect sizes in the observed cohort are sampled randomly from a population. Note that variance associated with members of w that are considered fixed is zero.

These analysis models are implemented (at least in part) in all major fMRI packages, including SPM [2], AFNI [50], FSL [51], BrainVoyager [52], and REST Toolkit [53].

Within this context, we focus on rs-fMRI data, which can be analyzed with a first order autoregressive model, AR(1), for a weakly stationary time series [54],

$$y_i = X\beta_i + e_i,\ e_i \sim N(0, \sigma_i^2 V) \tag{1}$$

where y_i is a vector of intensity at voxel i, X is the design matrix, β_i is a vector of regression parameters at voxel i, and e_i is a non-spherical error vector. The correlation matrix V is estimated using Restricted Maximum Likelihood (ReML) and β is estimated on the whitened data (i.e., the Ordinary Least Square – OLS – approach). Alternatively, a robust estimator (e.g., the "Huber" M-estimator [55]) may be applied after whitening. Both the OLS and Huber methods are available within the SPM software [29]. Herein, we used the Huber method with the tuning constant chosen for 95% asymptotic efficiency when the distribution of observation error is Gaussian distribution [56].

2.2   Assessment of Inference with Simulation

When a true effect is known, specificity and sensitivity of an inference method may be calculated based on thresholding statistical parametric maps. Specificity and sensitivity may be generalized across p-value thresholds using area under-the curve (AUC) metrics, which are commonly applied in machine learning. Additionally, the accuracy of parameter estimates may be explicitly computed through mean squared error (or another appropriate metric) between the true and estimated parameters. When the classical assumptions hold and errors can be reasonably approximated by well-defined mathematical models, simulating datasets is straightforward and easily interpretable. These simulations readily demonstrate that robust inference measures suffer from reduced power compared with the classic tests (e.g., Figure 2A).

When imaging, physiological, or reconstruction artifacts are prevalent, simulating realistic data becomes a bit of an art form. By definition, the alternative noise distribution is unknown *a priori* (otherwise, one could either properly whiten the data such that classic assumptions would hold or use an inference metric optimal for the known noise structure). With one interpretation of artifact structure, a robust inference method would be superior (Figure 2C), whereas with a similar one, a classical approach is preferable (Figure 2B). Inter-modality and multivariate approaches further complicate proper simulation of noise / artifact distributions. Therefore, we posit that quantitative, comparative assessment of robust/alternative inference methods based on simulation data is inherently limited, and true empirical quantification is preferable.

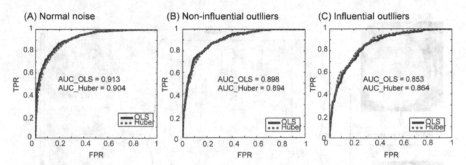

Fig. 2. The relative performance of classic (e.g., ordinary least squared - OLS) and robust (e.g., "Huber"-ized OLS) is strongly dependent on the degree of non-normality of the underlying data

The simulation in Figure 2 follows an exceptionally simple model,

$$y = x\beta + \epsilon \tag{2}$$

where x is a random vector with 20 points that are simulated from a uniform distribution between (0,2) and ϵ is an error vector distributed as a unit normal (**A**). One thousand Monte Carlo simulations were performed for each for three experiments (corresponding to plots **A, B, C**). For the first 500 Monte Carlo simulations, $\beta = 0$, and $\beta = 0.8$ for the next 500. To simulate non-influential and influential outliers, the x values were sorted. For non-influential outliers (**B**), two observed y values with median x values are increased to twice their original values to correspond to artifacts in middle-intensity regions. For influential outliers (**C**), two observed y values with low x values (second and third lowest) are increased to twice their original values to correspond to artifacts in low intensity regions.

2.3   Monte Carlo Assessment of Inference

Empirical characterization of inference performance when the true value is unknown is a circular problem – to quantify error, one must have a baseline against which to compare, but, to compute a baseline from empirical data, one needs an estimator. The SIMEX [28] approach offers a seemingly implausible, but extraordinarily powerful, shortcut around the issue of unknown ground truth. The theoretical core of SIMEX is that the expected value of an estimator diverges smoothly with increasing noise level; therefore, the mean degree of corruption can be estimated by extrapolating a trend of divergence when synthetic noise is added to empirical data. Assuming that the statistical methods under consideration are consistent (i.e., that estimates improve with increasing information), one can use the marginal sensitivity to information loss (e.g., increasing noise) to compute and expected estimator bias based on synthetic noise and a *single* dataset. We have successfully applied SIMEX in a medical imaging context to quantify empirical bias in diffusion tensor imaging (DTI) [57, 58]. In the context of this study, it is not reasonable to add noise because the noise distributions are uncertain — especially in the context of outliers.

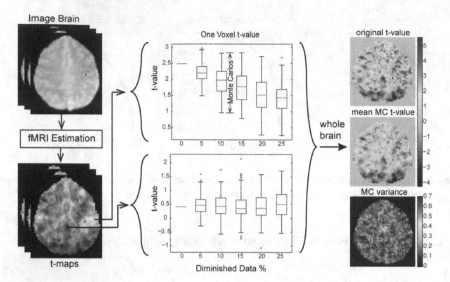

Fig. 3. Illustration of resilience with on two separate voxels of one rs-fMRI dataset

If we apply the SIMEX assumption of smooth convergence to the problem of imaging inference with unknown noise / artifact distributions, we can probe the marginal reduction in sensitivity of an estimator by *removing* data as we have shown in [27]. We define resilience as the ability of an inference method to maintain a consistent parametric map estimate despite a reduction in data. Over the time course of an rs-fMRI experiment (5-10 mins), the active brain regions vary. Hence, reproducibility of inferences based on sampled time periods is not meaningful. Therefore, we focus on randomly diminishing random data samples as opposed to structured temporal resampling. Note that pre-processing steps must be adapted to address random data removal; specifically, the high-pass filters and the estimated covariance matrix must be modified. For the high-pass filter, we created the filters, remove the time points that do not exist, and then apply the filtering. For the covariance estimation, we adjust the starting point of the estimated covariance in ReML by removing the positions corresponding to the non-existed time points. Subsample examples for one voxel t-value are displayed in **Figure 3.**

2.4   Resilience

An intuitive way to assess the resilience of an inference method to a reduction in data might be to calculate the absolute slope of the mean t-value (across Monte Carlo simulations) as a function of data size (i.e., the slope of the linear drop in Figure 3). However, this method will result in higher slope when the t-value with all data is high versus the t-value with all data is low. Such an approach will strongly depend on the true effect size. Hence, it is important to also consider the variance of the estimated parametric maps – we have advocated evaluating the resilience in terms of *consistency* and *variance*.

Consistency assesses the bias of the computed parametric map of the decimated data relative to the same map computed with complete data. *A priori,* one would expect to see small reductions in parametric map values between the complete and decimated datasets due to power loss, but there would be few large changes as both classical and robust inference methods are reasonably unbiased. We summarize consistency by pooling information across all in-brain voxels using linear regression:

$$\overline{t_{subsamples}} = \beta \times t_{all-data} + \epsilon \tag{3}$$

where $t_{all-data}$ is the estimated t-value from all data, $\overline{t_{subsamples}}$ is the mean t-value of all subsamples (across Monte Carlo iteration) and β is the pooled consistency (Figure 4). ϵ is assumed to be Gaussian distributed, so OLS is used. If the inference method is consistent, the slope β should be closed to one and the fitting error would be small. The value of $\beta_{mean} - 1$ can be viewed as a reflection of bias with the sign indicates positive or negative bias and the R-squared can assess the goodness of fit.

The variance of the estimated statistical maps under decimation reflects how resistant an estimation method is to outliers. If a method is affected by outliers, the variance will increase because the outliers may appear in some subsamples while not in others. To compare the resistance of two estimation methods, we plot their variance inside the brain as shown in Figure 5. We pool information across the brain by computing the slope β_{var} of all observation. If two methods are equal, the slope is close to one. If the slope is larger than one, the method on the x-axis is better; on the contrary, if the slope is smaller than one, the method on the y-axis is better.

Small reductions in data result in approximately linear reductions in t-value (due to smooth loss of power – not shown), so we advocate focusing on a specified diminished data size (e.g., randomly diminished by 10% and 20%) rather than on a large number of different data decimations. Simulation experiments (not shown) indicate that approximately 50 Monte Carlo simulations for each decimation level results in

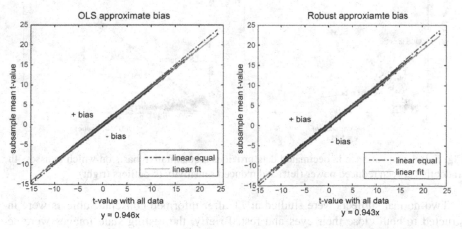

Fig. 4. Propensity for bias is assessed through *consistency* – i.e., the slope between the parametric map with all data and with the mean value estimated with decimated data

stable resilience characterizations when applied to rs-fMRI data. The choice of decimation levels and number of Monte Carlo simulations should be validated for each
imaging inference context.

3   Methods

3.1   Empirical Data

For illustrative purposes, we consider three distinct datasets.

An example healthy subject rs-fMRI requiring at 3T was downloaded from
http://www.nitrc.org/projects/nyu_trt/ (197 volumes, FOV = 192 mm, flip θ = 90°,
TR/TE = 2000/25 ms, 3x3x3 mm, 64x64x39 voxels) [59]. Prior to analysis, all images were corrected for slice timing artifacts and motion artifacts using SPM8 (University College London, UK). All time courses were low pass filtered at 0.1 Hz using
a Chebychev Type II filter, spatially normalized to Talairach space, spatially
smoothed with an 8 mm FWHM Gaussian kernel, linearly detrended, and de-meaned.
Two voxels inside the right primary motor cortex for each subject were manually
selected as the region of interest (ROI) by experienced researchers through exploring
the unsmoothed images and comparing with the standard atlas. The design matrix for
the general linear model was defined as the ROI time courses, the six estimated motion parameters, and one intercept. To create whole-brain connectivity maps, every
labeled brain voxel underwent linear regression using the design matrix followed by a
one sided t-test ($\beta > 0$) on the coefficient for the ROI time courses.

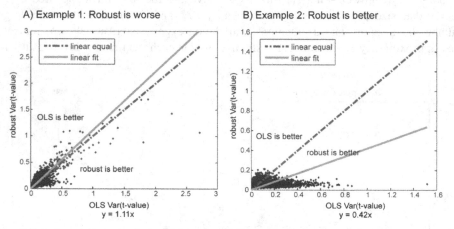

Fig. 5. Relative variance in decimated data provides a quantitative basis on which to assess the
tradeoffs between reduced power (left) and reduced sensitivity to outliers (right)

Two normal subjects were studied at 7T after informed consent. Subjects were in-
structed to both close their eyes and rest. Briefly, the resting state images were acquired for 500s using single shot gradient echo EPI (500 volumes, FOV = 192mm,
flip θ = 53.8°, TR/TE = 1000/28ms, SENSE factor = 3.92, full k-space acquisition,

resolution 2x2x2mm, 96x96x13 voxels). Prior to analysis, all images were corrected for slice timing artifacts and motion artifacts using SPM8 (University College London, UK). All voxels' time courses were low pass filtered at 0.1Hz using a Chebychev Type II filter, linearly detrended, and de-meaned. A single voxel along the right primary motor cortex was manually selected as the seed voxel. The design matrix for the general linear model was defined as the seed voxel time course, the six estimated motion parameters and the intercept. Each voxel's BOLD time course underwent linear regression of the design matrix to create connectivity maps.

3.2   Comparative Analysis of Classical and Robust Inference

rs-fMRI analysis was performed on each dataset in SPM8 using ordinary "OLS" and robust regression "Huber" methods (§2.1). For each decimation level (10% and 20%), 50 Monte Carlo simulations were perform. For each Monte Carlo simulation, a subset of either 90% or 80% of the total data was randomly selected, the OLS and Huber estimation methods were applied, and the parametric maps were stored. Consistency was assessed between the mean of the decimated maps and the map using all data, while the relative variance was assessed between Monte Carlo simulations with each method. For the resilience variance metrics, OLS was on the x-axis and Huber on the y-axis. Note that both OLS and Huber were fit to the same randomize decimation of the data. Representative statistical parametric maps from OLS and robust regression are displayed in Figure 6. The results of one 3T fMRI and two 7T fMRIs are shown in Table 2.

Next, we illustrate how the qualitative metrics may be used for selection of inference method.

- For subject 1, the consistency estimates are similar and close to zero for both OLS and Huber, while the R-squared values are high. This indicates that neither method is particularly biased by the decimation process. The variance metric for both 10% and 20% decimation is negative, which indicates that OLS was more resilient than Huber.
  - — *Conclusion:*   Robust inference is not necessary; OLS is preferable.
- For subject 2, the consistency estimates are similar and close to zero for both OLS and Huber, and the R-squared values are high. Hence, neither method is particularly biased by the decimation process. The variance metric for both 10% and 20% decimation is positive, which indicates that Huber was more resilient than OLS.
  - — *Conclusion:* Robust inference yields higher resilience and should be used.
- For subject 3, the consistency estimates are similar and close to zero for both OLS and Huber, but the R-squared values are notably lower at 20% decimation. Hence, neither method is particularly biased by the 10% decimation process, but 20% decimation is likely less stable. The variance metric for 10% decimation is marginally positive while the variance metric for the 20% decimation is negative. The mixed results indicate that neither method is clearly superior and that care data inspection is warranted.
  - — *Conclusion:* Robust inference may be desirable, but OLS could be suitable.

Table 2. Evaluation of inference methods on three dataset

| | Percent Decimation | Inference Method | Consistency | | Variance |
			$\beta_{mean} - 1$	R^2	$1 - \beta_{var}$
Subj 1 (3T)	10%	OLS	-0.016	0.992	-0.113
		Huber	-0.018	0.991	
	20%	OLS	-0.050	0.984	-0.179
		Huber	-0.049	0.981	
Subj 2 (7T)	10%	OLS	-0.054	0.999	0.579
		Huber	-0.057	0.999	
	20%	OLS	-0.119	0.997	0.280
		Huber	-0.120	0.995	
Subj 3 (7T)	10%	OLS	-0.051	0.995	0.029
		Huber	-0.049	0.995	
	20%	OLS	-0.115	0.964	-0.106
		Huber	-0.107	0.968	

4   Discussion

The answer to the question, "Do we really need robust and alternative inference methods for brain MRI?" is unequivocally, "Sometimes."

Simulations can be constructed to demonstrate that classical assumptions are sufficient or insufficient (Figure 2); it is very difficult to assess the stability of the robust/non-robust decision to variations in outliers as "Anything that can go wrong will go wrong" in imaging. Hence, creating representative artifact-prone distributions is a substantial endeavor. It is possible to acquire a massive reproducibility dataset (e.g., the 45 repeated DTI scans each consisting of 33 volumes over 3 days [60]) and use this dataset to produce a highly robust ground truth estimate. Given such data, one may map artifact distributions. However, such acquisitions are exceedingly resource intensive and generalization of the spatial-temporal properties of rare artifacts to other datasets is questionable. Furthermore, the endurance of a volunteer willing to be extensively scanned would likely be different than a clinical or typical subject; hence, motion induced artifacts would likely be quite different in the populations.

The proposed resilience consistency and variance metrics provide a quantitative basis on which to judge the tradeoffs between improved power when classical assumptions are met and reduced susceptibility to outliers based on empirical data. As these metrics are available for *individual* datasets, one could evaluate suitability of particular inference mechanisms on initial pilot data, on case studies, or as part of multi-level analysis.

Implementation of this approach requires the ability to decimate (remove) data randomly, loop over multiple possible data subsets, and calculate summary measures of the resulting statistical fields. With other study design, we must carefully consider the appropriate mechanisms by which to decimate data – for example, with task-based fMRI we could randomly remove observations, remove equally random observations across tasks, or structure the sampling to preserve aspects of the original structure in the randomly decimated data. We note that the engineering required to augment analysis software to more easily work around missing data has the added benefit that it will enable more targeted exclusion of outliers and finer grained quality control. With modern multi-core and cluster environments, a 50-100 fold increase in the computational burden of a traditional analysis is not typically problematic for off-line analysis. For example, the experiments presents one OLS analysis takes approximately 39s and one Huber analysis takes 6250s. With proper parallelization, the total wait time would not be substantively longer than the time for a single robust analysis.

In conclusion, statistical theories characterizing finite sample statistical behavior are undergoing rapid and exciting developments in the statistical community. These statistical methods, encompassing SIMEX, boot strap, and Monte Carlo approaches, offer the potential to understand both the uncertainty *and bias* in metrics estimated from imaging data. Given the abundance of computational power generally available, these methods can now be feasibly applied on routine basis.

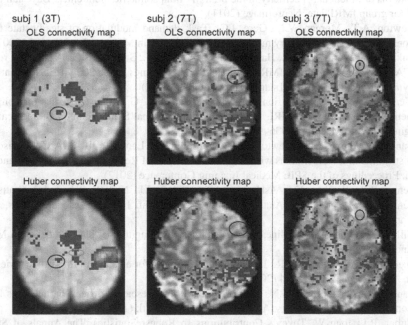

Fig. 6. Propensity for bias is assessed through *consistency* – i.e., the slope between the parametric map with all data and with the mean value estimated with decimated data

Acknowledgement. This research was supported in part by grants NIH N01-AG-4-0012, NIH 1R03EB012461, NIH 5R01EB000461, and NIH 5T32EB03817. We are grateful for the assistance of Allen Newton, Robert Barry, and Victoria Morgan.

References

1. Matthews, P.M., Honey, G.D., Bullmore, E.T.: Applications of fMRI in translational medicine and clinical practice. Nature reviews. Neuroscience 7, 732–744 (2006)
2. Friston, K.: Statistical Parametric Mapping: The Analysis of Functional Brain Images. Academic Press (2006)
3. Lustig, M., Donoho, D.L., Santos, J.M., Pauly, J.M.: Compressed Sensing MRI (A look at how CS can improve on current imaging techniques). IEEE Signal Processing Magazine 25, 72–82 (2008)
4. Vaughan, J.T., Garwood, M., Collins, C.M., Liu, W., DelaBarre, L., Adriany, G., Andersen, P., Merkle, H., Goebel, R., Smith, M.B., Ugurbil, K.: 7T vs. 4T: RF power, homogeneity, and signal-to-noise comparison in head images. Magnetic Resonance in Medicine: Official Journal of the Society of Magnetic Resonance in Medicine / Society of Magnetic Resonance in Medicine 46, 24–30 (2001)
5. Luo, W.L., Nichols, T.E.: Diagnosis and exploration of massively univariate neuroimaging models. NeuroImage 19, 1014–1032 (2003)
6. Nichols, T.E., Holmes, A.P.: Nonparametric permutation tests for functional neuroimaging: a primer with examples. Human Brain Mapping 15, 1–25 (2002)
7. Lashkari, D., Sridharan, R., Vul, E., Hsieh, P.J., Kanwisher, N., Golland, P.: Search for patterns of functional specificity in the brain: A nonparametric hierarchical Bayesian model for group fMRI data. NeuroImage (2011)
8. Newton, A.T., Morgan, V.L., Gore, J.C.: Task demand modulation of steady-state functional connectivity to primary motor cortex. Human Brain Mapping 28, 663–672 (2007)
9. Lukic, A.S., Wernick, M.N., Hansen, L.K., Anderson, J., Strother, S.C.: A spatially robust ICA algorithm for multiple fMRI data sets. In: Proceedings of the 2002 IEEE International Symposium on Biomedical Imaging, pp. 839–842 (2002)
10. Meriaux, S., Roche, A., Thirion, B., Dehaene-Lambertz, G.: Robust statistics for nonparametric group analysis in fMRI. In: 3rd IEEE International Symposium on Biomedical Imaging: Nano to Macro, pp. 936–939 (2006)
11. Yang, X., Holmes, M.J., Newton, A.T., Morgan, V.L., Landman, B.A.: A Comparison of Distributional Considerations with Statistical Analysis of Resting State fMRI at 3T and 7T. In: Proceedings of the SPIE Medical Imaging Conference (2012)
12. Penny, W.D., Friston, K.J., Ashburner, J.T., Kiebel, S.J., Nichols, T.E. (eds.): Statistical Parametric Mapping: The Analysis of Functional Brain Images. Academic Press, New York (2006)
13. Gill, P.S.: A robust mixed linear model analysis for longitudinal data. Statistics in Medicine 19, 975–987 (2000)
14. Diedrichsen, J., Shadmehr, R.: Detecting and adjusting for artifacts in fMRI time series data. NeuroImage 27, 624–634 (2005)
15. Launer, R.L., Wilkinson, G.N.: United States. Army Research Office. Mathematics Division.: Robustness in statistics. Academic Press, New York (1979)
16. Huber, P.J.: John W. Tukey's Contributions to Robust Statistics. The Annals of Statistics 30, 1640–1648 (2002)
17. R Development Core Team: R: A language and environment for statistical computing. R Foundation for Statistical Computing, Vienna (2008)
18. Friston, K.J., Stephan, K.E., Lund, T.E., Morcom, A., Kiebel, S.: Mixed-effects and fMRI studies. NeuroImage 24, 244–252 (2005)

19. Pinheiro, J.C., Liu, C., Wu, Y.N.: Efficient Algorithms for Robust Estimation in Linear Mixed-Effects Models Using the Multivariate t Distribution. Journal of Computational and Graphical Statistics 10, 249–276 (2001)
20. Bluemink, J.J., Andreychenko, A., van Lier, A.L., Phillippens, M., Lagendijk, J.J., Luijten, P.R., van den Berg, C.A.: 7T Imaging of the head and neck region: B0 and B1+ challenges. In: ISMRM (2011)
21. Uğurbil, K.: BRAIN IMAGING at 3T and CHALLENGES at 7. In: ISMRM (2006)
22. Gold, G.E.: Clinical Protocol Challenges in MSK High Field (3T and 7T). In: ISMRM (2011)
23. Garrett, M.A., Holmes, H.T., Nolte, F.S.: Selective buffered charcoal-yeast extract medium for isolation of nocardiae from mixed cultures. Journal of Clinical Microbiology 30, 1891–1892 (1992)
24. Graves, N.M., Ludden, T.M., Holmes, G.B., Fuerst, R.H., Leppik, I.E.: Pharmacokinetics of felbamate, a novel antiepileptic drug: application of mixed-effect modeling to clinical trials. Pharmacotherapy 9, 372–376 (1989)
25. Dalton, J.E., Pederson, S.L., Blom, B.E., Holmes, N.R.: Diagnostic errors using the Short Portable Mental Status Questionnaire with a mixed clinical population. Journal of Gerontology 42, 512–514 (1987)
26. Abbasi, K., Demant, P., Festenstein, H., Holmes, J., Huber, B., Rychikova, M.: Mouse mixed lymphocyte reactions and cell-mediated lympholysis: genetic control and relevance to antigenic strength. Transplantation Proceedings 5, 1329–1337 (1973)
27. Yang, X., Landman, B.A.: Quantitative Evaluation of Statistical Inference in Resting State Functional MRI. In: Medical Image Computing and Computer Assisted Intervention, MICCAI (2012)
28. Carroll, R.J., Ruppert, D., Stefanski, L.A., Crainiceanu, C.: Measurement error in nonlinear models: a modern perspective. CRC Press (2006)
29. Yang, X., Beason-Held, L., Resnick, S.M., Landman, B.A.: Biological parametric mapping with robust and non-parametric statistics. NeuroImage 57, 423–430 (2011)
30. Yang, X., Beason-Held, L., Resnick, S.M., Landman, B.A.: Robust Biological Parametric Mapping: An Improved Technique for Multimodal Brain Image Analysis. In: Proceedings - Society of Photo-Optical Instrumentation Engineers, vol. 7962, p. 79623X (2011)
31. Yang, X., Lauzon, C.B., Crainiceanu, C., Caffo, B., Resnick, S.M., Landman, B.A.: Biological parametric mapping accounting for random regressors with regression calibration and model II regression. NeuroImage 62, 1761–1768 (2012)
32. Yang, X., Lauzon, C.B., Crainiceanu, C., Caffo, B., Resnick, S.M., Landman, B.A.: Massively Univariate Regression Accounting For Random Regressors. In: Joint Statistical Meetings, JSM (2011)
33. Yang, X., Lauzon, C.B., Crainiceanu, C., Caffo, B., Resnick, S.M., Landman, B.A.: Accounting for Random Regressors: A Unified Approach to Multi-modality Imaging. In: MICCAI 2011 Workshop of Multi-Modal Methods (2011)
34. Landman, B., Huang, A., Gifford, A., Vikram, D., Lim, I., Farrell, J., Bogovic, J., Hua, J., Chen, M., Jarso, S., Smith, S., Joel, S., Mori, S., Pekar, J., Barker, P., Prince, J., van Zijl, P.: Multi-Parametric Neuroimaging Reproducibility: A 3T Resource Study. NeuroImage 4, 2854–2866 (2011)
35. Friston, K., Holmes, A., Worsley, K., Poline, J., Frith, C., Frackowiak, R.: Statistical parametric maps in functional imaging: a general linear approach. Human Brain Mapping 2, 189–210 (1994)
36. Worsley, K.J., Friston, K.J.: Analysis of fMRI time-series revisited–again. NeuroImage 2, 173–181 (1995)

37. Bullmore, E., Brammer, M., Williams, S.C.R., Rabehesketh, S., Janot, N., David, A., Mellers, J., Howard, R., Sham, P.: Statistical methods of estimation and inference for functional MR image analysis. Magnetic Resonance in Medicine 35, 261–277 (1996)
38. Locascio, J.J., Jennings, P.J., Moore, C.I., Corkin, S.: Time series analysis in the time domain and resampling methods for studies of functional magnetic resonance brain imaging. Human Brain Mapping 5, 168–193 (1997)
39. Ruttimann, U.E., Unser, M., Rawlings, R.R., Rio, D., Ramsey, N.F., Mattay, V.S., Hommer, D.W., Frank, J.A., Weinberger, D.R.: Statistical analysis of functional MRI data in the wavelet domain. IEEE Transactions on Medical Imaging 17, 142–154 (1998)
40. Lange, N., Zeger, S.L.: Non-linear Fourier time series analysis for human brain mapping by functional magnetic resonance imaging. Appl. Stat-J. Roy. St. C 46, 1–19 (1997)
41. Katanoda, K., Matsuda, Y., Sugishita, M.: A spatio-temporal regression model for the analysis of functional MRI data. NeuroImage 17, 1415–1428 (2002)
42. Worsley, K.J., Liao, C.H., Aston, J., Petre, V., Duncan, G.H., Morales, F., Evans, A.C.: A general statistical analysis for fMRI data. NeuroImage 15, 1–15 (2002)
43. Bowman, F.D.: Spatio-temporal modeling of localized brain activity. Biostatistics 6, 558–575 (2005)
44. Bowman, F.D.: Spatiotemporal models for region of interest analyses of functional neuroimaging data. J. Am. Stat. Assoc. 102, 442–453 (2007)
45. Ombao, H., Shao, X.F., Rykhlevskaia, E., Fabiani, M., Gratton, G.: Spatio-Spectral Analysis of Brain Signals. Stat. Sinica 18, 1465–1482 (2008)
46. Kang, H., Ombao, H., Linkletter, C., Long, N., Badre, D.: Spatio-spectral mixed effects model for functional magnetic resonance imaging data. Journal of American Statistical Association (in press, 2012)
47. Genovese, C.R.: A Bayesian time-course model for functional magnetic resonance imaging data. J. Am. Stat. Assoc. 95, 691–703 (2000)
48. Bowman, F.D., Caffo, B., Bassett, S.S., Kilts, C.: A Bayesian hierarchical framework for spatial modeling of fMRI data. NeuroImage 39, 146–156 (2008)
49. Yue, Y., Loh, J.M., Lindquist, M.A.: Adaptive spatial smoothing of fMRI images. Stat. Interface 3, 3–13 (2010)
50. Saad, Z.S., Chen, G., Reynolds, R.C., Christidis, P.P., Hammett, K.R., Bellgowan, P.S., Cox, R.W.: Functional imaging analysis contest (FIAC) analysis according to AFNI and SUMA. Human Brain Mapping 27, 417–424 (2006)
51. Smith, S.M., Jenkinson, M., Woolrich, M.W., Beckmann, C.F., Behrens, T.E., Johansen-Berg, H., Bannister, P.R., De Luca, M., Drobnjak, I., Flitney, D.E., Niazy, R.K., Saunders, J., Vickers, J., Zhang, Y., De Stefano, N., Brady, J.M., Matthews, P.M.: Advances in functional and structural MR image analysis and implementation as FSL. NeuroImage 23(suppl. 1), S208–S219 (2004)
52. Goebel, R.: BrainVoyager - Past, present, future. NeuroImage 62, 748–756 (2012)
53. Song, X.W., Dong, Z.Y., Long, X.Y., Li, S.F., Zuo, X.N., Zhu, C.Z., He, Y., Yan, C.G., Zang, Y.F.: REST: a toolkit for resting-state functional magnetic resonance imaging data processing. PloS one 6, e25031 (2011)
54. Friston, K.J., Penny, W., Phillips, C., Kiebel, S., Hinton, G., Ashburner, J.: Classical and Bayesian inference in neuroimaging: theory. NeuroImage 16, 465–483 (2002)
55. Huber, P.J., Ronchetti, E.: MyiLibrary: Robust statistics. Wiley Online Library (1981)
56. Holland, P.W., Welsch, R.E.: Robust regression using iteratively reweighted least-squares. Communications in Statistics-Theory and Methods 6, 813–827 (1977)

57. Lauzon, C.B., Asman, A.J., Crainiceanu, C., Caffo, B.C., Landman, B.A.: Assessment of Bias for MRI Diffusion Tensor Imaging Using SIMEX. In: Fichtinger, G., Martel, A., Peters, T. (eds.) MICCAI 2011, Part II. LNCS, vol. 6892, pp. 107–115. Springer, Heidelberg (2011)

58. Lauzon, C.B., Crainiceanu, C., Caffo, B.C., Landman, B.A.: Assessment of bias in experimentally measured diffusion tensor imaging parameters using SIMEX. Magnetic Resonance in Medicine: Official Journal of the Society of Magnetic Resonance in Medicine / Society of Magnetic Resonance in Medicine (2012)

59. Shehzad, Z., Kelly, A., Reiss, P.T., Gee, D.G., Gotimer, K., Uddin, L.Q., Lee, S.H., Margulies, D.S., Roy, A.K., Biswal, B.B.: The resting brain: unconstrained yet reliable. Cerebral Cortex 19, 2209 (2009)

60. Landman, B.A., Farrell, J.A., Jones, C.K., Smith, S.A., Prince, J.L., Mori, S.: Effects of diffusion weighting schemes on the reproducibility of DTI-derived fractional anisotropy, mean diffusivity, and principal eigenvector measurements at 1.5T. NeuroImage 36, 1123–1138 (2007)

Sparse Patch-Based Label Fusion
for Multi-Atlas Segmentation

Daoqiang Zhang[1,2], Qimiao Guo[1,2], Guorong Wu[1], and Dinggang Shen[1]

[1] Dept. of Radiology and BRIC, University of North Carolina at Chapel Hill, NC 27599
[2] Dept. of Computer Science and Engineering, Nanjing University of Aeronautics
and Astronautics, Nanjing 210016, China
{dqzhang,qimiaoguo}@nuaa.edu.cn, {grwu,dgshen}@med.unc.edu

Abstract. Patch-based label fusion methods have shown great potential in
multi-atlas segmentation. It is crucial for patch-based labeling methods to determine appropriate graphs and corresponding weights to better link patches in
the input image with those in atlas images. Currently, two independent steps are
performed, i.e., first constructing graphs based on the fixed image neighborhood and then computing weights based on the heat kernel for all patches in the
neighborhood. In this paper, we first show that many existing label fusion methods can be unified into a graph-based framework, and then propose a novel
method for simultaneously deriving both graph adjacency structure and graph
weights based on the sparse representation, to perform multi-atlas segmentation.
Our motivation is that each patch in the input image can be reconstructed by the
sparse linear superposition of patches in the atlas images, and the reconstruction
coefficients can be used to deduce both graph structure and weights simultaneously. Experimental results on segmenting brain anatomical structures from
magnetic resonance images (MRI) show that our proposed method achieves
significant improvements over previous patch-based methods, as well as other
conventional label fusion methods.

1   Introduction

Automatic and accurate image segmentation is a critical step for many clinical studies
in computational anatomy, including pathology detection and brain parcellation, etc.
Recently, multi-atlas based segmentation methods have shown great success in segmenting brain into anatomical structures. There are two major steps in multi-atlas
based segmentation, i.e., image registration and label fusion. In the first step, it registers each atlas image to the input image and further warps the corresponding label
map by following the same estimated deformation field. Then, in the second step, it
combines the multiple propagated labels from different atlases to obtain the final labels of the input image by some heuristics. We focus on label fusion in this study.

A number of label fusion strategies have been proposed for multi-atlas based segmentation. For example, majority voting (MV) and weighted MV are widely used in
medical image segmentation. In [1], various weighting strategies were categorized
into two groups, i.e., global weighted voting and local weighted voting, and it was

P.-T. Yap et al. (Eds.): MBIA 2012, LNCS 7509, pp. 94–102, 2012.
© Springer-Verlag Berlin Heidelberg 2012

shown that the local weighted voting method outperforms the global one when segmenting high-contrast brain structures. Recently, besides weighting, some more advanced learning techniques have also been developed for further improving performance of label fusion. In [2], a probabilistic label fusion method was proposed to explicitly model the relationship between the atlas and the input image. In [3], a regression-based label fusion method was proposed to use the correlations between results from different atlases. In [4], a labeling confidence was estimated based on forward and backward k-nearest neighbor search to guide the subsequent sequential label fusion.

On the other hand, most of the above label fusion methods only consider one candidate on each atlas image when labeling a voxel in the input image, under the implicit assumption that the input and atlas images should be well registered, i.e., through a non-rigid registration. More recently, inspired by the success of non-local strategy and patch-based method in imaging applications, e.g., image denoising [5], patch-based label fusion that does not require any non-rigid registration was independently proposed in [6] and [7], respectively. Here, the main idea is to allow multiple candidates (usually in the neighborhood) on each atlas image and to aggregate them based on non-local mean. It is crucial for the patch-based label fusion method to determine the appropriate graphs and corresponding weights to better link patches in the input image with patches in the atlas images. At present, the graph construction processes are generally divided into two independent steps, i.e., first manually constructing graphs based on the fixed image neighborhood and then computing weights based on the heat kernel for all patches in the neighborhood.

In this paper, we show that many existing label fusion methods, including the patch-based method, can be unified into a graph-based framework, with differences in different definitions on the graph adjacency structure and graph weights. Furthermore, we propose a novel graph construction method for patch-based label fusion by using sparse representation. Here, our motivation is that each patch in the input image can be reconstructed by the sparse linear superposition of patches in the atlas images. Then, the reconstruction coefficients, which can be gotten by solving an l_1-norm regularized linear regression problem, will be used to deduce the graph adjacency structure and the graph weights simultaneously. It is worth noting that due to the use of l_1-norm, a lot of coefficients will have zero values, i.e., sparse patches are selected for subsequent label fusion. To the best of our knowledge, no previous works have used sparse representation for multi-atlas label fusion, although it has achieved great successes on a number of other applications such as face recognition [8]. We will apply our proposed sparse patch-based label fusion method for segmenting brain anatomical structures from magnetic resonance images (MRI).

2   Graph-Based Framework for Label Fusion

We follow the notations in [7]. Let A be an anatomy textbook (or atlas) containing a set of atlas images and label maps, denoted as $\{(I_i, L_i), i = 1, \ldots, n\}$. Given an input image I, we construct a weighted graph G_i between voxels x of input image I and voxels y of each atlas image I_i, along with corresponding weight $w_i(x, y)$, for $(x, y) \in \Omega^2$ where Ω denotes the image domain. Once we have obtained the graph weights, we can perform label fusion for voxel x of input image I as below:

$$L(x) = \frac{\sum_{i=1}^{n} \sum_{y \in \Omega} w_i(x, y) L_i(y)}{\sum_{i=1}^{n} \sum_{y \in \Omega} w_i(x, y)}, \forall x \in \Omega. \tag{1}$$

We will show that many existing label fusion methods, e.g., majority voting (MV), and patch-based method (PBM), can be derived from Eq. 1, by using different definitions for graph weights.

1) Majority Voting (MV): We can get the label fusion rule for majority voting from Eq. 1, if we define the following graph weights:

$$w_i^{MV}(x, y) = \begin{cases} 1, & \forall (x, y) \in \Omega^2 \text{ and } x = y; \\ 0, & otherwise. \end{cases} \tag{2}$$

2) Patch-Based Method (PBM): We can get the label fusion rule for patch-based method from Eq. 1, if we define the following graph weights:

$$w_i^{PBM}(x, y) = \begin{cases} g\left(\dfrac{\sum_{x' \in P_I(x),\, y' \in P_{I_i}(y)} \left(I(x') - I_i(y') \right)^2}{h_p} \right), \\ \qquad \forall (x, y) \in \Omega^2 \text{ and } y \in N_i(x); \\ 0, \qquad otherwise. \end{cases} \tag{3}$$

Where $N_i(x)$ denotes the neighborhood of voxels x in the atlas image I_i; $P_I(x)$ and $P_{I_i}(y)$ denote the patch centered at voxel x in the input image I and the patch centered at voxel y in the atlas image I_i; g is a smoothing kernel function (in PBM, the heat kernel $g(z) = e^{-z}$ was used), and h_p is the kernel width.

It is worth noting that the constructed graph and its corresponding weights essentially determine the label fusion rule of a certain method, which inspires us to seek other graph construction ways in order for devising new label fusion methods.

3   Sparse Patch-Based Method

Inspired from the discriminating power of sparse representation which has been validated on other tasks such as face recognition, we propose to reconstruct each patch in the input image by the sparse linear superposition of patches in the atlas images. Then, the reconstruction coefficients of those patches are used to deduce the graph adjacency structure and the graph weights simultaneously.

Following the notations in Section 2, given a set of atlas images and label maps $\{(I_i, L_i), i = 1, \dots, n\}$, for each voxel x of input image I and each voxel $y \in N_i(x)$ in atlas image I_i, we want to automatically optimize the weight $w_i(x, y)$ based on sparse representation.

Denote $A_y^i \triangleq col(\{I_i(\mathbf{y}') | \mathbf{y}' \epsilon P_{I_i}(\mathbf{y})\})$ as a patch vector corresponding to $P_{I_i}(\mathbf{y})$, and $b_x \triangleq col(\{I(\mathbf{x}') | \mathbf{x}' \epsilon P_I(\mathbf{x})\})$ as a patch vector corresponding to $P_I(\mathbf{x})$, where col is an operator which aligns all elements in a set into a column vector. Then, for each $\mathbf{x} \in \Omega$, we optimize the following objective function to get the graph weights $w_i(\mathbf{x}, \mathbf{y})$, for each $\mathbf{y} \in N_i(\mathbf{x})$ and $i = 1, \ldots, n$:

$$\min_{\{w_i(x,y)\}} \frac{1}{2} \left\| \sum_{i=1}^{n} \sum_{y \in N_i(x)} A_y^i w_i(\mathbf{x}, \mathbf{y}) - b_x \right\|_2^2 + \lambda \sum_{i=1}^{n} \sum_{y \in N_i(x)} |w_i(\mathbf{x}, \mathbf{y})|. \quad (4)$$

The intuition of Eq. 4 is to sparsely reconstruct the patch vector b_x in the input image using by patch vectors A_y^i in the atlas images. Specifically, the function of the first term of Eq. 4 is to minimize the reconstruction error, while the second term, which is equivalent to the l_1-norm, requires a sparse solution. The regularization parameter λ balances the relative contributions of the two terms and also controls the 'sparsity' of the linear model.

Furthermore, Eq. 4 can be simplified into the following equivalent form:

$$\min_{w_x} \frac{1}{2} \|Aw_x - b_x\|_2^2 + \lambda \|w_x\|_1. \quad (5)$$

where $w_x \triangleq col(\{w_i(\mathbf{x}, \mathbf{y}) | \mathbf{y} \epsilon N_i(\mathbf{x}), i \epsilon \{1, 2, \ldots, n\}\})$, and A is defined as $A \triangleq row(\{A_y^i | \mathbf{y} \epsilon N_i(\mathbf{x}), i \epsilon \{1, 2, \ldots, n\}\})$ where row is an operator which aligns all elements in a set into a (block) row vector. Note that since A_y^i is a column vector, aligning A_y^i with the operator row will lead to a matrix A. Eq. 5 is a standard l_1-norm optimization problem (with the same form as the Lasso method [9]), which can be efficiently solved by a number of existing optimization software [10]. It is worth nothing that a non-negative constraint is required on weight $w_i(\mathbf{x}, \mathbf{y})$ in this study.

Once we have obtained the graph weights $w_i(\mathbf{x}, \mathbf{y})$ by solving Eq. 4 (or 5), we can perform the label fusion process using Eq. 1, to get the propagated label $L(\mathbf{x})$ for each voxel $\mathbf{x}$ in the input image I. Note that generally $L(\mathbf{x})$ takes a continuous value, e.g., a value between 0 and 1 for binary segmentation (i.e., two classes with labels 0 and 1). We focus on binary segmentation in this paper. To get the final label, we use the following equation, for each $\mathbf{x} \in \Omega$:

$$\Gamma(\mathbf{x}) = \begin{cases} 1, & L(\mathbf{x}) \geq 0.5; \\ 0, & otherwise. \end{cases} \quad (6)$$

4   Experiments

In this section, we evaluate the performance of our proposed sparse-patch based method (SPBM) on segmenting brain anatomical structures, i.e., region-of-interests (ROIs), from the MR brain images of NA0-NIREP database [11]. We compare our method with other label fusion methods, including majority voting (MV), local weighted voting (LWV), STAPLE [12], and patch-based method (PBM) [6, 7].

4.1   Dataset and Experimental Settings

The NA0-NIREP dataset [11] used for evaluation consists of 16 annotated MR images, including 8 normal adult males and 8 females. The 16 MR images have been manually segmented into 32 ROIs. The MR images were obtained in a General Electric Signa scanner operating at 1.5 Tesla, using the following protocol: SPGR/50, TR 24, TE 7, NEX 1 matrix 256×192, FOV 24 cm.

For evaluation, a random sampling of approximate two thirds (i.e., 11) of the total 16 MR images in NA0-NIREP dataset are used as atlases and the rest 5 images are used as input images. 10 independent runs are performed and the averaged results are reported. We segment the input images using different multi-atlas label fusion methods, and then measure their performances using the Dice overlap, defined as $Dice(S_a, S_b) = 2|S_a \cap S_b|/(|S_a| + |S_b|)$, where the symbol $\cap$ denotes the overlapping voxels between the two segmentations, and $|S|$ denotes the number of voxels of the corresponding segmentation.

In LWV, PBM and our SPBM, there is a common parameter, i.e., the size of neighborhood region N or N_i. In our experiments, a neighborhood size of $5 \times 5 \times 5$ is used for all the three algorithms. On the other hand, both PBM and SPBM have another common parameter, i.e., the size of patches P_I and P_{I_i}. In our experiments, following [7], a small size of patches (i.e., $3 \times 3 \times 3$ voxels) is used for both methods. Besides, both LWV and PBM adopt the heat kernel, and the corresponding kernel widths h_w and h_p are estimated based on the minimal distances between region $N(x)$ and regions $N_i(x)$ ($i = 1, ..., n$), and between patch $P_I(x)$ and patches $P_{I_i}(y)$ ($y \in N_i(x)$ and $i = 1, ..., n$), for LWV and PBM, respectively. Similar strategy has also been used in [6]. We use the SLEP software [10] to solve the l_1-norm optimization in Eqs. 4-5, and the parameter λ is set as $0.01\lambda_{max}$, where λ_{max} is automatically computed by the program, and it denotes the maximal value of λ, above which shall lead to the zero solution.

4.2   Comparison on Segmentation Results

We first compare the segmentation results of different multi-atlas label fusion algorithms on NA0-NIREP. It is worth noting that we focus on binary segmentation, and thus in our experiments for each method we perform 32 independent binary segmentations corresponding to 32 ROIs. At each segmentation corresponding to a certain ROI, we set the (ground truth) label of a voxel as 1 if it belongs to the ROI, and 0 otherwise. Table 1 gives the segmentation results measured by Dice overlap using five different methods on different ROIs of brain.

As can be seen from Table 1, our SPBM method achieves the best performance among all five methods on segmenting nearly all brain ROIs. Specifically, it outperforms MV, STAPLE and LWV on all 32 brain ROIs, and PBM on 30 of 32 ROIs. We also compute the averaged Dice overlap of different methods across 32 ROIs, and the results are 53.6%, 56.9%, 68.0%, 73.6% and 75.6%, for MV, STAPLE, LWV, PBM and SPBM, respectively. These results show that in average our method achieves 2.0 percent improvement over the conventional PBM, and both patch-based method (including PBM and SPBM) significantly outperform the other label fusion methods, which validate the advantage of using the one-to-many correspondence strategy in the patch-based methods over the use of conventional one-to-one correspondence strategy in the non-patch-based methods. Tables 1 also indicates that by considering the image information through local weighting, LWV achieves a big improvement than MV and STAPLE which do not use image information in label fusion, but is still much inferior to the patch-based methods (including both PBM and SPBM) due to the use of one-to-one correspondence.

Tables 1 also show that there exist great differences on performances of five methods across different ROIs. For example, the differences between results on L insula gyrus (one of the best segmented ROI) and those on L postcentral gyrus (one of the worst segmented ROI) are 30.1%, 22.6%, 22.4%, 21.5% and 21.8%, for MV, STAPLE, LWV, PBM and SPBM, respectively. Clearly, these results show that segmenting the latter brain structure is more challenging than segmenting the former brain structure.

Finally, in Fig. 1 we visually plot the segmentation results of five methods on segmenting *L insula gyrus*. For comparison, we also show the original image and corresponding ground truth. As can be seen from Fig. 1, our SPBM method achieves the best visual quality of segmentation results among the five methods.

4.3   Comparison on Graph Weights

In this experiment, we compare the graph weights gotten by different graph-based label fusion methods. Because the graphs constructed by MV and LWV are very simple (i.e., one-to-one correspondence), we only compare the graph weights constructed from two patch-based methods, i.e., PBM and SPBM. To this end, in Fig. 2, we plot the graph weights constructed by both PBM and SPBM methods, for a 'positive' input patch (i.e., centered voxel has a label of 1) on segmenting *L insula gyrus*. In Fig. 2, red lines denote the weights for 'positive' patches from 11 atlas images, while blue lines denote those for 'negative' patches (i.e., centered voxel has a label of 0), and the green lines denote the separation lines between different atlas images.

As can be seen from Fig. 2, PBM obtains a dense graph even after the pre-selection of patches. This is because in some (especially smooth) regions, there may exist a number of adjacent patches that have high similarities to the input patch, and thus it is difficult to get a sparse graph through threshold on similarities. In contrast, SPBM get a very sparse graph by explicitly imposing the 'sparsity' constraint into the objective function. On the other hand, Fig. 2(b) indicates that SPBM also achieves a discriminating power by using sparse representation, which has been validated on other tasks, e.g., face recognition [8]. Specifically, Fig. 2(b) shows that the graph weights of SPBM for the current input patch are dominated by 'positive' patches. This

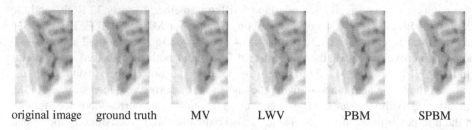

original image   ground truth   MV   LWV   PBM   SPBM

Fig. 1. Visual views on segmentation results of five different label fusion algorithms on *L insula gyrus*

spontaneously-emerged discriminating power is very helpful for subsequent labeling, as shown in above results.

Table 1. Segmentation results on different ROIs of brain, measured by Dice overlap (%) using five different algorithms. Results are presented in (left hemisphere - right hemisphere).

Brain ROIs	MV	STAPLE	LWV	PBM	SPBM
Occipital lobe	52.1 - 55.2	58.5 - 61.7	69.3 - 74.9	73.6 - 79.6	**77.3 - 81.2**
Cingulated gyrus	59.4 - 61.0	62.5 - 64.7	70.0 - 71.5	72.9 - 75.5	**75.7 - 77.0**
Insula gyrus	65.6 - 69.0	64.0 - 67.1	74.3 - 76.3	77.8 - 80.3	**82.3 - 84.0**
Temporal pole	59.7 - 65.4	62.0 - 65.9	73.2 - 78.0	76.6 - 81.6	**78.6 - 81.9**
Superior temporal gyrus	48.0 - 43.8	52.5 - 52.9	62.6 - 64.3	67.2 - 70.0	**73.1 - 72.2**
Infero emporal region	59.9 - 59.8	60.5 - 59.8	73.3 - 76.2	76.8 - 80.7	**80.1 - 80.9**
Parahippocampal gyrus	64.6 - 70.4	61.2 - 63.7	73.4 - 77.5	77.3 - 82.1	**79.9 - 82.5**
Frontal pole	62.8 - 62.5	63.6 - 58.9	75.3 - 74.7	**81.0 - 81.6**	80.6 - 79.6
Superior frontal gyrus	52.6 - 53.0	55.7 - 55.1	69.7 - 69.5	74.4 - 74.6	**76.0 - 75.3**
Middle frontal gyrus	53.4 - 48.7	55.3 - 55.1	68.2 - 65.9	72.7 - 70.7	**74.9 - 71.7**
Inferior gyrus	47.2 - 44.8	49.7 - 53.6	64.1 - 62.8	69.9 - 67.8	**71.7 - 69.5**
Orbital frontal gyrus	61.9 - 61.6	62.4 - 61.6	74.6 - 73.3	79.9 - 77.4	**81.3 - 78.1**
Precentral gyrus	39.1 - 37.7	52.1 - 48.4	61.9 - 62.3	66.1 - 67.6	**70.0 - 69.6**
Superior parietal lobule	42.5 - 46.2	49.8 - 51.9	62.4 - 64.2	67.3 - 69.4	**69.8 - 72.2**
Inferior parietal lobule	49.7 - 50.6	53.4 - 54.8	64.3 - 67.8	68.9 - 73.0	**72.4 - 73.3**
Postcentral gyrus	35.5 - 30.5	41.4 - 41.8	51.9 - 55.6	56.3 - 63.4	**60.5 - 65.7**

5   Conclusion

In this paper we proposed a novel sparse patch-based method (SPBM) for multi-atlas label fusion, based on sparse representation. We also show that the patch-based methods as well as many existing methods can be unified into a graph-based label fusion framework, with different ways for graph construction. Different from the conventional patch-based method (PBM) which constructs a graph and computes weights based on similarities between patches in the input image and the atlas images, our method automatically obtains the graph and weights by solving l_1 optimization. Our experiments on segmenting brain anatomical structures on NA0-NIREP dataset show

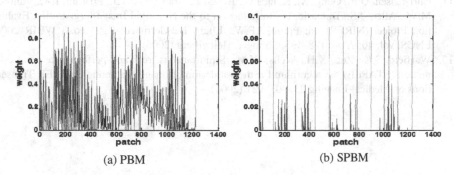

(a) PBM   (b) SPBM

Fig. 2. Comparison of the graph weights constructed by PBM (a) and SPBM (b)

that SPBM achieves up to 5.9 (and 2.0 in average) percent improvements over PBM, and significantly outperforms other label fusion methods.

References

1. Artaechevarria, X., Munoz-Barrutia, A., Ortiz-de-Solorzano, C.: Combination strategies in multi-atlas image segmentation: application to brain MR data. IEEE Transactions on Medical Imaging 28, 1266–1277 (2009)
2. Sabuncu, M.R., Yeo, B.T., Van Leemput, K., Fischl, B., Golland, P.: A generative model for image segmentation based on label fusion. IEEE Transactions on Medical Imaging 29, 1714–1729 (2010)
3. Wang, H., Suh, J.W., Das, S.R., Pluta, J., Altinay, M., Yushkevich, P.: Regression-based label fusion for multi-atlas segmentation. In: CVPR, pp. 1113–1120 (2011)
4. Zhang, D., Wu, G., Jia, H., Shen, D.: Confidence-Guided Sequential Label Fusion for Multi-atlas Based Segmentation. In: Fichtinger, G., Martel, A., Peters, T. (eds.) MICCAI 2011, Part III. LNCS, vol. 6893, pp. 643–650. Springer, Heidelberg (2011)
5. Coupe, P., Yger, P., Barillot, C.: Fast non local means denoising for 3D MR images. Med. Image Comput. Comput. Assist. Interv. 9, 33–40 (2006)
6. Coupe, P., Manjon, J.V., Fonov, V., Pruessner, J., Robles, M., Collins, D.L.: Patch-based segmentation using expert priors: application to hippocampus and ventricle segmentation. NeuroImage 54, 940–954 (2011)
7. Rousseau, F., Habas, P.A., Studholme, C.: A supervised patch-based approach for human brain labeling. IEEE Transactions on Medical Imaging 30, 1852–1862 (2011)
8. Wright, J., Yang, A.Y., Ganesh, A., Sastry, S.S., Ma, Y.: Robust face recognition via sparse representation. IEEE Transactions on Pattern Analysis and Machine Intelligence 31, 210–227 (2009)
9. Tibshirani, R.: Regression shrinkage and selection via the lasso. Journal of the Royal Statistical Society Series B 58, 267–288 (1996)
10. Liu, J., Ji, S., Ye, J.: SLEP: Sparse learning with efficient projections. Arizona State University (2009)

11. Christensen, G.E., Geng, X., Kuhl, J.G., Bruss, J., Grabowski, T.J., Pirwani, I.A., Vannier, M.W., Allen, J.S., Damasio, H.: Introduction to the Non-rigid Image Registration Evaluation Project (NIREP). In: Pluim, J.P.W., Likar, B., Gerritsen, F.A. (eds.) WBIR 2006. LNCS, vol. 4057, pp. 128–135. Springer, Heidelberg (2006)
12. Warfield, S.K., Zou, K.H., Wells, W.M.: Simultaneous truth and performance level estimation (STAPLE): an algorithm for the validation of image segmentation. IEEE Transactions on Medical Imaging 23, 903–921 (2004)

How Many Templates Does It Take for a Good Segmentation?: Error Analysis in Multiatlas Segmentation as a Function of Database Size

Suyash P. Awate, Peihong Zhu, and Ross T. Whitaker

Scientific Computing and Imaging (SCI) Institute, University of Utah

Abstract. This paper proposes a novel formulation to model and analyze the statistical characteristics of some types of segmentation problems that are based on combining label maps / templates / atlases. Such segmentation-by-example approaches are quite powerful on their own for several clinical applications and they provide prior information, through spatial context, when combined with intensity-based segmentation methods. The proposed formulation models a class of *multiatlas* segmentation problems as *nonparametric regression* problems in the high-dimensional space of images. The paper presents a systematic analysis of the nonparametric estimation's *convergence behavior* (i.e. characterizing segmentation *error* as a function of the *size* of the multiatlas database) and shows that it has a specific analytic form involving several parameters that are fundamental to the specific segmentation problem (i.e. chosen anatomical structure, imaging modality, registration method, label-fusion algorithm, etc.). We describe how to estimate these parameters and show that several brain anatomical structures exhibit the trends determined analytically. The proposed framework also provides per-voxel confidence measures for the segmentation. We show that the segmentation error for large database sizes can be *predicted* using small-sized databases. Thus, small databases can be exploited to predict the database sizes required ("how many templates") to achieve "good" segmentations having errors lower than a specified tolerance. Such cost-benefit analysis is crucial for designing and deploying multiatlas segmentation systems.

1 Introduction and Background

The strategy of segmenting an image using other examples of similar segmentations has lead to various approaches in a spectrum of clinical applications over the last two decades. This paper considers segmentation methods, e.g. [1,5,11], using a combination of (i) a set of *template* images that depict the anatomy and (ii) a set of tissue probability maps or *segmentations* that give, for each template, the true probability of each voxel belonging to a specific anatomical structure. A pair comprising a template image and its true segmentation is termed an *atlas*. For segmenting structures in biomedical images where boundary parts of the anatomy are *not* readily apparent in the image data, atlases can infuse crucial prior information, strongly influenced by anatomical context, and thereby complement solely-data-driven segmentation methods.

P.-T. Yap et al. (Eds.): MBIA 2012, LNCS 7509, pp. 103–114, 2012.

For segmenting anatomical structures having weakly-visible boundaries, atlas-based methods leverage information within the spatial configuration of those surrounding structures whose boundaries *are* well defined in the image. This relies on the assumption that the geometry (i.e. location, pose, size, and shape) of the weakly-visible structure is a function of the geometry of these surrounding structures. Subsequently, atlas-based segmentation methods register pre-segmented template images to match the *target* image containing the structure we want to segment. Assuming reliable matching of the surrounding structures, registration methods yield a deformation to best match the weakly-visible structure of interest. Subsequently, template segmentations are deformed to the target.

Large collections of medical images, and associated expert-defined segmentations, are becoming ubiquitous as public resources, and within specific clinical practices. This has lead to *multiatlas*, nonparametric atlas, or label-fusion approaches [1,2,5,10,11,13,15,16] to segmentation that leverage information in the entire database of atlases. Multiatlas approaches can exploit methods for fast selection [18] of a small subset of templates that are most similar to the target. They independently register the selected templates to the target and, then, deform database segmentations to the target space. A weighted average [1] of the deformed segmentations produces a nonparametric estimate of the segmentation of the target. Instead of using the entire database, the carefully selected subset produces better estimates, as shown for brain [1] and cardiac [5] images. The proposed theoretical framework and the results shed light on this behavior, indicating that an optimal subset size depends on the database size.

The spirit of the proposed framework differs significantly from that of methods focussing on estimating rater-performance parameters (particularly, rater bias) [17] and the parameters' confidence intervals [4] or compensating for inter-voxel label correlations [15]. Unlike such methods, the proposed approach models and predicts segmentation error as a function of database size and provides per-voxel confidence measures on the segmentation.

This paper makes many contributions. It proposes a novel statistical nonparametric regression framework to model a class of multiatlas segmentation approaches and analyze the *convergence* behavior of segmentation error with respect to database size. It shows that the error convergence rate as a function of database size has an analytic form with parameters fundamental to the segmentation problem. By measuring these parameters, it characterizes multiatlas segmentation problems (i.e. chosen anatomical structure, imaging modality, etc.) and a class of approaches (i.e. registration algorithm, label-fusion algorithm, etc.) in terms of (i) the complexity of the function mapping the geometry of (clearly-visible) surrounding structures to the geometry of the structure of interest, (ii) the inherent anatomical randomness in the structure's geometry, (iii) number of atlases available in the database, and (iv) some algorithm parameters. In this way, the framework offers new methods to evaluate the efficacy of a particular database of atlases, modality, algorithm, etc. It can provide per-voxel confidence measures for segmentations. We demonstrate that the segmentation error for large database sizes can be *predicted* using small-sized databases.

Thus, small databases can be exploited to predict the database sizes required ("how many templates") to achieve "good" segmentations having errors lower than a specified tolerance. Such cost-benefit analysis is crucial for designing and deploying multiatlas segmentation systems.

2   Methods

This section presents a novel statistical framework, relying on *nonparametric regression*, to model and analyze a class of multiatlas segmentation approaches.

Consider the problem of estimating the unknown segmentation for a target image, using a database of atlases (templates and their segmentations). Treating each atlas as a *member of a family of atlases* under constrained diffeomorphisms (e.g. constrained under limited deformation norm), we first transform the database to factor out a diffeomorphism between the geometrical configurations of anatomical structures within the target and each template; better matches of the two geometries would usually lead to better matches of the segmentations. We assume that multiatlas segmentation methods can compute an optimal smooth diffeomorphism using image registration on the raw intensities or on derived geometry-capturing features and, later, deform each template and segmentation, in the database, to the target-image physical space. Thus, we propose to (i) model multiatlas segmentation as a regression problem where the *independent variable* represents the *deformed template images* and the *dependent variable* represents the *deformed segmentation images* and (ii) analyze the rate of convergence of the error in multiatlas segmentation with respect to increasing database sizes to characterize the difficulty for a specific segmentation problem.

2.1   Statistical Modeling and Analysis of Multiatlas Segmentation

Consider a vector random variable F that models a (deformed) biomedical image with V voxels. Observed images $f \in \mathbb{R}^V$ are drawn from the probability density function (PDF) $P(F)$. For a specific anatomical structure in the image, let S be a V-dimensional vector random variable modeling the (deformed) true probabilistic-segmentation image. Segmentations s are drawn from $P(S)$. Let $S[v]$ denote the random variable at the v-th component of S (i.e. voxel v in image); $\forall s \forall v, s[v] \in [0, 1]$. Assume that the joint random variable (F, S) has a PDF $P(F, S)$ capturing dependencies between images f and segmentations s.

Consider a *database* $a^M \triangleq \{(f_m, s_m)\}_{m=1,\cdots,M}$ of M atlases, i.e. *template* images $\{f_m\}_{m=1,\cdots,M}$ paired with their *true segmentations* $\{s_m\}_{m=1,\cdots,M}$, where each observed image pair (f_m, s_m) is drawn independently from the PDF $P(F, S)$. For a given *target* image f_0 whose true segmentation s_0 is *unknown*, we get an estimate $\hat{s}_0$ of the true segmentation, using database a^M.

We treat the multiatlas segmentation problem as that of statistical *non-parametric regression* [8,14]. Let $r(F)$ be a regression function of S (dependent variable) on F (independent variable). We choose $r(F)$ as the regression function that minimizes the mean squared error (MSE) *risk function* $E_{P(F,S)}$

$[\|S - r(F)\|^2]^r = E_{P(F)}\left[E_{P(S|F)}[\|S - r(F)\|^2]\right]$. For any target f, the MSE-minimizing regression function is the conditional expectation $r(f) \triangleq E_{P(S|f)}[S]$. Let $\hat{r}(F, a^M)$ be an estimator of $r(F)$.

We want to characterize the behavior of conditional-expectation regression estimators over (i) varying images $f \sim P(F)$ and (ii) varying databases a^M comprising M image pairs. Hence, we treat the database as a random variable $\mathcal{A}^M$, assume a joint PDF $P(F, S, \mathcal{A}^M)$, and then define a new MSE function:

$$\mathrm{MSE}(M) \triangleq E_{P(F,S,\mathcal{A}^M)}[\|S - \hat{r}(F, \mathcal{A}^M)\|^2] = E_{P(F)}[\mathrm{MSE}(M, F)], \text{ where} \quad (1)$$

$$\mathrm{MSE}(M, f) \triangleq E_{P(S|f)}[\|S - r(f)\|^2] + E_{P(\mathcal{A}^M|f)}[\|r(f) - \hat{r}(f, \mathcal{A}^M)\|^2]$$
$$+ E_{P(S,\mathcal{A}^M|f)}[2(S - r(f)) \cdot (r(f) - \hat{r}(f, \mathcal{A}^M))]. \quad (2)$$

The second term in the $\mathrm{MSE}(M, f)$ expression leads to $E_{P(F)}E_{P(\mathcal{A}^M|F)}[\|r(F) - \hat{r}(F, \mathcal{A}^M)\|^2]$, which is the mean *integrated* squared error associated with regression estimators [14]. We consider $P(\mathcal{A}^M|F) = P(\mathcal{A}^M)$.

Let $r(f)[v]$ denote the v-th component of $r(f)$ and let $\hat{r}(f, \mathcal{A}^M)[v]$ denote the v-th component of $\hat{r}(f, \mathcal{A}^M)$. Then, the linearity of expectation gives:

$$\mathrm{MSE}(M, f) = \sum_{v=1}^{V} \mathrm{MSE}(M, f)[v], \text{ where} \quad (3)$$

$$\mathrm{MSE}(M, f)[v] = E_{P(S|f)}\left[(S[v] - r(f)[v])^2\right] + E_{P(\mathcal{A}^M|f)}\left[(r(f)[v] - \hat{r}(f, \mathcal{A}^M)[v])^2\right]$$
$$+ E_{P(S,\mathcal{A}^M|f)}\left[2(S[v] - r(f)[v])(r(f)[v] - \hat{r}(f, \mathcal{A}^M)[v])\right]. \quad (4)$$

We now analyze all three terms in the expression for $\mathrm{MSE}(M, f)[v]$:

1. For the conditional-expectation regression function $r(f)$, the first term is the variance of the conditional PDF $P(S[v]|f)$. This term (i) depends on the inherent (beyond human control) randomness in the segmentation, at voxel v, given image data f and (ii) is independent of the estimator $\hat{r}(f, \mathcal{A}^M)$.
2. The second term relates to the quality of approximation of the estimator $\hat{r}(f, \mathcal{A}^M)$ to the true conditional-expectation regression function $r(f)$. This term depends on the database size M and the characteristics of the marginal distribution $P(F)$ and the regression function $r(\cdot)$ in the locality of f [8]. This term equals the sum of the *squared bias* and *variance of the estimator*.
3. The third term vanishes because it is equal to $E_{P(\mathcal{A}^M)}E_{P(S|\mathcal{A}^M,f)}[2(S[v] - r(f)[v])(r(f)[v] - \hat{r}(f, \mathcal{A}^M)[v])]$ where the inner expectation is zero (decomposition of random variable $S[v] - \hat{r}(F, \mathcal{A}^M)[v]$).

Thus, $\mathrm{MSE}(M, f)[v]$ is the sum of the variance of the conditional PDF, the squared bias of the estimator, and the variance of the estimator:

$$\mathrm{MSE}(M, f)[v] = \mathrm{Var}(S[v]|f) + \mathrm{Bias}^2(\hat{r}(f, \mathcal{A}^M)[v]) + \mathrm{Var}(\hat{r}(f, \mathcal{A}^M)[v]). \quad (5)$$

We now choose a specific regression estimator. A consistent estimator for the conditional-expectation regression function $r(f)$ is the *generalized k-nearest-neighbor* (kNN) estimator [12] $\hat{r}(f, a^M)$:

$$\hat{r}(f, a^M)[v] \triangleq \left\{ \sum_{m=1}^{M} s_m[v] w\left(\frac{g(f_m, f)}{R_k}\right) \right\} / \left\{ \sum_{m=1}^{M} w\left(\frac{g(f_m, f)}{R_k}\right) \right\}, \quad (6)$$

where $g(\cdot, \cdot)$ is some distance metric in the space of f, R_k is the distance between f and its k-th nearest neighbor in the set $\{f_m\}_{m=1,\cdots,M}$, and $w(\cdot) : \mathbb{R} \to \mathbb{R}$ is a bounded non-negative *generalized* weight function satisfying $\int w(u) du = 1$ and $w(u) = 0$ for $\|u\| > 1$. In this paper, $w(u)$ is constant $\forall u : \|u\| \leq 1$.

For the class of generalized kNN estimators [12],

$$\text{Bias}(\hat{r}(f, \mathcal{A}^M)[v]) \approx \phi\big(r(\cdot)[v], P(F), f, D\big) \, (k/M)^{2/D}; \quad (7)$$

$$\text{Var}(\hat{r}(f, \mathcal{A}^M)[v]) \approx \psi\big(w(\cdot), D\big) \, \text{Var}(S[v]|f) \, (1/k), \quad (8)$$

where (i) D is the dimension of the independent variable; (ii) $\phi\big(r(\cdot)[v], P(F), f, D\big)$ depends on the values and differential properties of the PDF $P(F)$ in the locality of the fixed image f, the local differential properties of the v-th component of the true regression function $r(\cdot)$, and dimension D; (iii) $\psi\big(w(\cdot), D\big)$ depends on the chosen weight function $w(\cdot)$ and the dimension D. Indeed, the kNN estimator converges to the true conditional-expectation regression function asymptotically as the database size $M \to \infty$ and the number of nearest neighbors $k \to \infty$ at an appropriate rate such that $(k/M) \to 0$.

It is important to note that the rate of convergence of the bias and variance depends on (i) the dimensionality D associated with the independent random variable F, (ii) the values and the differential properties of the PDF $P(F)$ of images, and (iii) the differential properties of the regression function $r(f)$.

2.2 Practical Interpretation Using the Statistical Analysis

This section leverages the theory described in Section 2.1 to get practically useful measures of the difficulty of multiatlas segmentation for a specific segmentation problem. It describes how to empirically characterize the typical behavior of the regression-based segmentation scheme for an anatomical structure of interest.

Empirically Computing MSE: For a chosen k and database size M, we propose to empirically compute MSE(M) in Equation 1 by: (i) Monte-Carlo sampling of target images f to compute $E_{P(F)}[\cdot]$, (ii) for each f, Monte-Carlo sampling of databases a^M, from a large database with size $N > M$, to compute $E_{P(\mathcal{A}^M|f)}[\cdot]$, and (iii) computing the MSE terms at each voxel v and summing them over all voxels. We repeat this process for a range of M values.

Parametric Form for MSE: When the class of signals F is unconstrained, D equals the number of image voxels, which is typically very large. However, consistent with empirical evidence in the signal-processing literature that the intrinsic dimension [9] of real-world multivariate data is far less than the number of variables, we consider D as the *intrinsic dimension* of the independent variable (template images) and estimate it empirically. Note that each voxel v can have a different value for the intrinsic dimension D_v.

Tracing our way back, we (i) substitute Equations (7) and (8) for voxelwise regression estimator's bias and variance, respectively, into Equation (5), (ii) substitute that into Equation (3), and (iii) substitute the resulting equation into Equation (1). This gives the following parametric forms for the MSEs:

$$\text{MSE}(M)[v] = \alpha_v + \beta_v\big(k/M\big)^{4/D_v} + \gamma_v(1/k) = \delta_v + \beta_v\big(k/M\big)^{4/D_v}, \text{ where}$$

$$\alpha_v = E_{P(F)}\big[\text{Var}(S[v]|F)\big], \beta_v = E_{P(F)}\big[\phi^2\big(r(\cdot)[v], P(F), F, D_v\big)\big],$$

$$\gamma_v = E_{P(F)}\big[\text{Var}(S[v]|F)\psi\big(w(\cdot), D_v\big)\big], \delta_v = \alpha_v + \gamma_v/k. \tag{9}$$

$$\text{MSE}(M) = \alpha + \beta\big(k/M\big)^{4/D} + \gamma(1/k) = \delta + \beta\big(k/M\big)^{4/D}, \text{ where}$$

$$\alpha = \sum_{v=1}^{V} \alpha_v, \beta \approx \sum_{v=1}^{V} \beta_v, \gamma = \sum_{v=1}^{V} \gamma_v, \delta = \alpha + \gamma/k. \tag{10}$$

These equations captures the characteristics of a specific segmentation problem and approach through parameters α, δ, β, D, whose significance we describe next:

1. α denotes the intrinsic randomness in the segmentations s as a function of the image data f. α is independent of the regression estimator and hence is the lowest possible achievable MSE.
   δ closely relates to α and captures the lowest possible MSEs for the chosen generalized-kNN estimator (i.e. $w(\cdot)$) and k, which is achieved when the database size $M \to \infty$. As $M \to \infty$, we make the kNN estimator converge to the true conditional expectation, by letting k go to ∞ at such a rate so that $(k/M) \to 0$; in that case, $\delta \to \alpha$.
   Assuming that f lies in a Euclidean space, at each voxel, $\psi\big(w(\cdot), D_v\big) = c(D_v)\int w^2(u)du$, where $c(D_v)$ is the volume of the unit sphere in D_v dimensions [12]. For the chosen kNN scheme with constant $w(\cdot)$ within the unit sphere, $\psi\big(w(\cdot), D_v\big) = 1$, $\alpha_v = \gamma_v = \delta_v/(1+1/k)$, and $\alpha = \gamma = \delta/(1+1/k)$.
2. β represents the overall complexity of multiatlas segmentation in terms of the (i) differential properties of the true regression function $r(f)$ and (ii) values and differential properties of the image PDF $P(F)$. For example, $r(\cdot)$ is harder to estimate when β is increased when: (i) larger gradients and curvatures in $r(\cdot)$ lead to larger values of ϕ; (ii) around a target f_0, low values of $P(F)$ make it harder to obtain databases comprising sufficiently-many templates near f_0; (iii) around a target f_0, locally-varying $P(F)$ leads to databases where the templates near f_0 pull the segmentation estimate towards that for the local higher-probability templates.
3. D in the exponent represents the overall intrinsic dimension associated with the entire anatomical structure. Larger D increases the difficulty of multiatlas segmentation by requiring estimation of a higher-dimensional regressor.

Parameter Estimation $(\alpha, \beta, \delta, D)$: To estimate parameters δ, β, D (for a specific segmentation problem and approach) we (i) empirically evaluate

MSE(M_j) for a range of database sizes M_j (e.g. $M_1 = 10$, $M_{j+1} = M_j + 10$) and then (ii) solve a weighted nonlinear least-squares curve-fitting problem

$$\arg \min_{\delta, \beta, D} \sum_j W_j \|\mathrm{MSE}(M_j) - \delta - \beta (k/M_j)^{4/D}\|^2, \qquad (11)$$

where weights W_j are the computed variances of the squared errors for each M_j. Interestingly, effects of changing k are absorbed by changes in δ and β, leaving D unchanged. As described before, for chosen kNN estimator, $\alpha = \delta/(1 + 1/k)$. Parameter estimates for any voxel v are obtained by curve fitting to MSE(M_j)[v].

3   Experiments and Results on a Clinical Database

This section describes some practical considerations and shows results on a large clinical database. The results demonstrate the validity of the proposed model for multiatlas segmentation and the utility of the proposed analysis in clinical applications. Section 3.1 shows that several anatomical structures in the brain exhibit the parametric trends determined by the model, which in turn shows that the model is well-suited for real applications. Section 3.2 shows that the segmentation error for large database sizes can be predicted using small-sized databases. Thus, small databases can be exploited to predict the database sizes required to achieve a specified maximum tolerable MSE in segmentation.

Practical Considerations: The proposed formulation is based on the independent variable being the deformed templates in the *entire* database. However, multiatlas approaches require only a few most-similar templates (k in kNN) and registration between the target and thousands of templates in a large database can be very expensive. Thus, this paper uses an extremely-fast approximate search for similar templates relying on affine registration followed by spatial pyramid matching on coded geometry-capturing features (canny edges clustered and coded based on orientation and curvature) [18]. This implicitly induces a distance metric in the space of deformed images f, underlying kNN regression. The fast lookup makes multiatlas schemes viable for large databases. Next, we compute the optimal deformations, between each selected template and the target, using constrained diffeomorphic registration using [7].

Clinical Database: We evaluate the proposed methods on a large clinical database obtained from the National Alliance for Medical Image Computing (www.na-mic.org) comprising 186 T1 MR brain images (dimensions $\approx$ $256{\times}256{\times}240$; voxel size $\approx 1^3\mathrm{mm}^3$) with expert segmentations for the caudate, putamen, thalamus, hippocampus, and globus pallidus in both hemispheres.

3.1   Error Convergence in Multiatlas Segmentation in Brain MRI

We selected 20 random target images f. For each f, we performed 50 random Monte-Carlo simulations of databases $a^M, \forall M$. We chose $k = 10$. Figure 1(a) shows MSE values (divided by the average size of the structure in the database),

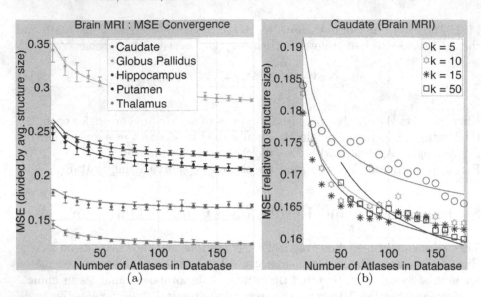

Fig. 1. MSE Convergence for Subcortical Structures in Brain MR images.
(a) The dots and the error bars show MSE(M_j) and the standard deviation, respectively, (divided by the average true size of structures in database) for $k = 10$. The parametric fitted curves are shown by solid lines. Table 1 gives the parameter values. (b) shows MSEs and fitted curves for the caudate (as an example) for varied k.

Table 1. Parameters indicating difficulty of multiatlas segmentation and the underlying convergence behavior (of segmentation MSE with increasing database sizes M_j) for anatomical structures in brain MR images (using 186 atlases)

Parameters	Caudate	Globus Pallidus	Hippocampus	Putamen	Thalamus
δ: randomness	0.15	0.26	0.20	0.18	0.11
β: complexity	0.03	0.10	0.06	0.08	0.03
D: dimension	10.1	10.0	10.0	10.0	10.0

and fitted curves, for various database sizes. Corresponding structures in the left and right brain hemisphere structures are combined.

The size-normalized MSE values relate to Dice, both measuring degree of (dis)similarity relative to size. While the Dice measure takes values in $[0, 1]$, size-normalized MSE takes values in $[0, \eta]$ where η is twice the ratio of (i) the size of the largest structure in the database to (ii) the average size of the structure in the database. For example, for thalamus segmentation, using the largest database $M = 186$, averaged over 20 target images, Dice = 0.91 and MSE = 0.11.

Table 1 shows the parameters underlying the fitted curves. Values for δ (inherent randomness) indicate the lowest possible MSE achievable with $k = 10$ and the chosen generalized-kNN estimator. Values for β (regression complexity) and D (intrinsic dimension) indicate (i) the size of databases needed to achieve small MSEs, e.g. MSE closer to δ, and (ii) the amount of *benefit*, in terms of

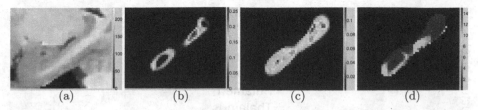

Fig. 2. Parameter values *per voxel* for multiatlas hippocampus segmentation from T1 MR images. **(a)** MR image, sagittal slice with voxels $\{v\}$. **(b)** $\delta_v \equiv$ inherent randomness. **(c)** $\beta_v \equiv$ complexity of regression function. **(d)** $D_v \equiv$ *intrinsic* dimension.

a decrease in MSE, obtained for the *cost* of an increase in database size. Such cost-benefit analyses are crucial for designing clinical support systems. Interestingly, the range of our estimates for D, for probabilistic segmentations, is similar to that found for fuzzy digit images [9] and texture [3,6].

The globus pallidus has probably the weakest boundaries and is the most difficult to segment (for its very small size) leading to the highest values for MSE, δ, β, D. The hippocampus is the second most difficult to segment probably because of its elongated thin shape and small size. The thalamus gives the lowest MSEs probably due to its large size, despite the part of its boundary next to the gray matter being quite weak.

Figure 1(b) shows MSEs and fitted curves for the caudate (as an example) for varied k. Consistent with the theory of kNN-estimator convergence (Section 2), large k leads to lower MSE for large database sizes M, but can increase MSE for lower M. Indeed, for the kNN estimator to converge asymptotically to the true conditional expectation, as M increases, k must increase at an appropriate rate [8]. Thus, Figure 1(b) is consistent with the regression theory in the sense that the MSE-minimizing k does depend on the database size M.

Figure 2 shows a hippocampus and parameter values associated with curves fitted to MSE values obtained at each voxel, i.e. without the summation $\sum_v(\cdot)$ for δ, β in Equation 10. Zero values for MSE and δ for voxels well inside or well outside the hippocampus indicate the ease of segmentation for such voxels. Voxels where the segmentation is the most difficult (highest β, D; high δ) lie near the hippocampus head (near the amygdala; very low contrast) and the tail (perhaps larger shape variability leads to inaccurate registration). As described in Section 2.2, for the chosen kNN estimator and $k = 10$, $\alpha = \delta/(1+1/k) = \delta/1.1$.

3.2   Predicting Error Convergence Using Small Databases of Atlases

Figure 3 shows the results of experiments where we first randomly picked 40 atlases from the brain database, then computed MSE values for $M_j = 10, 20, 30, 40$ using the 40-atlas database, and finally fitted the parametric curves for these 4 values of M_j. We then compare these fitted curves to the fitted curves in Figure 1 that were obtained using the full-sized database. Figure 3 shows that the curves using small-sized databases predict the MSEs at large database sizes quite well.

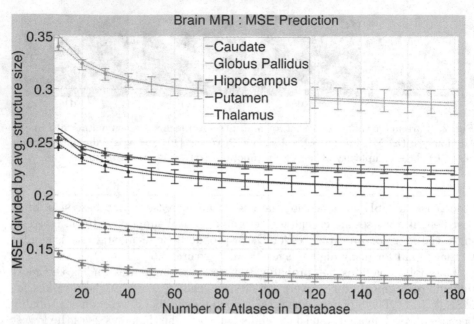

Fig. 3. Predicting MSE for Large Database Sizes using Small Databases.
MSEs (dot ≡ mean value; error bar ≡ standard deviation) and fitted curves (dashed
lines; error bars ≡ standard deviation on the fitted curve) using small databases (40
atlases) compared with the fitted curves (solid lines) using large databases in Figure 1.

Table 2. Parameters obtained using small-sized databases (each with 40 atlases)
of **brain MR** images. The numbers indicate the mean and standard deviation (in
parenthesis) of the parameters over different randomly selected 40-sized atlas databases.

Parameters	Caudate	Globus Pallidus	Hippocampus	Putamen	Thalamus
δ: randomness	0.15 (0.01)	0.26 (0.01)	0.21 (0.01)	0.19 (0.01)	0.11 (0.01)
β: complexity	0.03 (0.01)	0.08 (0.02)	0.05 (0.01)	0.06 (0.01)	0.04 (0.01)
D: dimension	10.1 (0.05)	10.0 (0.03)	10.0 (0.03)	10.1 (0.06)	10.0 (0.02)

Table 2 shows the mean and standard deviation of the parameters estimated
using random 40-sized databases for brain MR images. It shows that these parameter estimates, using 40-sized databases, are very close to the parameters
estimated using the full 186-sized database in Table 1.

Figure 3 and Table 2 show that the error-convergence curves as well as the
underlying parameters predicted using small-sized databases are a good approximation to those observed using much larger databases. Thus, small databases,
which require fewer expert segmentations and lesser time and effort to construct,
can be exploited to predict the much-larger database sizes required to achieve a
specified maximum tolerable error in segmentation. Such cost-benefit analysis is
crucial for designing and deploying multiatlas segmentation systems, potentially
comprising a few thousand atlases.

4   Discussion and Conclusions

This paper presents a new statistical modeling and analysis framework for measuring the *difficulty* of multiatlas segmentation (for a specific anatomical structure, imaging modality, registration method, label-fusion strategy, etc.) in terms of the convergence behavior of segmentation error as a function of database size. It captures these properties using parameters fundamental to the underlying nonparametric regression and extends the analysis to give per-voxel estimates. It shows results using a large clinical database. Furthermore, it shows that small databases, requiring expert segmentations of only a small number of atlases, can be exploited to make valid predictions of the (much-larger) database sizes required to achieve a specified maximum tolerable error in segmentation.

Future work will deal with empirically determining how small can atlas databases be before they start losing their power of predicting MSE convergence for much larger database sizes. Some preliminary evidence indicates that the prediction needs significantly fewer atlases (perhaps just 15 or 20) than those used in this paper. Another interesting aspect unexplored in this paper is the applicability of the proposed framework to anatomical structures outside the brain where our initial experiments are quite promising.

The experiments in this paper use simple averaging for label fusion even though the proposed theoretical framework relies on generalized-kNN regression and thus allows for generalized weighting schemes. Some recent approaches to label fusion have found that generalized weighting schemes can perform better [16]. In the future, the proposed framework can be exploited to analyze approaches with sophisticated weighting schemes.

Recent works [2,10,13] in multiatlas segmentation have found improvements in performance by using local averaging approaches where the tissue probability at a voxel is determined by using only that information in the (registered) atlases which lies within the locality of that voxel. The proposed framework can be extended to model local label fusion by modeling a separate regression problem at each voxel in the image, i.e. the set of k nearest neighbors can be different at each voxel and will be determined by local similarities between the target and the templates, instead of global similarities proposed in this paper. Indeed, this is an important part of future work. Nevertheless, this paper makes significant contributions by establishing a brand new principled theoretical framework for modeling and analysis. Furthermore, this paper shows how the proposed framework coupled with a small set of atlases (requiring few expert segmentations) can be utilized to predict the much-larger database sizes ("cost") required to achieve a specified maximum tolerable error ("benefit") in segmentation. Such "cost-benefit" analysis is crucial for designing and deploying multiatlas segmentation systems comprising, potentially, several hundreds or thousands of atlases.

Acknowledgments. The authors gratefully acknowledge the support of this work through the National Alliance for Medical Image Computing (NAMIC) and the NIH/NCRR Center for Integrative Biomedical Computing (CIBC) grant P41-RR12553.

References

1. Aljabar, P., Heckemann, R., Hammers, A., Hajnal, J., Rueckert, D.: Multi-atlas based segmentation of brain images: Atlas selection and its effect on accuracy. NeuroImage 46(3), 726–738 (2009)
2. Artaechevarria, X., Munoz-Barrutia, A., Ortiz-de-Solorzano, C.: Combination strategies in multi-atlas image segmentation: application to brain MR data. IEEE Trans. Med. Imaging 28(8), 1266–1277 (2009)
3. Carter, K., Raich, R., Hero, A.: On local intrinsic dimension estimation and its applications. IEEE Trans. Signal Proc. 58(2), 650–663 (2010)
4. Commonwick, O., Warfield, S.: Estimation of inferential uncertainty in assessing expert segmentation performance from STAPLE. IEEE Trans. Med. Imag. 29(3), 771–780 (2010)
5. Depa, M., Sabuncu, M.R., Holmvang, G., Nezafat, R., Schmidt, E.J., Golland, P.: Robust atlas-based segmentation of highly variable anatomy: Left atrium segmentation. In: MICCAI Workshop Stat. Atlases Comp. Models Heart, pp. 1–8 (2010)
6. Felsberg, M., Kalkan, S., Krueger, N.: Continuous dimensionality characterization of image structures. Image and Vision Computing 27(6), 628–636 (2009)
7. Ha, L., Kruger, J., Fletcher, T., Joshi, S., Silva, C.: Fast parallel unbiased diffeomorphic atlas construction on multi-graphics processing units. In: Euro. Symp. Parallel Graph. Vis., pp. 65–72 (2009)
8. Hardle, W.: Applied Nonparametric Regression. Cambridge Univ. Press (1990)
9. Hein, M., Audibert, J.Y.: Intrinsic dimensionality estimation of submanifolds. In: R^d. In: Int. Conf. Mach. Learn., pp. 289–296 (2005)
10. Isgum, I., Staring, M., Rutten, A., Prokop, M., Viergever, M., Ginneken, B.: Multi-atlas-based segmentation with local decision fusion - application to cardiac and aortic segmentation in CT scans. IEEE Trans. Med. Imag. 28(7), 1000–1010 (2009)
11. Lotjonen, J., Wolz, R., Koikkalainen, J., Thurfjell, L., Waldemar, G., Soininen, H., Rueckert, D.: ADNI: Fast and robust multi-atlas segmentation of brain magnetic resonance images. NeuroImage 49(3), 2352–2365 (2010)
12. Mack, Y.P.: Local properties of k-NN regression estimates. SIAM J. Alg. Disc. Meth. 2(3), 311–323 (1981)
13. Sabuncu, M., Yeo, B., van Leemput, K., Fischl, B., Golland, P.: A generative model for image segmentation based on label fusion. IEEE Trans. Med. Imaging 29(10), 1714–1729 (2010)
14. Takezawa, K.: Introduction to Nonparametric Regression. Wiley (2005)
15. Wang, H., Suh, J.W., Das, S., Pluta, J., Altinay, M., Yushkevich, P.: Regression-based label fusion for multi-atlas segmentation. IEEE Conf. Comp. Vis. Pattern Recog. 1, 1113–1120 (2011)
16. Wang, H., Suh, J.W., Pluta, J., Altinay, M., Yushkevich, P.: Optimal weights for multi-atlas label fusion. In: Int. Conf. Info. Proc. Med. Imag., pp. 73–84 (2011)
17. Warfield, S., Zou, K., Wells, W.: Validation of image segmentation by estimating rater bias and variance. Phil. Trans. Roy. Soc. 366(1874), 2361–2375 (2008)
18. Zhu, P., Awate, S.P., Gerber, S., Whitaker, R.: Fast Shape-Based Nearest-Neighbor Search for Brain MRIs Using Hierarchical Feature Matching. In: Fichtinger, G., Martel, A., Peters, T. (eds.) MICCAI 2011, Part II. LNCS, vol. 6892, pp. 484–491. Springer, Heidelberg (2011)

A Generative Model for Probabilistic Label Fusion of Multimodal Data

Juan Eugenio Iglesias[1], Mert Rory Sabuncu[1,*], and Koen Van Leemput[1,2,3,*]

[1] Martinos Center for Biomedical Imaging, MGH, Harvard Medical School, USA
[2] Department of Informatics and Mathematical Modeling, DTU, Denmark
[3] Departments of Information and Computer Science and of Biomedical
Engineering and Computational Science, Aalto University, Finland

Abstract. The maturity of registration methods, in combination with
the increasing processing power of computers, has made multi-atlas segmentation methods practical. The problem of merging the deformed label
maps from the atlases is known as label fusion. Even though label fusion
has been well studied for intramodality scenarios, it remains relatively
unexplored when the nature of the target data is multimodal or when its
modality is different from that of the atlases. In this paper, we review the
literature on label fusion methods and also present an extension of our
previously published algorithm to the general case in which the target
data are multimodal. The method is based on a generative model that
exploits the consistency of voxel intensities within the target scan based
on the current estimate of the segmentation. Using brain MRI scans acquired with a multiecho FLASH sequence, we compare the method with
majority voting, statistical-atlas-based segmentation, the popular package FreeSurfer and an adaptive local multi-atlas segmentation method.
The results show that our approach produces highly accurate segmentations (Dice 86.3% across 22 brain structures of interest), outperforming
the competing methods.

1   Introduction

Registration-based segmentation [1] is popular in brain image analysis because
the relatively low variability of this organ (compared to the mediastinal or ab-
dominal regions) allows for accurate registrations and therefore good segmentation results. The principle of registration-based segmentation is straightforward:
assuming that an image with manually labeled structures (henceforth an "atlas")
is available, this image can be spatially mapped or deformed (i.e., "registered")
to a different target image. The registration outputs a deformation field that can
be used to warp ("propagate") the atlas labels in order to obtain an estimate of
the labeling ("segmentation") of the target image.

Registering and propagating the labels from a single atlas achieves limited
accuracy because a single example cannot sufficiently represent the whole population of potential test data. This is a particularly limiting factor when pathology

---

* Both authors contributed equally.

P.-T. Yap et al. (Eds.): MBIA 2012, LNCS 7509, pp. 115–133, 2012.
© Springer-Verlag Berlin Heidelberg 2012

might be present in the images. A possible way of overcoming this limitation is using a statistical atlas, which models the intensity and/or label distribution in a population from a collection of atlases. For example, instead of a discrete label at each voxel, a statistical atlas has a vector of label probabilities representing the prior probability of observing a segmentation label at that location. Statistical atlases have two major advantages over using a single template: 1. the image is a summary of the population that was used to build the atlas and therefore it is more likely that a given target image can be successfully registered to it; and 2. the fact that the labels are probabilistic rather than deterministic can overcome, to some extent, inaccuracies in the registration.

Building a statistical atlas from a set of labeled images is computationally expensive: it is typically an iterative process which requires registering the images to the current estimate of the atlas, updating this estimate by averaging the warped images, registering the images again, and so on [2]. However, once the statistical atlas has been built, only one registration is required to propagate the label probabilities from the atlas to a target image. These propagated probabilities are usually interpreted as a Bayesian prior that, combined with a likelihood term (computed from the image intensities), provides posterior probabilities for the possible labels at each voxel location [3,4,5].

Even though probabilistic atlases have been successfully applied in brain MRI segmentation, they still have difficulties representing larger anatomical variations. A computationally taxing, though effective way of handling such cases is registering each available atlas to the target image independently. Even though this multiplies the registration time by the number of atlases N, one would hope that, if enough training data is available, at least one or two atlases will be registered successfully to the test image. The question is then how to automatically decide from which atlases the labels should be picked to render the final segmentation. We call this problem *label fusion*.

1.1 Label Fusion

The popularity of label fusion algorithms is rising mainly for two reasons. First, the maturity of registration algorithms allows them to produce excellent results. The second reason is that the increasing processing power of computers alleviates the high computational demand associated with this technique. Label fusion techniques are based on weighting the contributions of the atlases depending on their similarity to the target image after registration. There are two major families of label fusion techniques: those that allow the weights to change across spatial locations and whose that do not.

In global weighting methods, the weight of the contribution of each atlas to the segmentation is the same for every voxel of the target image. In "majority voting" [6], all atlas are weighted equally, independently of their similarity to the target image after registration. Therefore, the most frequent propagated label is selected at each voxel. The main limitation of this method is that, since atlases are equally weighted, underrepresented features in the training data are often outweighted by the more frequent variations. In "best atlas selection" [7], the labels are propagated only from the atlas which is most similar to the test image after warping. This represents a considerable waste of CPU time dedicated to registering atlases, whose labels are never used. SIMPLE (Langerak et al. [8]) computes a joint segmentation using majority voting, estimates the performance of the individual atlases given the current segmentation, defines weights based on the performances and finally uses these weights to update the estimated segmentation. The performances of the atlases and the fused segmentation are iteratively updated until convergence. In [9], global weights are defined based on the normalized mutual information (MI) of each atlas and the target image after registration.

Locally-weighted label fusion techniques achieve higher segmentation accuracy [10] by exploiting the fact that different atlases might have been correctly registered in different parts of the target image. Therefore, it makes sense to borrow labels from different atlases at different locations. STAPLE [11] weights the propagated labels according to an estimated accuracy level, while incorporating consistency constraints. However, it is limited by the fact that it does not consider the intensities of the target image in the segmentation. An ad-hoc fusion method is proposed by Isgum et al. in [12]. They compute the local weight of each atlas at each voxel as the inverse of the absolute intensity difference of the target and registered images. The weighting maps are convolved with a Gaussian kernel to ensure the smoothness of the output. A more principled version of this method is proposed by Sabuncu et al. in [13]. They define a generative model in which a discrete membership field specifies the index of the atlas from which the intensity and label where borrowed at each voxel. Variational expectation maximization is used to infer the most likely labels in this framework. The fusion weights are given by the posterior distribution of the membership field in light of the observed data.

Furthermore, local label fusion has been extended to a nonlocal framework by Coupé et al. in [14]. They compare the local appearance of the target volume with patches of the atlases centered not only at the voxel at hand but also at shifted locations, and use the resulting similarity metrics to weight the label corresponding to each patch. Because they explore the neighborhood of each voxel, they do not need the registration to be precise, hence a linear transform (which can be quickly optimized) rather than a deformable registration method can be used. Other recent works on label fusion have explored ways of improving the segmentation based on exploiting the correlations of the errors from the different atlases to enhance the fusion [15], using advanced similarity metrics derived from manifold learning for the weighting [16] and developing hierarchical schemes for the fusion depending on the local label confidence [17].

1.2 Label Fusion in Intermodal and in Multimodal Setups

There are certain scenarios, where we cannot assume consistency between the intensity values of the atlases and the target image. This is particularly a problem in MRI, in which the intensities depend heavily on the selected pulse sequence, imaging hardware and acquisition parameters. Even though histogram matching and intensity standardization techniques (such as [18]) can alleviate this problem, they are only applicable if the type of MRI contrast of the input images is the same (e.g., T1-weighted).

The intermodality [1] registration literature has coped with the issue of intensity variation mainly through metrics based on global MI. We will assume here that the registration of the atlases to the target image has already been solved. In case of multimodal target data, the registration can either use heuristics (e.g., using the average MI between the target and all the atlases) or estimate the true multichannel MI via high-dimensional histograms [19] or entropic spanning graphs [20].

Global label fusion approaches can be easily generalized to the inter / multimodal case using MI to compute global "distances" between images. This is the case for best template selection [7] and Cao et al.'s manifold learning approach [16]. For majority voting, SIMPLE and STAPLE, generalization is not even needed because they do not rely on the intensities of the images, and they are thus independent of the modalities or number of image channels of the data.

Local fusion approaches, which are the most appealing ones due to their excellent performance, are however harder to extend to inter- and multimodal scenarios: techniques that rely on computing local similarities by directly comparing image intensities (e.g., Isgum et al. [12]) cannot be used. In the multimodal case, if one of the channels matches the modality of the atlas, it would be possible to discard the rest of the channels and use a intramodal algorithm. However, this strategy is suboptimal in the sense that it does not consider data that might convey important information.

Another option would be to use MI or normalized cross correlation (NCC) to define local weights. However, both MI and NCC require a number of image samples for estimation, which represents a compromise between localization and metric reliability if it is to be computed at a certain voxel using the local neighborhood. Moreover, neither MI nor NCC decay very fast with poorly aligned images. Therefore, one typically needs to define a function that maps them to weights, enhancing the differences in metric values (e.g. $w = [NCC]^{\alpha}$, with $\alpha > 1$). Despite these disadvantages, this type of heuristics could be used to generalize the methods by Isgum et al., Coupé et al. [14] and Wang et al. [15] to intermodal and multimodal settings. Sabuncu et al.'s method [13], which produces excellent results in an intramodality brain MRI segmentation problem, relies on a principled generative model in which the intensity of the target image at a voxel location is assumed to be equal to the intensity of one of the deformed atlases at the same location plus Gaussian noise. This generative model was modified to accommodate the intermodality case in [21].

---

[1] Throughout the rest of this paper, we use "intermodality" to refer to the situation in which the atlases and the target image are from different modalities (or have different types of MRI contrast), and "multimodality" for the situation in which more than one image channel is available for the target image.

1.3 Contribution of This Paper

To the best of our knowledge, no prior work has been carried out that deals with how to carry out label fusion on multimodal data. In a previous conference paper [21], we presented a generative model for multi-atlas image segmentation across modalities. Rather than directly comparing the intensities of the registered atlases and the target image, we proposed exploiting the consistency of voxel intensities within the segmentation regions, as well as their relation with the propagated labels. Here we extend this framework to the multimodal case as well as present some improvements in the inference algorithm that yield improved segmentation results. In particular, we use expectation maximization (EM) rather than k-means to compute the estimates of the image intensity parameters.

The rest of the paper is organized as follows. Section 2.1 describes the generalization of the framework to multimodal data, as well as the improved inference algorithm based on EM. Section 3 presents the experimental setup, in which we use the proposed method and a number of competing algorithms (majority voting, FreeSurfer [22], statistical-atlas-based segmentation and a NCC-adaption of Isgum et al.'s algorithm) to segment brain MRI data from a multiecho FLASH sequence. Finally, Section 4 discusses the results and future directions of work and concludes the paper.

2 Methods

The proposed method relies on a generative model of image data. We first describe the model and then propose a method to carry out inference in order to obtain the segmentation corresponding to a target image.

2.1 Generative Model

The generative model displayed in Figure 1 (see corresponding equations in Table 1) was used in this study:

1. We assume that a set of N atlases (each with $\mathcal{L}$ different labels) has been registered to a common space (which is the space of the target scan). We name the propagated label maps $\{L_n\} = L_1, \ldots, L_N$. Rather than using the discrete propagated labels directly in the fusion, we assume that each voxel in the (deformed) atlases has an associated vector of label probabilities which is built through a logOdds model [23] with slope ρ. This model is described by Equation 1 in Table 1, where D_n^l is the signed distance transform corresponding to label l in atlas n; it is greater than zero inside the object, zero on the boundary, and less than zero outside. The logOdds model essentially replaces the discrete labels by smoother probability maps which can, to some extent, compensate for inaccuracies in the registration (in a similar way as statistical atlases).

Table 1. Equations corresponding to the graphical model in Figure 1(a)

1. $p(L(\mathbf{x}) = l | L_n) = \exp\left[\rho D_n^l(\mathbf{x})\right] / \sum_{l'=1}^{\mathcal{L}} \exp\left[\rho D_n^{l'}(\mathbf{x})\right]$

2. $M \sim \frac{1}{Z_\beta} \prod_{x \in \Omega} \exp\left(\beta \sum_{\mathbf{y} \in \mathcal{N}(\mathbf{x})} \delta(M(\mathbf{x}) = M(\mathbf{y}))\right)$

3. $L(\mathbf{x}) \sim p(L(\mathbf{x}) = l | L_{M(\mathbf{x})})$

4. $\mathbf{I}^*(\mathbf{x}) \sim (2\pi)^{-\frac{C}{2}} \left|\Sigma_{L(\mathbf{x})}\right|^{-\frac{1}{2}} \exp\left[-\frac{1}{2}(\mathbf{I}^*(\mathbf{x}) - \boldsymbol{\mu}_{L(\mathbf{x})})^{\mathrm{T}} \Sigma_{L(\mathbf{x})}^{-1}(\mathbf{I}^*(\mathbf{x}) - \boldsymbol{\mu}_{L(\mathbf{x})})\right]$

5. $\mathbf{I}(\mathbf{x}) = \mathbf{B}(\mathbf{x})\mathbf{I}^*(\mathbf{x})$, with $\mathbf{B}(\mathbf{x}) = \mathrm{diag}(\exp\left[-\sum_k \mathbf{b}_k \psi_k(\mathbf{x})\right])$

2. A discrete field of memberships M such that $M(\mathbf{x}) \in \{1, \dots, N\}$ is sampled from a Markov random field (MRF) parametrized by the smoothness constant β (Equation 2 in the table, where $\mathcal{N}(\mathbf{x})$ represents the 6-neighborhood of $\mathbf{x}$). Higher values of β encourage larger clusters of voxels with the same label. The field $M(\mathbf{x})$ indicates from which atlas the generated image borrows the information at each voxel location $\mathbf{x}$ in the image domain Ω.

3. From $\{L_n\}$ and M, the "real", underlying segmentation of the data $L(\mathbf{x})$ is generated by sampling at each voxel location $\mathbf{x}$ from the probability vector specified by atlas $L_{M(\mathbf{x})}$ at $\mathbf{x}$ (Equation 3 in the table).

4. Given the label of a voxel $L(\mathbf{x})$, the "real", underlying image intensity $\mathbf{I}^*(\mathbf{x})$ is sampled from a multivariate Gaussian distribution associated with that label (Equation 4 in Table 1). Each of the $\mathcal{L}$ Gaussians is described by a $C \times 1$ mean vector $\boldsymbol{\mu}_l$ and a $C \times C$ covariance matrix Σ_l (where C is the number of image channels). We assume a flat prior for the Gaussian parameters i.e., $p(\boldsymbol{\mu}_l) \propto 1$, $p(\Sigma_l) \propto 1$.

5. $\mathbf{I}^*(\mathbf{x})$ is corrupted by a multiplicative bias field $\mathbf{B}(\mathbf{x})$, which is modeled through a set of low-spatial-frequency basis functions $\{\psi_k(\mathbf{x})\}$ to yield the final observed intensities $\mathbf{I}(\mathbf{x})$ (Equation 5 in the table, where the exponential ensures that the field is non-negative). The bias field is described by the vectors of coefficients $\{\mathbf{b}_k\}$, where $\mathbf{b}_k = [b_{k,1}, \dots, b_{k,C}]^{\mathrm{T}}$ groups the C coefficients (one per channel) for basis function ψ_k. Note that we allow a different set of coefficients per image channel, i.e. we assume that the bias fields for the different channels are independent. As for the parameters of the Gaussian distributions, we also assume a flat prior for the bias field coefficients: $p(\{\mathbf{b}_k\}) \propto 1$. Henceforth, we use the variable Θ to refer to the whole set of intensity parameters i.e., $\Theta = \{\{\mathbf{b}_k\}, \{\boldsymbol{\mu}_l\}, \{\Sigma_l\}\}$ and $p(\Theta) \propto 1$.

It is worth to note that some segmentation methods are particular cases of this generative model. For example, by setting $\beta = 0$, $\rho \to \infty$, $\Sigma_l = \lim_{\alpha \to \infty} \alpha \mathbf{Id}$ (where $\mathbf{Id}$ is the identity matrix) we obtain majority voting. Setting $\beta \to \infty$ and $\rho \to \infty$ amounts to best atlas selection. Finally, making $\beta = 0$ gives a model which is very similar to statistical-atlas-based segmentation [3]. The main difference is that, instead of registering a pre-built statistical atlas (a parametric model), we have a nonparametric approach in which an atlas is constructed

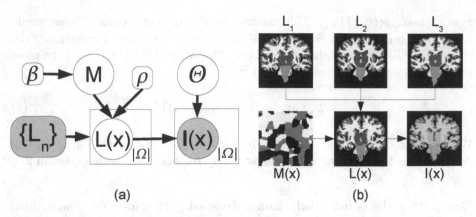

Fig. 1. a) Graphical model of the image generation process. Random variables are in circles and constants are in boxes. Observed variables are shaded. Plates indicate replication. b) Illustration of the generative process: three deformed atlases are combined through the membership field $M(\mathbf{x})$ to yield the labels $L(\mathbf{x})$. The image intensities $I(\mathbf{x})$ are obtained by sampling a Gaussian distribution for each label. We purposely chose the Gaussian parameters to make $I(\mathbf{x})$ resemble a T1-weighted MRI scan.

directly in target image space by registering all the atlases to the dataset to segment.

2.2   Segmentation Using Bayesian Inference

We can use Bayesian inference to compute the most likely segmentation by maximizing the posterior probability of the labels $L(\mathbf{x})$ given the available information, i.e., the image intensities $\mathbf{I}(\mathbf{x})$ and the deformed atlases $\{L_n\}$:

$$\widehat{L} = \operatorname*{argmax}_{L} p(L|I, \{L_n\}) = \operatorname*{argmax}_{L} \int_{\Theta} p(L, \Theta|I, \{L_n\}) d\Theta$$

$$= \operatorname*{argmax}_{L} \int_{\Theta} p(L|\Theta, I, \{L_n\}) p(\Theta|I, \{L_n\}) d\Theta \qquad (1)$$

In our previous conference paper, we attempted to maximize $p(L, \Theta|I, \{L_n\})$ with respect to $\{L, \Theta\}$, which was achieved with a coordinate ascent algorithm, i.e., alternatively optimizing for L and Θ. This is a k-means style algorithm. However, when we compute the most likely Θ, we are not interested in the labels L, hence a better strategy would be to integrate out L. This leads to the EM algorithm proposed in this paper, in which soft label assignments (rather than hard, like in k-means) are used to update Θ.

Looking at Equation 1, we see that it involves a high-dimensional integral over the parameters in Θ. However, we can make the assumption that the statistical distribution of these parameters given the observed data I and $\{L_n\}$ is sharp, i.e., $p(\Theta|I, \{L_n\}) \approx \delta(\Theta - \widehat{\Theta})$, where $\delta(\cdot)$ is Kronecker's delta and

$\widehat{\Theta} = \mathrm{argmax}_{\Theta}\, p(\Theta|I, \{L_n\})$. This assumption can be quite realistic, since we do not expect the values of Θ to deviate much from $\widehat{\Theta}$ without considerably decreasing the likelihood of the model. Then, the integral disappears and the most likely labels are (approximately) given by:

$$\widehat{L} \approx \mathrm{argmax}_{L}\, p(L|\widehat{\Theta}, I, \{L_n\}) \qquad (2)$$

We will first discuss how to obtain the optimal estimate of $\widehat{\Theta}$. Then, we will describe a method to compute the most likely segmentation with Equation 2.

Computing the Most Likely Image Intensity Parameters: The optimal point estimate of the image intensity parameters Θ is given by:

$$\widehat{\Theta} = \mathrm{argmin}_{\Theta} \left(- \log p(I|\Theta, \{L_n\})\right) \qquad (3)$$

$$= \mathrm{argmin}_{\Theta} \left(- \log \left[\sum_{L}\sum_{M} p(I, L, M|\Theta, \{L_n\})\right]\right) \qquad (4)$$

where we have used $p(\Theta) \propto 1$. Equation 4 is computationally intractable due to the sum over all possible membership fields $\sum_{M}$, which does not factorize over voxels. Instead, we use variational EM (VEM) to minimize an upper bound. We define the free energy J as:

$$J = - \log p(I|\Theta, \{L_n\}) + KL[q(M)||p(M|I, \Theta, \{L_n\})] \qquad (5)$$

$$= -H(q) - \sum_{M} q(M) \log p(I, M|\Theta, \{L_n\}) \qquad (6)$$

where $H(\cdot)$ is Shannon's entropy, $KL(\cdot||\cdot)$ is the Kullback-Leibler divergence and $q(M)$ is a statistical distribution over M, which approximates the posterior probability $p(M|I, \Theta, \{L_n\})$. The free energy J is a bound of the target function to minimize (Equation 3) because the KL divergence is nonnegative. The standard computational trick in VEM is to assume that $q(M)$ factorizes:

$$q(M) = \prod_{\mathbf{x}\in\Omega} q_x(M(\mathbf{x})),$$

which eventually makes the intractable sum tractable. The idea is to minimize J by iteratively optimizing for $q(M)$ (expectation or E step) and Θ (maximization or M step):

- *E step:* to optimize J for $q(M)$, it is easier to work with Equation 5, since the only term depending on $q(M)$ is the KL divergence. We have

$$\hat{q} = \underset{q}{\operatorname{argmin}} \sum_M q(M) \log \frac{q(M)}{p(M|I, \Theta, \{L_n\})}$$

$$= \underset{q}{\operatorname{argmin}} \sum_M q(M) \log \frac{q(M)}{p(M) \sum_L p(I|L, \Theta) p(L|M, \{L_n\})}$$

$$= \underset{q}{\operatorname{argmin}} \left(\sum_{\mathbf{x} \in \Omega} \sum_{n=1}^{N} q_x(n) \log q_x(n) - \beta \sum_{\mathbf{x} \in \Omega} E_{q_x} \left[\sum_{\mathbf{y} \in \mathcal{N}(\mathbf{x})} q_y(M(\mathbf{x})) \right] - \ldots \right.$$

$$\left. \ldots - \sum_{\mathbf{x} \in \Omega} \sum_{n=1}^{N} q_x(n) \log \left[\sum_{l=1}^{\mathcal{L}} p(I(\mathbf{x})|\Theta_l) p(L_{M(\mathbf{x})} = l) \right] \right)$$

Building the Lagrangian with a multiplier for the constraint $\sum_n q_x(n) = 1$ and taking derivatives with respect to q_x, we obtain:

$$q_x(M(\mathbf{x})) = \frac{\exp\left[\beta \sum_{\mathbf{y} \in \mathcal{N}(\mathbf{x})} q_y(M(\mathbf{x}))\right] \sum_{l=1}^{\mathcal{L}} p(I(\mathbf{x})|\Theta_l) p(L_{M(\mathbf{x})}(\mathbf{x}) = l)}{\sum_{n=1}^{N} \left(\exp\left[\beta \sum_{\mathbf{y} \in \mathcal{N}(\mathbf{x})} q_y(n)\right] \sum_{l'=1}^{\mathcal{L}} p(I(\mathbf{x})|\Theta_{l'}) p(L_n(\mathbf{x}) = l')\right)},$$

$$(7)$$

which can be solved with fixed point iterations. Note that the constraint $q_x \geq 0$ is implicitly enforced due to the nonnegative nature of probabilities and of the exponential function.

– *M step:* to optimize J with respect to Θ, we focus on Equation 6 instead (since the entropy does not depend on Θ):

$$\hat{\Theta} = \underset{\Theta}{\operatorname{argmax}} f(\Theta) = \underset{\Theta}{\operatorname{argmax}} \sum_{\mathbf{x} \in \Omega} \sum_{n=1}^{N} q_x(n) \log \left(\sum_{l=1}^{\mathcal{L}} [p(I(\mathbf{x})|\Theta_l) p(L_n(\mathbf{x}) = l)] \right).$$

$$(8)$$

Here, one must be careful with the scaling of the Gaussian probability density function:

$$p(\mathbf{I}(\mathbf{x})|\Theta_l) = \exp\left[\sum_{c=1}^{C} \sum_k b_{k,c} \psi_k(\mathbf{x})\right] \mathcal{G}(\mathbf{I}^*(\mathbf{x}); \boldsymbol{\mu}_l, \boldsymbol{\Sigma}_l)$$

where $\mathcal{G}$ is the probability density function of the multivariate Gaussian distribution. Taking matrix derivatives of Equation 8 with respect to $\boldsymbol{\mu}_l$ and $\boldsymbol{\Sigma}_l$ (see [24]), we obtain the following update equations:

$$\boldsymbol{\mu}_l \leftarrow \frac{\sum_{\mathbf{x} \in \Omega} w_l(\mathbf{x}) \mathbf{I}^*(\mathbf{x})}{\sum_{\mathbf{x} \in \Omega} w_l(\mathbf{x})}, \quad \boldsymbol{\Sigma}_l \leftarrow \frac{\sum_{\mathbf{x} \in \Omega} w_l(\mathbf{x}) (\mathbf{I}^*(\mathbf{x}) - \boldsymbol{\mu}_l)(\mathbf{I}^*(\mathbf{x}) - \boldsymbol{\mu}_l)^{\mathrm{T}}}{\sum_{\mathbf{x} \in \Omega} w_l(\mathbf{x})}$$

$$(9)$$

where

$$w_l(\mathbf{x}) = \sum_{n=1}^{N} q_x(n) \frac{p(\mathbf{I}(\mathbf{x})|\Theta_l)p(L_n(\mathbf{x}) = l)}{\sum_{l'=1}^{\mathcal{L}} p(\mathbf{I}(\mathbf{x})|\Theta_{l'})p(L_n(\mathbf{x}) = l')}$$

For the bias field parameters $\{b_k\}$, the derivatives of the target function in Equation 8 are:

$$\frac{\partial f}{\partial \mathbf{b}_k} = \sum_{\mathbf{x}\in\Omega} \psi_k(\mathbf{x}) \sum_{n=1}^{N} \frac{\sum_{l=1}^{\mathcal{L}} p(\mathbf{I}(\mathbf{x})|\Theta_l)p(L_m(\mathbf{x}) = l) \left[\mathbf{Id} - \mathbf{\Sigma}_l^{-1}(\mathbf{I}^*(\mathbf{x}) - \boldsymbol{\mu}_l)\mathbf{I}^{*T}(\mathbf{x})\right]}{\sum_{l'=1}^{\mathcal{L}} p(\mathbf{I}(\mathbf{x})|\Theta_{l'})p(L_m(\mathbf{x}) = l')}$$

(10)

and we use a quasi-Newton algorithm with line search (BFGS [25]) to numerically find the optimum. Because the bias field has a low number of degrees of freedom, the first iteration of the VEM algorithm already produces a relatively good estimate of the coefficients. Therefore, the BFGS algorithm converges very quickly (one or two steps) in successive iterations.

Computing the Final Segmentation: Once we have the estimate $\widehat{\Theta}$, computing the most likely segmentation in Equation 2 is straightforward. Replacing the posterior probability of M by its approximation $q(M)$ in Equation 2, we have:

$$\widehat{L} \approx \operatorname*{argmax}_L p(L|I,\widehat{\Theta},\{L_n\}) \approx \sum_M p(L|M,I,\widehat{\Theta},\{L_n\})q(M)$$

$$= \prod_{\mathbf{x}\in\Omega} \sum_{n=1}^{N} q_x(n) \frac{p(I(\mathbf{x})|\widehat{\Theta}_{L(\mathbf{x})})p(L_n(\mathbf{x}) = L(\mathbf{x}))}{\sum_{l'=1}^{\mathcal{L}} p(I(\mathbf{x})|\widehat{\Theta}_{l'})p(L_n(\mathbf{x}) = l')}$$

Since this expression factorizes over voxels, the most likely label at location $\mathbf{x}$ is just:

$$\widehat{L}(\mathbf{x}) = \operatorname*{argmax}_l \sum_{n=1}^{N} q_x(n) \frac{p(I(\mathbf{x})|\widehat{\Theta})p(L_n(\mathbf{x}) = l)}{\sum_{l'=1}^{\mathcal{L}} p(I(\mathbf{x})|\widehat{\Theta}_{l'})p(L_n(\mathbf{x}) = l')}$$

(11)

The complete segmentation algorithm is summarized in Table 2.

3   Experiments and Results

3.1   Datasets

We used two different datasets in this study, one for training and one for testing. The training dataset (i.e., the atlases) consists of 39 T1-weighted scans acquired with a MP-RAGE sequence in a 1.5T scanner with the following parameters: TR=9.7ms, TE=4.ms, TI=20ms, flip angle = 10°, 1 mm. isotropic resolution.

Table 2. Summary of the proposed multimodal label fusion framework

I. Compute the most likely image intensity parameters: 0. Initialize $q_x(n) = 1/N$, $\Sigma_l = \lim_{\alpha \to \infty} \alpha \mathbf{Id}$ (equivalent to majority voting). 1. Update q with Equation 7 until convergence. 2. Update means and variances with Equation 9. 3. Update the bias field using the derivatives in Equation 10. 4. Go to 1 until convergence. II. Compute the most likely segmentation for each voxel using Equation 11 and the latest estimate of q from step I.1.

Thirty-six brain structures were manually delineated by expert human raters using the protocol described in [26]. We note that these are the same subjects that were used to construct the probabilistic atlas in FreeSurfer [22]. As in [21,13], rather than using all 36 structures in the evaluation, we consider a representative subset here: left and right white matter (WM), cerebral cortex (CT), lateral ventricle (VE), cerebellum white matter (CWM), cerebellum cortex (CCT), thalamus (TH), caudate (CA), putamen (PU), pallidum (PA), hippocampus (HP) and amygdala (AM).

The test dataset [27] consists of eight multimodal brain MRI scans acquired with a multiecho FLASH sequence in a 1.5T scanner with the following parameters: TR=20ms, TE = minimum, flip angle = $\{3°, 5°, 20°, 30°\}$, 1 mm. isotropic resolution. There are therefore $C = 4$ channels available, one per value of flip angle. The lowest flip angles produce PD-weighted images, whereas the higher angles yield T1-weighted data. The same set of 36 structures was labeled using the same protocol. These manual annotations were drawn on the images corresponding to the largest flip angles, i.e., T1-weighted scans.

3.2 Preprocessing

All the scans from both datasets were first skull-stripped using ROBEX [28]. For the test dataset, we only used the T1-weighted volume as input to the skull stripping module. The training images were then deformed to the test images using a nonlinear, symmetric, diffeomorphic registration method (ANTS [29], version 1.9). For the registration metric, we used the mean mutual information (computed with 32 bins) between the four fixed images (i.e., the four flip angles) and the moving image. The executed command was:

```
ANTS 3 -m MI[fix1,mov1,0.25,32] ... -m MI[fix4,mov4,0.25,32]
      -r Gauss[3,0] -t SyN[0.25] -i 11x51x51x15 -o output
```

The resulting warps were used to deform the distance transforms of the different labels and atlases D_n^l, which are in turn used to compute label probabilities for each voxel of the target image to segment with Equation 1 in Table 1.

In addition to registering the atlases to the target images (used in label fusion), we built a single probabilistic atlas via an iterative, unbiased approach [2]

126   J.E. Iglesias, M.R. Sabuncu, and K. Van Leemput

as described as follows. First, we used the FreeSurfer pipeline to obtain intensity-standardized images. The atlases were then spatially normalized by registering with a population template image (which was the average intensity image computed based on the latest registrations). Since the images were intensity normalized, we used cross correlation as the registration similarity metric. Hence, this time the command was:

```
ANTS 3 -m CC[fix,mov,1,5] -r Gauss[3,0] -t SyN[0.25]
       -i 11x51x51x15 -o output
```

After a round of registration (where all atlases were registered with the current template), the template was updated as the average intensity image. Then, the atlases were re-registered to the template and this whole cycle was iterated until the intensity template converged. The final warps were then used to deform the corresponding manual annotations and compute label probabilities for each voxel in the statistical atlas as:

$$p(L(\mathbf{x}) = l) = (1/N) \sum_{n=1}^{N} \delta(L_n(\mathbf{x}) = l). \tag{12}$$

The obtained template was registered to the test images using the mean mutual information metric, as described above. The resulting deformations were used to propagate the label probabilities of Equation 12 to the target image space.

3.3 Experimental Setup

We used the $N = 39$ atlases to segment the eight multimodal volumes using a number of competing approaches:

– Majority voting. Rather than using discrete labels (i.e., $\rho = \infty$ in the logOdds model), we use $\rho = 1$, which is shown in [13] to constitute a better prior by introducing some "fuzziness", which can partially compensate for inaccurate registration. The performance of majority voting marks the accuracy that can be reached with registration only.
– The statistical atlas, which was constructed by co-registering the atlases as described in Section 3.2. The algorithm to obtain the segmentation given the (registered) statistical atlas is very similar to our method in Section 2.2. We actually used the same implementation assuming a single atlas for which the label probabilities are not given by the logOdds model, but by Equation 12 instead. The basis for the bias field model $\{\psi_l(\mathbf{x})\}$ was set to a third-degree polynomial, which, in 3D, yields 20 coefficients per image channel. Rather than iterating through all voxels in the estimation of the bias field (Equations 8 and 10), we only used a randomly selected subset (10% of the total number of voxels $|\Omega|$) to speed up the algorithm. The estimate will still be reliable thanks to the low number of degrees of freedom of the field.

- An ad-hoc locally-weighted label fusion method. To estimate the local similarity, we computed the 10th power of the NCC of the two images in a $7 \times 7 \times 7$ voxel window around the location of interest. We also considered using MI instead of NCC, but NCC performed better in pilot experiments and also has the advantage that it can efficiently be computed using integral images [30]. Since four channels are available for the target image to analyze, we simply took the average NCC of the four. The coefficient of the exponential (10) was coarsely tuned based on visual inspection of the results on a T1-weighted MRI scan of the first author's brain, preprocessed in the same way as the test data.
- The proposed framework. We used $\rho = 1.0$, $\beta = 0.75$, which we borrowed from [13]. A third-order polynomial was again used for the bias field modeling, using 10% of the available image data for the estimation. The iterative EM algorithm was stopped when no parameter in Θ changed more than 0.1% or when the maximal number of iterations (set to 25) was reached.
- Finally, it is also interesting to segment the data using only one of the channels in order to estimate the benefit of using all four channels. As a representative, state-of-the-art method, we used FreeSurfer to segment the T1-weighted channel (i.e., flip angle = 30°). Using FreeSurfer also has the advantage that it was trained on the same training data used in this study, enabling a fair comparison. Moreover, the fact that it uses the same set of labels facilitates the comparison with the other methods.

In order to evaluate the accuracy of the aforementioned approaches, we used the popular Dice coefficient (Dice $= 2|A \cap M|/[|A| + |M|]$), where A and M denote the automatic and manual segmentations, respectively; and $|\cdot|$ denotes the volume.

3.4   Results

Figures 2 and 3 display, for each hemisphere, the boxplots for the Dice overlaps corresponding to the structures of interest listed in Section 3.1. The mean Dice scores for each hemisphere are listed in Table 3. Table 4 displays p-values corresponding to paired t-tests comparing the different competing methods with the proposed algorithm. Finally, Figures 4 and 5 show sample segmentations from the different methods.

FreeSurfer is the one of the best performers only in the cortex. For the other structures, it is consistently inferior to the other methods, which take advantage of the multimodal nature of the target images. It is important to mention that the T1-weighted volume, which is the one we feed to the FreeSurfer pipeline, has relatively poor white matter / gray matter contrast (see for instance Figure 4), which explains the low Dice overlaps produced by this method compared with previously reported results (e.g. [13]).

Majority voting, thanks to the good performance of the registration method and the large number of atlases, outperforms FreeSurfer and also the method based on a single statistical atlas. Even though the statistical atlas produces

Table 3. Mean Dice scores (in %) across the 11 structures of interest for each method: left hemisphere (top row), right hemisphere (middle), and both combined (bottom)

Method	FreeSurfer	Stat.atlas	Maj.Vot.	Ad-hoc NCC	This study
Left hemisphere	82.4	84.4	85.4	85.6	86.4
Right hemisphere	83.2	84.1	85.1	85.4	86.1
Both	82.8	84.3	85.2	85.5	86.3

Table 4. p values corresponding to paired t-tests comparing the Dices scores from the different methods with those from the proposed approach

Method	FreeSurfer	Stat.atlas	Maj.Vot.	Ad-hoc NCC
Left hemisphere	$4.1 \cdot 10^{-19}$	$2.3 \cdot 10^{-11}$	$2.3 \cdot 10^{-6}$	$1.6 \cdot 10^{-4}$
Right hemisphere	$9.4 \cdot 10^{-12}$	$5.0 \cdot 10^{-11}$	$1.4 \cdot 10^{-4}$	$9.6 \cdot 10^{-3}$
Both	$7.9 \cdot 10^{-29}$	$5.0 \cdot 10^{-21}$	$1.9 \cdot 10^{-9}$	$8.9 \cdot 10^{-6}$

better results for the cortices of the cerebrum and the cerebellum, which are very difficult to register, it performs considerably worse in the subcortical structures. In this case, the flexibility of having the 39 atlases registered independently represents an advantage over the single registration of the statistical atlas.

When the locally-computed NCCs are used to assign different weights to the atlases at each voxel, a small (Dice increment 0.3%) but significant ($p < 10^{-5}$) improvement is achieved. When we use the generative model proposed here, we obtain as good results as the statistical atlas on the cortices, significantly outperforming the other multi-atlas methods (majority voting and NCC-based). Furthermore, the proposed method also provides slightly better results majority voting and the NCC-based algorithm for the subcortical structures.

Sample segmentations are displayed in Figures 4 and 5. The segmentations are in general poor in the cortex (red label), but quite accurate for the subcortical structures. The arrows pinpoint the typical mistakes made by the other methods as explained above. In Figure 4, FreeSurfer makes quite a few mistakes around the lateral ventricle (in purple) and in the cerebellum. The statistical atlas, next to mistakes in the ventricle, also displays a leak in the hippocampal label (yellow). Majority voting cannot capture the large ventricle, which is anatomically infrequent. The ad-hoc locally-weighted model produces a poor segmentation for the caudate nucleus (light blue). The proposed algorithm, on the other hand, provides a robust segmentation across all structures.

In figure 5, FreeSurfer (next to oversegmenting the cortex) severely undersegments the thalamus. The statistical atlas undersegments the left and right pallidum (dark blue), whereas majority voting shows some problems with the cortex. So does the ad-hoc NCC method, which also undersegments the right caudate nucleus (oversegmenting the right lateral ventricle). Again, the proposed algorithm produces the most accurate segmentation across the different structures.

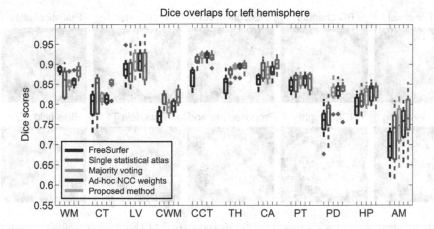

Fig. 2. Boxplot of Dice overlap scores corresponding to the 11 structures of interest for the left hemisphere; see Section 3.1 for the abbreviations. Horizontal box lines indicate the three quartile values. Whiskers extend to the most extreme values within 1.5 times the interquartile range from the ends of the box. Samples beyond those points (outliers) are marked with crosses.

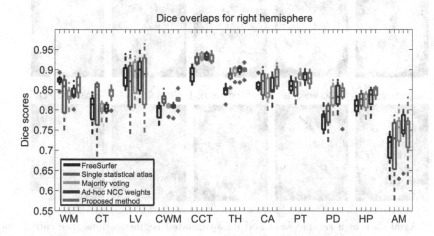

Fig. 3. Boxplot of Dice overlap scores corresponding to the 11 structures of interest for the right hemisphere; see caption of Figure 2

4 Discussion

In this paper we have presented a multimodal label fusion scheme that does not make any assumptions about the relation between the intensities of the deformed atlases and the target images. Instead, the framework uses a principled generative model to take advantage of the consistency of intensities within image

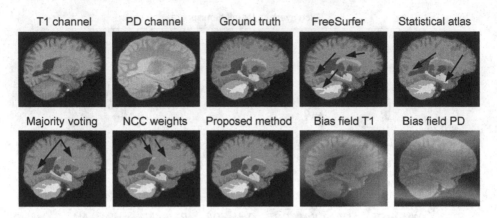

Fig. 4. Sagittal slice of a sample scan: input data (two of the four channels), ground truth, outputs from the different algorithms, and bias fields estimated by our method (blue=0.85, red=1.15). The arrows point to mistakes made by the different algorithms.

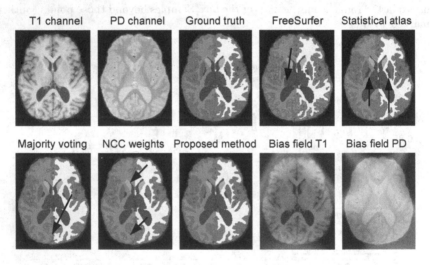

Fig. 5. Axial slice of a sample scan and its automated segmentations (see caption of Figure 4)

regions. This is done by assuming that the intensities corresponding to each label follow a multivariate Gaussian distribution. The results show that the presented approach outperforms: 1. majority voting, which does not consider the intensities of the target images; 2. FreeSurfer, a state-of-the-art segmentation tool that only takes advantage of one of the channels of the target data; 3. using a single statistical atlas (which takes advantage of all the channels); and 4. a heuristic rule for locally weighted label fusion.

The proposed method has the disadvantage that the Gaussian intensity distribution assumption might break down because of the nature of the data or if two structures with different intensity profiles share the same label. For example one might only be interested in one structure such as the hippocampus, in which case a single Gaussian might not be an appropriate model for the background intensities. One possible solution would be to use a mixture of Gaussians. In this case, one must be careful because excessive flexibility in the intensity model might lead to leaks in the segmentation.

Another disadvantage of the presented framework is that the parameters β and ρ are fixed by the user. It would be desirable to allow the inference method to handle them automatically, either by computing point estimates (as we did with Θ here) or integrating them out. Exploring this direction, as well as incorporating the registration into the framework (rather than considering it a preprocessing step) remains as future work.

Acknowledgements. This research was supported by NIH NCRR (P41-RR14075), NIBIB (R01EB006758, R01EB013565, 1K25EB013649-01), NINDS (R01NS052585), NIH 1KL2RR025757-01, Academy of Finland (133611), TEKES (ComBrain), Harvard Catalyst, and financial contributions from Harvard and affiliations.

References

1. Rohlfing, T., Brandt, R., Menzel, R., Russakoff, D., Maurer, C.: Quo vadis, atlas-based segmentation? Handbook of Biomedical Image Analysis, pp. 435–486 (2005)
2. Joshi, S., Davis, B., Jomier, M., Gerig, G.: Unbiased diffeomorphic atlas construction for computational anatomy. NeuroImage 23, S151–S160 (2004)
3. Ashburner, J., Friston, K.: Unified segmentation. Neuroimage 26, 839–851 (2005)
4. Van Leemput, K., Maes, F., Vandermeulen, D., Suetens, P.: Automated model-based tissue classification of MR images of the brain. IEEE Transactions on Medical Imaging 18(10), 897–908 (1999)
5. Thomas Yeo, B., Sabuncu, M., Desikan, R., Fischl, B., Golland, P.: Effects of registration regularization and atlas sharpness on segmentation accuracy. Medical Image Analysis 12(5), 603–615 (2008)
6. Heckemann, R., Hajnal, J., Aljabar, P., Rueckert, D., Hammers, A.: Automatic anatomical brain MRI segmentation combining label propagation and decision fusion. NeuroImage 33(1), 115–126 (2006)
7. Rohlfing, T., Brandt, R., Menzel, R., Maurer, C.: Evaluation of atlas selection strategies for atlas-based image segmentation with application to confocal microscopy images of bee brains. NeuroImage 21(4), 1428–1442 (2004)
8. Langerak, T., Van Der Heide, U., Kotte, A., Viergever, M., Van Vulpen, M., Pluim, J.: Label fusion in atlas-based segmentation using a selective and iterative method for performance level estimation (simple). IEEE Transactions on Medical Imaging 29(12), 2000–2008 (2010)
9. Klein, S., van der Heide, U., Lips, I., van Vulpen, M., Staring, M., Pluim, J.: Automatic segmentation of the prostate in 3D MR images by atlas matching using localized mutual information. Medical Physics 35, 1407 (2008)

10. Artaechevarria, X., Muñoz-Barrutia, A., Ortiz-de Solorzano, C.: Combination strategies in multi-atlas image segmentation: Application to brain MR data. IEEE Transactions on Medical Imaging 28(8), 1266–1277 (2009)
11. Warfield, S., Zou, K., Wells, W.: Simultaneous truth and performance level estimation (staple): an algorithm for the validation of image segmentation. IEEE Transactions on Medical Imaging 23(7), 903–921 (2004)
12. Isgum, I., Staring, M., Rutten, A., Prokop, M., Viergever, M., van Ginneken, B.: Multi-atlas-based segmentation with local decision fusion application to cardiac and aortic segmentation in ct scans. IEEE Transactions on Medical Imaging 28(7), 1000–1010 (2009)
13. Sabuncu, M., Yeo, B., Van Leemput, K., Fischl, B., Golland, P.: A generative model for image segmentation based on label fusion. IEEE Transactions on Medical Imaging 29(10), 1714–1729 (2010)
14. Coupé, P., Manjón, J., Fonov, V., Pruessner, J., Robles, M., Collins, D.: Nonlocal Patch-Based Label Fusion for Hippocampus Segmentation. In: Jiang, T., Navab, N., Pluim, J.P.W., Viergever, M.A. (eds.) MICCAI 2010, Part III. LNCS, vol. 6363, pp. 129–136. Springer, Heidelberg (2010)
15. Wang, H., Suh, J., Das, S., Pluta, J., Craige, C., Yushkevich, P.: Multi-atlas segmentation with joint label fusion. IEEE Transactions on Pattern Analysis and Machine Intelligence (in press, 2012)
16. Cao, Y., Yuan, Y., Li, X., Turkbey, B., Choyke, P., Yan, P.: Segmenting Images by Combining Selected Atlases on Manifold. In: Fichtinger, G., Martel, A., Peters, T. (eds.) MICCAI 2011, Part III. LNCS, vol. 6893, pp. 272–279. Springer, Heidelberg (2011)
17. Zhang, D., Wu, G., Jia, H., Shen, D.: Confidence-Guided Sequential Label Fusion for Multi-atlas Based Segmentation. In: Fichtinger, G., Martel, A., Peters, T. (eds.) MICCAI 2011, Part III. LNCS, vol. 6893, pp. 643–650. Springer, Heidelberg (2011)
18. Nyul, L., Udupa, J., Zhang, X.: New variants of a method of MRI scale standardization. IEEE Transactions on Medical Imaging 19(2), 143–150 (2000)
19. Staring, M., van der Heide, U., Klein, S., Viergever, M., Pluim, J.: Registration of cervical MRI using multifeature mutual information. IEEE Transactions on Medical Imaging 28(9), 1412–1421 (2009)
20. Sabuncu, M., Ramadge, P.: Using spanning graphs for efficient image registration. IEEE Transactions on Image Processing 17(5), 788–797 (2008)
21. Iglesias, J., Sabuncu, M., Van Leemput, K.: A generative model for multi-atlas segmentation across modalities. In: IEEE ISBI, pp. 888–891 (2012)
22. FreeSurfer: http://surfer.nmr.mgh.harvard.edu
23. Pohl, K., Fisher, J., Shenton, M., McCarley, R., Grimson, W., Kikinis, R., Wells, W.: Logarithm Odds Maps for Shape Representation. In: Larsen, R., Nielsen, M., Sporring, J. (eds.) MICCAI 2006. LNCS, vol. 4191, pp. 955–963. Springer, Heidelberg (2006)
24. Petersen, K., Pedersen, M.: The matrix cookbook (2008)
25. Nocedal, J., Wright, S.: Numerical optimization. Springer (1999)
26. Caviness Jr., V., Filipek, P., Kennedy, D.: Magnetic resonance technology in human brain science: blueprint for a program based upon morphometry. Brain Dev. 11(1), 1–13 (1989)
27. Fischl, B., Salat, D., van der Kouwe, A., Makris, N., Ségonne, F., Quinn, B., Dale, A.: Sequence-independent segmentation of magnetic resonance images. Neuroimage 23, S69–S84 (2004)

28. Iglesias, J., Liu, C., Thompson, P., Tu, Z.: Robust brain extraction across datasets and comparison with publicly available methods. IEEE Transactions on Medical Imaging 30(99), 1617–1634 (2011)
29. Avants, B., Epstein, C., Grossman, M., Gee, J.: Symmetric diffeomorphic image registration with cross-correlation: Evaluating automated labeling of elderly and neurodegenerative brain. Medical image analysis 12(1), 26–41 (2008)
30. Viola, P., Jones, M.: Rapid object detection using a boosted cascade of simple features. In: CVPR 2001 vol. 1, pp. 511–518

Spatial Normalization of Diffusion Tensor Images with Voxel-Wise Reconstruction of the Diffusion Gradient Direction

Wei Liu[1,2], Xiaozheng Liu[1,2], Xiaofu He[2], Zhenyu Zhou[2], Ying Wen[2], Yongdi Zhou[1], Bradley S. Peterson[2], and Dongrong Xu[2,*]

[1] Key Laboratory of Brain Functional Genomics, & Key Laboratory of Magnetic Resonance, East China Normal University, Shanghai 200062, China
[2] MRI Unit, Columbia University Department of Psychiatry, New York State Psychiatric Institute, Unit 74, New York, NY 10032, U.S.A.

Abstract. We propose a reconstructed diffusion gradient (RDG) method for spatial normalization of diffusion tensor imaging (DTI) data that warps the raw imaging data and then estimates the associated gradient direction for reconstruction of normalized DTI in the template space. The RDG method adopts the backward mapping strategy for DTI normalization, with a specially designed approach to reconstruct a specific gradient direction in combination with the local deformation force. The method provides a voxel-based strategy to make the gradient direction align with the raw diffusion weighted imaging (DWI) volumes, ensuring correct estimation of the tensors in the warped space and thereby retaining the orientation information of the underlying structure. Compared with the existing tensor reorientation methods, experiments using both simulated and human data demonstrated that the RDG method provided more accurate tensor information. Our method can properly estimate the gradient direction in the template space that has been changed due to image transformation, and subsequently use the warped imaging data to directly reconstruct the warped tensor field in the template space, achieving the same goal as directly warping the tensor image. Moreover, the RDG method also can be used to spatially normalize data using the Q-ball imaging (QBI) model.

Keywords: diffusion weighed imaging, backward mapping, tensor reorientation.

1 Introduction

Diffusion tensor imaging (DTI) is an advanced medical technology for studying brain structure[1]. Spatial normalization is required to establish correspondences across the individuals for group studies. Because the tensor data contain not only the magnitude information but also information of spatial orientation, normalization of DTI needs not only warping of the data to the correspondence location to match the target dataset (template) but also adjustment of the orientation of the diffusion tensors (DTs)

---

* Corresponding author.

P.-T. Yap et al. (Eds.): MBIA 2012, LNCS 7509, pp. 134–146, 2012.

properly to retain the consistence between the tensors and the relative anatomical structures[2].

In order to ensure tensor orientations to be accurate after image transformation, Alexander et al. proposed a finite-strain (FS) reorientation strategy that estimates the rotation component from the deformation field (DF)[2]. The preservation of principal direction (PPD) method was also proposed to reorient tensors by estimating the spatial transformation of the tensor along its principal eigenvectors[2]. The PPD method is more effective than FS method because the effects of shear and scale are properly considered. However the performance of PPD method relies on the accuracy and robustness of principal component estimation in the noisy DTI data. Based on these two reorientation methods, several improved algorithms were proposed in recent years [3, 4]. All these methods depend on a forward mapping (DF defined in the subject space pointing to the template space) strategy. It is known that warping using forward mapping will generate seams and consequently artifacts in the warped tensor images. A seamless warping (SW) method therefore has been offered to address this issue of quality downgrading [5]. But this method needs to calculate a bijection that is in essence a pair of one-to-one forward and backward mapping (defined the template space pointing to the subject space), which is very time-consuming.

Because DTI images are artificially reconstructed based on diffusion weighted imaging (DWI) data, an alternative approach to normalize DTI images is actually to normalize diffusion weighted (DW) images and then reconstruct DTI data using the warped DW images. Although all the voxels in one DWI volume share the same identical gradient direction in the original space, this universal gradient direction throughout the DWI volume will no longer be universally the same but will change individually for each voxel, if the DWI volume is deformed to a different space, particularly when the deformation is nonlinear, which is always the case. Therefore, any warping that involves local deformation needs to properly adjust the gradient direction that is associated to a particular voxel for correctly estimating the tensor data in a warped space. However, adjusting the gradient direction following the deformation process is complicated, and depends on the local force received by a vector of this direction. For example, if the local deformation shows a shearing effect, it will generate different effects on tilting the gradient vectors that originally point to different orientations (Fig.1). If the gradient vectors are oriented parallel to the direction of shearing force, they will receive no rotation effect (Fig.1B). On the contrary, the gradient vectors not originally parallel to the direction of the shearing force need to be rotated appropriately (Fig.1D). Therefore we need to consider the original directional configuration of the gradient direction in relation to the local deformation to determine a tensor's final setting.

Whereas the tensor model assumes one single orientation of underlying fibers, Q-ball imaging (QBI) is a widely used model for processing multiple intravoxel fiber orientations, based on high angular resolution imaging (HARDI) data[6, 7]. QBI represents underlying fiber orientation using orientation distribution function (ODF), which is modeled on the basis of spherical harmonics (SH) [8, 9]. Similar to the spatial normalization of DTI, spatial normalization of QBI data using ODF also inevitably involves the issue of appropriate reorientation of the gradient associated with the

DWI data. Because QBI data are also estimated from the DWI data (which are specially termed as HARDI data), the adjustment of gradient directions can reasonably employ the same strategy as that developed for conventional DWI data.

The approaches proposed by Ingalhalikar are along these lines. The work proposed to rotate gradient vectors based on a rotation matrix estimated using the PPD method[10, 11], which rotated the associated gradient and could be applied directly to higher order models like the Q-ball model. However, this method inherited the shortages of the PPD method, as discussed above. Moreover, its FS strategy was problematic in theory as it extracts a rotation component anyway independent of the original tensor's orientation, thereby violating the principle we just discussed (Fig. 1).

We introduce a novel method called Reconstructed Diffusion Gradient (RDG) for spatial normalization of DTI via normalizing DWI data with two distinct features: (1) This algorithm adopts the standard backward mapping strategy to figure out the implicit information for reorientation of a specific spatial direction in combination with the local deformation force; (2) This algorithm directly calculates new gradient vectors in the template space instead of complex computations for local affine matrix or rotation matrix. Therefore, our strategy of reconstructing new gradient directions is completely different from all published methods thus far. Moreover, because the proposed method tackles the DWI data instead of the estimated DTs, it works not only for the DTI data but also for QBI data.

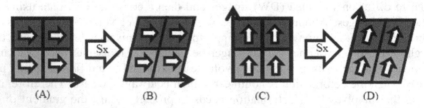

(A)   (B)   (C)   (D)

Fig. 1. A schematic illustration of how different gradient directions prescribe different effects from the same spatial transformations applied to DW images. (A),(C) are two original DW images acquired along the gradient directions as shown by the arrows. (B),(D) are the spatially transformed images and the associated gradient directions after sheared by a horizontal force (Sx). We can see that a gradient direction originally parallel to the shear force will remain unchanged (A,B), while a nonparallel direction will be tilted (C,D). Therefore, gradient vectors may receive different rotations even when they are under the same shearing force.

2   Method

We propose a generalized approach for spatial transformation of the tensor fields based on a backward DF that maps voxel-wise correspondence from a template space T to an individual subject space I. First, we normalize the baseline image S0 (b=0 s/mm^2) from I to that of T using any available tools that were developed for normalizing scalar images [12-15], and thus obtain a backward DF *def* defined in T projecting correspondence back to I. Subsequently, we use this *def* to normalize each volume of the DWI dataset in the same space I to the template space. Suppose F is the local deformation at a voxel from I to T, for a grid point (x,y,z) in T defined in Cartesian coordinate system, the corresponding point-to-point relationship between I and T can be represented as $def(x, y, z) \xrightarrow{F} (x, y, z)$, where $def(x, y, z)$ is the corresponding location in I. $def(x, y, z)$ can be obtained by retrieving the vector in def defined at (x, y, z) in T. Note $def(x,y,z)$ in I may not be at a grid point.

Each raw DWI volume (in I) is associated to a particular gradient direction $\vec{G}_{ori}$. It is a standard routine procedure to normalize the DWI data to the space T using the def we just obtained. Our additional step is now to obtain the reconstructed version of $\vec{G}_{ori}$ in T so that the new gradient direction in T is associated appropriately with the measure at each voxel of the warped DWI in T, as if the DWI data were acquired directly in T. To simplify the discussion, we first consider the procedure in 2D case, in which $\vec{G}_{ori}$ is the unit gradient vector started from point $def(x, y)$ in I, and the location (x, y) in T should take the DWI value at $def(x, y)$ with an adjusted unit gradient vector $\vec{G}_T$ rooted at (x, y) pointing to (x_{GT}, y_{GT}) (Fig.2). Therefore, in space I:

$$def((x, y) + \vec{G}_T) = def(x_{GT}, y_{GT}) = def(x, y) + \vec{G}_{ori} \tag{1}$$

In Eq. (1), $def(x, y) + \vec{G}_{ori}$ represents the end point of the original gradient vector rooted at location $def(x,y)$, corresponding to the end point of $(x,y) + \vec{G}_T$ in T. To sample locally at the current point location under consideration, we modify Eq. (1) to:

$$def((x, y) + \tilde{k}\vec{G}_T) = def(x, y) + k\vec{G}_{ori} \tag{2}$$

where k is a very small constant in I and $\tilde{k}$ is the corresponding constant in T. The relationship between k and $\tilde{k}$ is decided by the local deformation. Now we can use the def to calculate the corresponding location $(x, y) + \tilde{k}\vec{G}_T$ in T, in which the vector $\vec{G}_T$ defines the orientation of the new gradient. Thus, the point location $(x, y) + \tilde{k}\vec{G}_T$ implicitly contained in def is what we need to find out, thus to know the final orientation of the new gradient.

Assuming def is smooth and topology-preserved (which is always true), we could then obtain the exact location $(x, y) + \tilde{k}\vec{G}_T$, by solving an interpolation defined on the locations in the neighborhood of $def(x, y)$ in space I. For an arbitrary point M in T, the issue is simply to find its corresponding location P in I, based on def. This process is straightforward when def is defined on a continuous domain. However, def is discrete in practice which has definition only on grid points in T. We therefore need a way to find M that satisfies $def(M)=P$.

Back to the 3D case and supposing $M = (x, y, z) + \tilde{k}\vec{G}_T$, we have:

$P = def(M) = def(x, y, z) + k\vec{G}_{ori}$. We can estimate M by minimizing the expected value of $\|P - def(M)\|^2$:

$$M' = \arg \min_{M} E\{\|P - def(M)\|^2\}. \tag{3}$$

where M is $(x_{GT}, y_{GT}, z_{GT}) = (x, y, z) + k\vec{G}_T$, and $def(M)$ could be calculated by any interpolation methods. We adopt trilinear interpolation for convenience in this work.

A shortened Fletcher version of the Levenberg-Maquardt algorithm [16] is applied to estimate M from Eq.(3). This algorithm is an iterative procedure that gradually approaches a numerical solution to M by minimizing the errors, projecting location M in space T to P in space I via def. M' is the estimation of (x_{GT}, y_{GT}, z_{GT}) in T, thus the estimated unit gradient direction in T is $\vec{G}_T = Norm(M' - (x, y, z))$. *Norm* means to normalize its parameter to a unit vector.

Once $\vec{G}_T$ is reconstructed at each voxel, the warped DWI data associated to the new gradient vectors can be used to directly estimate tensors in T in a voxel-wise manner, using the linear least square fitting method [17]. The estimated DTI field thus forms the warped DTI in T, achieving the same goal of warping the original tensor field to the template space.

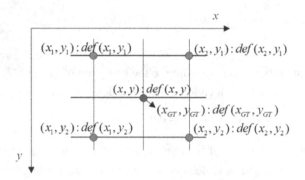

Fig. 2. A 2D illustration of gradient vector field in template space T. (x_1, y_1, x_2, y_2) defines a local neighborhood in T that encompasses the small gradient vector $\vec{G}_T$ rooted at (x,y), i.e., $(x_{GT}, y_{GT}) = (x, y) + \tilde{k} \cdot \vec{G}_T$, where $\tilde{k}$ is a small constant.

The RDG method warps DWI data and reconstructs their associated gradients. This method works for both single tensor model and QBI model. In brief, we summarize the steps of our framework as follows (Fig. 3): (1) Establish a voxel-wise correspondence between the subject and template spaces by normalizing the S0-images of the corresponding DWI datasets in the two spaces, generating a backward DF. (2) Reconstruct in the template space a new gradient for each voxel of each DWI volume, using our RDG method. (3) Warp the DWI dataset using the backward DF to the template space and estimate a tensor or ODF at each voxel using the newly reconstructed gradient table in the warped template space. Note that each voxel in the template space has its own gradient table, containing N new gradients if it involves N DWI volumes.

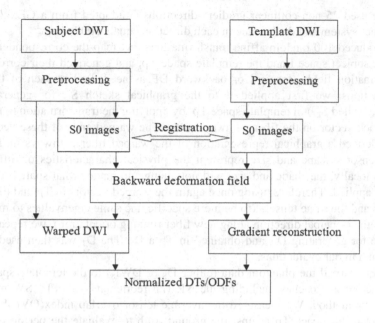

Fig. 3. The framework of using our RDG method for normalization of a DTI or QBI dataset

3   Simulation and Experiments

In this section, we designed a set of experiments using synthetic and real data to assess the effectiveness of our proposed method.

3.1   Simulation

In the simulation, we wanted to demonstrate using simulated data that our method can properly reorient tensors in the procedure of DTI normalization. We synthesized an anisotropic tensor field on a 3D lattice, following a well-received schema for simulating DTs [18-20]. We first drew a graphical sketch S_k two series of vectors in a subject space I, representing two fiber pathways. The fiber pathways were not parallel but did not intersect with each other. Taking the vectors as the directions of principal eigenvector, we synthesized a tensor field D_S in the subject space. Each voxel on these pathways was assigned with particular phantom values as defined below without involving   any partial volume effect. Fiber pathway 1: S0 = 100.00 for baseline image data, DT = 0.001 × [0.9697 1.7513 0.8423 0.0 0.0 0.0] mm^2/s for the tensors; Fiber pathway 2: S0 = 83.3 mm^2/s, DT = 0.001 × [1.5559 1.1651 0.8423 0.3384 0.0 0.0] mm^2/s.   The 3×3 symmetric tensor is depicted in the form of [D_{xx} D_{yy} D_{zz} D_{xy} D_{xz} D_{yz}]. We then generated the simulated DWI data (DWI$_S$) in space I using the Stejskal-Tanner equation at each voxel k as follows:

$$S(k) = S_0(k)e^{-bG^T D(k)G}.$$ (4)

where we used 25 non-collinear gradient directions G adopted from a GE 3.0 Tesla MR scanner system and the b-value in each direction equals 1000 s/mm^2.

We produced 100 random affine transformations that map the correspondence between the subject space I and the template space Tp, and generated their corresponding deformation fields (forward or backward DF as needed). For each of the 100 transformations, we first applied it to the graphical sketch S_k, for generating a warped S_k (called S_{kT}) in template space Tp, by applying the transformation to the two ends of each vector on the fiber pathways in S_k. The warped ends of these vectors in Tp thus defined a graphical representation of the warped fiber pathways in Tp. Because a tensor's shape and size represent the physical characteristics of diffusivity measured locally, the shape and size will not change no matter what spatial transformation is applied. Therefore, using once again the warped vectors in Tp and the same S0 values and the same tensors (to be more specific, the same eigenvalues to maintain shape but the principal direction along new fiber running orientation), we repeated the procedure for generating D_S, and obtained in Tp a D_T. The D_T was then used as the ground truth in our evaluations.

We then warped the phantom data (either D_S or DWI_S) to the template space Tp, using different approaches, including the NR (no reorientation), PPD, SW methods and also our method. We measured the average tensor overlap index(OVL)[21]   at each voxel in the space Tp against the ground truth to evaluate the performance of these methods:

$$OVL = \frac{\sum_{i=1}^{3} \lambda_i \lambda_i {}'(e_i \cdot e_i {}')^2}{\sum_{i=1}^{3} \lambda_i \lambda_i {}'} \tag{5}$$

where λ_i, e_i and $\lambda_i {}', e_i {}'$ denote the eigenvalue-eigenvector pair of two tensors (one from the ground truth, and the other from the result generated by the method being evaluated) . The OVL is 0 when there is no overlap (meaning the two tensors are totally different) and is 1 for complete overlap between the three principal axes of the diffusion tensors(meaning the two tensors are identical). We repeated this procedure for all 100 transformations and averaged the OVL at each voxel over the 100 repetitions.

3.2   Real Data Experiment

In this experiment using real data, we assessed the effectiveness of our reorientation strategy for preserving the topology of fiber tracts. Because the ability of recovering fiber pathways in a deformed space is a crucial indicator of the excellence of an approach for spatial normalization of DTI data, we performed tractography in both the original and the normalized DTI data, and compared the topology of the recovered fibers.

We acquired DTI datasets from the brains of six healthy adult volunteers, using a GE 3.0 Tesla MR scanner system, the acquisition parameters for the DWI volumes were: b-value = 1000 s/mm^2; 25 non-collinear gradient directions; image resolution = 0.9375×0.9375×2.5mm^3; TR/TE = 15700/80 ms. The DWI datasets were corrected for motion and eddy current artifacts using FSL 4.0 (*http://fsl.fmrib.ox.ac.uk/fsl/fdt/*). Written consents were obtained from these volunteers.

To evaluate the DTI normalization within the group, one of the DWI dataset was arbitrarily designated as the template, and the rest five datasets were spatially normalized to this selected template using the backward DFs that were computed based on the baseline image S0 extracted from the template and the S0 images from the other individuals. The DFs were generated using the coregistration procedure provided in the Statistical Parametric Map (SPM) (*http://www.fil.ion.ucl.ac.uk/spm/software/spm8/*) software package.

We calculated the color-encoded fractional anisotropy (FA) from the warped DT images for visual examination of the directional alignment in white matter (WM). Furthermore, we also visually evaluated the topology and alignment of fiber bundles in WM. In addition, we quantitatively evaluated the consistency (alignment) of two WM structures in the template and normalized data , by measuring the distance between 2 fiber bundles, following the method described in [4]. The distance d between two fiber bundles F and G is defined as:

$$\frac{1}{|F|+|G|}(\sum_{F_i \in F} \min_{G_j \in G} d(F_i, G_j) + \sum_{G_j \in G} \min_{F_i \in F} d(F_i, G_j)) \qquad (6)$$

where, $\min_{G_j \in G} d(F_i, G_j)$ is the distance between fiber F_i and the fiber in G that is closest to F_i, and similarly $\min_{F_i \in F} d(F_i, G_j)$ is the distance between fiber G_j and the fiber in F that is closest to G_i; |F| and |G| are the counts of fibers in F and G, respectively. When the two fiber bundles are identical and perfectly aligned, the distance d is zero.

In these examinations, we used a region-of-interest (ROI) on corpus callosum (CC) splenium for fiber tracking because it is one of the most important WM structures in human brain, which contains the best organized and visible fiber bundles connecting two hemispheres. The ROI was a 10×10×10 volume (pixel size) and all tracked fibers passing through this seeding region were preserved for visual and quantitative alignment comparisons. We used BioImage Suite (http://bioimagesuite.research.yale.edu/) for fiber tracking, which employs a fourth-order Runge-Kutta method [22] for fiber reconstruction. The tracking parameters were: step length = 0.25; fiber filtering: FA (0.2-1.0); mean diffusivity (MD) (0-10); fiber length (10-100mm); fiber max angle (45 degree).

4   Results

4.1   Simulation

As we expected, tensor orientation was far away from the ground truth in the results generated using the NR method. All the other reorientation methods generated results with improved consistency, which is not surprising because we know that the orientation of a DT must be adjusted in a deformed procedure. The average OVL over the 100 transformed results along with tensor reorientation showed that PPD, SW and our method produced more accurate results than did the NR method (Table 1). Basically, the NR method is not right in principle and needs to be abandoned, although the amount of orientation adjustment is often only slight as the local deformation is usually not large, making the results using NR always appear to be almost correct. Among all the other three methods that involved a strategy for tensor reorientation, PPD provided an improvement of accuracy at 24.45%, SW 24.83%, and our RDG method 25.73% (Table 1). Our RDG method outperformed other methods in that it not only provided the highest average OVL but also the smallest standard deviation, demonstrating that the performance of the RDG method is relatively more stable.

Table 1. The comparison of average tensor overlap (OVL) over the 100 transformed datasets. The improvememt referes to the increased consistency of tensors over that offered by the NR method. Our method yields the highest OVL and smallest standard deviation(STD).

	NR	PPD	SW	Our method
OVL	0.7436	0.9254	0.9282	0.9349
STD	0.2144	0.1036	0.1248	0.0653
Improvement		24.45%	24.83%	25.73%

4.2   Experiments

Visual inspection showed that our RDG method achieved better accuracy in tensor orientations than those of the competing methods(Fig. 4).

The examination of alignment of the WM structure demonstrated that using RDG method improved the accuracy in every dataset (Fig.5). The RDG method yielded the most accurate results in the comparison of distance between the fiber bundles in the individual CCs from the 5 warped datasets and that of the CC from the template (Fig. 6). Moreover, the overall topology of the recovered fiber bundles generated using RDG appeared to be the most similar one to those reconstructed from the template (Fig. 5E), preserving similar branches and twigs with similar thickness.

5   Discussion

We have proposed a method for warping DTI dataset that directly reconstructs tensors in template space using warped DWI data with reconstructed gradient direction at each voxel. More importantly, the reconstruction of the gradient directions is implemented based on a novel strategy that employs a single backward DF. Therefore, our DTI warping and normalization framework is capable of using a single backward DF to efficiently warp tensor fields with the tensors correctly adjusted to the truth in a deformed space. This mechanism had never been possible in the past, due to the intrinsic constrains that inherited in the process of warping DTI datasets. We evaluated

the performance of our RDG method against other popular methods using both synthetic and real DTI data and found that the RDG method offers best improvement in
aligning WM structures.

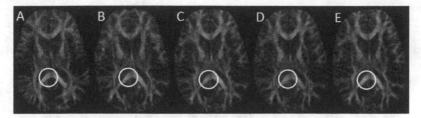

Fig. 4. A visual comparison of the color-encoded fractional anisotropy (FA) map from one
typical dataset normalized to the template. (A) The template; (B) The normalized result using
the NR method; (C) The normalized result using the PPD method; (D) The normalized result
using the SW method; (E) The normalized result using our RDG method. Our method had
better alignment of white mater tracts with the template and also achieved a smoother result
comparing with other methods. Note particularly the difference highlighted in the white circles
around the splenium region where it showed the result using our RDG method best matched the
template.

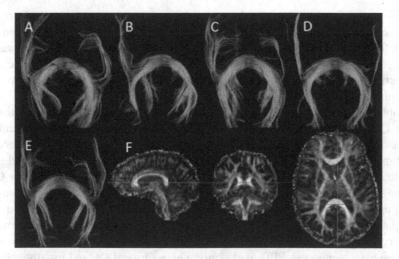

Fig. 5. A typical example demonstrating the comparison of tensor reorientation. A: the fiber
bundle in the template dataset; B-E: the fiber bundle from the NR, PPD, SW and RDG; F: the
central seed in the volume ($10 \times 10 \times 10$ pixel^3). Note that the fiber bundle from our method had
the highest similarity with the fiber bundle in the template data.

The key of our RDG method is the reconstruction of the gradient direction in a
voxel-wise manner, it therefore works directly on raw DWI data instead of the reconstructed tensors. Although working in this way requires all DWI data need to be preserved, it avoids errors in estimating the tensors in the original space to be propagated
to the template space in the warping process. In particular, warping a tensor field

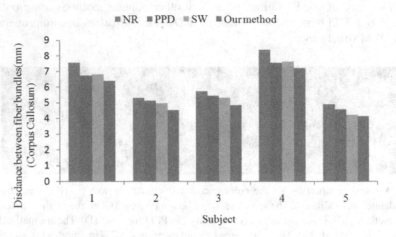

Fig. 6. The statistical comparison fiber alignment based on fiber tracts tracked using ROI defined at the splenium of corpus callosum. The statistics was generated from the results of five warped subjects (the horizontal axis), normalized to the template space using different methods for tensor reorientation.

requires special considerations on how to calculate a tensor at a non-grid point, as tensors are not defined in a regular Cartesian space. Our method is free from such worries. This may be one of the reasons that account for the improvement of warping accuracy offered by our RDG method. However, this advantage is at the price of reconstructing and maintaining an individual gradient table for every individual voxel in the template space.

Notably, the RDG method is capable of processing data acquired using either the DTI or QBI model. Once the individual DWI volumes are warped to the template space and the gradient tables associated with the DWI voxels are reconstructed, we can estimate tensors using conventional DTI model or ODFs using QBI model in the template space, achieving the same effect of warping the estimated tensors or ODFs from the individual space to the template space. This RDG method thus has provided also an approach for warping QBI data, which was a challenging task. Note that the PPD approach also works for reconstruction of gradient directions by estimating the necessary component of rotation using either DTI and QBI data[10, 11]. However, just as we have mentioned, PPD works only with a forward DF and usually generates seams in the warped results, which may significantly degrade the quality of the warped images[5]. Moreover, the PPD approach is also sensitive to noise while DTI data are always quite noisy. In contrast, our method uses backward DF and directly estimates the gradient vectors based on the backward DF without the complex computation of rotation matrix.

In our experiments, we found that FA values were generally decreased in the results warped to the template space. Because the warping procedure involves an interpolation for the DWI data, the DF and consequently also the gradient directions, smoothing effects are thus unavoidable. We adopted a straightforward strategy of trilinear interpolation. More accurate strategies, for example, 3D interpolations, perhaps can help to reduce the smoothing effects thus introduced in the warping procedure using backward DF. Our future work will need to carefully evaluate the available interpolation strategies, and find the one best suitable for our purpose by inspecting the dependency of our method on these interpolation strategies.

On the other hand, our method requires reconstruction of the warped tensor field in the template space using warped DWI data and gradient directions that are reconstructed in the template space. However, the nonlinear deformation that normalizes the image from the subject space to the template space T also deforms the sampling schema, making an optimal one no longer optimal in T when the data need to be reconstructed. That is to say, although the gradient table in the raw data space are noncollinear and optimal, the new gradient table thus reconstructed in the template space may probably no longer optimal. Moreover, although the DWI data were sampled on an optimal lattice in the original space, warped DWI data in T are transferred and sampled from the original space relying on a deformed sampling schema defined by the nonlinear DF. This could be another reason why we observed general decreases in FA values.

Acknowledgement. This research was supported in part by grants from Shanghai Commission of Science and Technology Grant # 10440710200, NIBIB Grant 1R03EB008235-01A1, NIMH Grant 5R01MH082255-03, NIEHS Grant 1 R01 ES01557901 A2/ A2S109. China National 985 Program, , Shanghai Key Laboratory of MR, Open Project Grant Support , two Grants from East China Normal University School of Psychology & Cognitive Neuroscience.

Reference

1. Basser, P.J., Mattiello, J., LeBihan, D.: MR diffusion tensor spectroscopy and imaging. Biophysical Journal 66, 259–267 (1994)
2. Alexander, D.C., Pierpaoli, C., Basser, P.J., Gee, J.C.: Spatial transformations of diffusion tensor magnetic resonance images. IEEE Transactions on Medical Imaging 20, 1131–1139 (2001)
3. Yeo, B.T., Vercauteren, T., Fillard, P., Peyrat, J.M., Pennec, X., Golland, P., Ayache, N., Clatz, O.: DT-REFinD: diffusion tensor registration with exact finite-strain differential. IEEE Transactions on Medical Imaging 28, 1914–1928 (2009)
4. Zhang, H., Yushkevich, P.A., Alexander, D.C., Gee, J.C.: Deformable registration of diffusion tensor MR images with explicit orientation optimization. Medical Image Analysis 10, 764–785 (2006)
5. Xu, D., Hao, X., Bansal, R., Plessen, K.J., Peterson, B.S.: Seamless warping of diffusion tensor fields. IEEE Transactions on Medical Imaging 27, 285–299 (2008)
6. Frank, L.R.: Anisotropy in high angular resolution diffusion-weighted MRI. Magn. Reson. Med. 45, 935–939 (2001)
7. Tuch, D.S., Reese, T.G., Wiegell, M.R., Makris, N., Belliveau, J.W., Wedeen, V.J.: High angular resolution diffusion imaging reveals intravoxel white matter fiber heterogeneity. Magn. Reson. Med. 48, 577–582 (2002)
8. Descoteaux, M., Angelino, E., Fitzgibbons, S., Deriche, R.: Regularized, fast, and robust analytical Q-ball imaging. Magn. Reson. Med. 58, 497–510 (2007)

9. Descoteaux, M., Angelino, E., Fitzgibbons, S., Deriche, R.: Apparent diffusion coefficients from high angular resolution diffusion imaging: estimation and applications. Magn. Reson. Med. 56, 395–410 (2006)
10. Ingalhalikar, M.A., Magnotta, V.A., Kim, J., Alexander, A.L.: A comparative study of diffusion tensor field transformations. In: Proc. SPIE Medical Imaging 2011, vol. 7259, pp. 72591Y–72591Y-8 (2009)
11. Ingalhalikar., M.A.: Spatial normalization of diffusion models and tensor analysis. vol. Ph.D. University of Iowa (2009)
12. Ashburner, J., Friston, K.J.: Nonlinear spatial normalization using basis functions. Hum. Brain. Mapp. 7, 254–266 (1999)
13. Ashburner, J., Neelin, P., Collins, D.L., Evans, A., Friston, K.: Incorporating prior knowledge into image registration. NeuroImage 6, 344–352 (1997)
14. Shen, D.G.: Image registration by local histogram matching. Pattern Recognition 40, 1161–1172 (2007)
15. Shen, D.G., Davatzikos, C.: HAMMER: Hierarchical attribute matching mechanism for elastic registration. IEEE Transactions on Medical Imaging 21, 1421–1439 (2002)
16. Fletcher, R.: A modified Marquardt subroutine for nonlinear least squares. Harwell Report 6799 (1971)
17. Basser, P.J., Mattiello, J., LeBihan, D.: Estimation of the effective self-diffusion tensor from the NMR spin echo. J. Magn. Reson. B 103, 247–254 (1994)
18. Wang, Z., Vemuri, B.C., Chen, Y., Mareci, T.H.: A constrained variational principle for direct estimation and smoothing of the diffusion tensor field from complex DWI. IEEE Transactions on Medical Imaging 23, 930–939 (2004)
19. Christiansen, O., Lee, T.M., Lie, J., Sinha, U., Chan, T.F.: Total variation regularization of matrix-valued images. Int. J. Biomed. Imaging, 27432 (2007)
20. Alexander, D.C., Pierpaoli, C., Basser, P.J., Gee, J.C.: Techniques for spatial normalization of diffusion tensor images. In: Proc. SPIE Medical Imaging, vol. 3919, pp. 470–481 (2000)
21. Basser, P.J., Pajevic, S.: Statistical artifacts in diffusion tensor MRI (DT-MRI) caused by background noise. Magn. Reson. Med. 44, 41–50 (2000)
22. Hult, J.: A fourth-order Runge-Kutta in the interaction picture method for, simulating supercontinuum generation in optical fibers. Journal of Lightwave Technology 25, 3770–3775 (2007)

Automatic Population HARDI White Matter Tract Clustering by Label Fusion of Multiple Tract Atlases[*]

Yan Jin[1], Yonggang Shi[1], Liang Zhan[1], Junning Li[1], Greig I. de Zubicaray[2],
Katie L. McMahon[2], Nicholas G. Martin[3], Margaret J. Wright[3],
and Paul M. Thompson[1]

[1] Laboratory of Neuro Imaging, Department of Neurology, David Geffen School of Medicine,
University of California, Los Angeles, Los Angeles, CA 90095, USA
{yjin,yshi,lzhan,jli,thompson}@loni.ucla.edu
[2] University of Queensland, Brisbane St. Lucia, QLD 4072, Australia
{greig.dezubicaray,katie.mcmahon}@uq.edu.au
[3] Queensland Institute of Medical Research, Herston, QLD 4029, Australia
{nick.martin,margiew}@qimr.edu.au

Abstract. Automatic labeling of white matter fibres in diffusion-weighted brain
MRI is vital for comparing brain integrity and connectivity across populations,
but is challenging. Whole brain tractography generates a vast set of fibres
throughout the brain, but it is hard to cluster them into anatomically meaningful
tracts, due to wide individual variations in the trajectory and shape of white
matter pathways. We propose a novel automatic tract labeling algorithm that
fuses information from tractography and multiple hand-labeled fibre tract atlases. As streamline tractography can generate a large number of false positive fibres, we developed a top-down approach to extract tracts consistent with known
anatomy, based on a distance metric to multiple hand-labeled atlases. Clustering
results from different atlases were fused, using a multi-stage fusion scheme.
Our "label fusion" method reliably extracted the major tracts from 105-gradient
HARDI scans of 100 young normal adults.

1 Introduction

Diffusion tensor magnetic resonance imaging (DT-MRI) recovers the local profile of
water diffusion in tissues, yielding information on white matter (WM) integrity and
connectivity that is not available from standard anatomical MRI. Recently, DT-MRI
has been extended to more sophisticated models of the local diffusion process, such as
high angular resolution diffusion imaging (HARDI [1]) and diffusion spectrum imaging. These advances allow more accurate reconstruction of fibres that mix and cross.
WM fibres may be recovered using tractography methods that fit a path through the
directional diffusion data at each voxel. Due to its speed, the streamline technique has

---

[*] This study was supported by Grant RO1 HD050735 from the National Institutes of Health
(NIH) and Grant 496682 from the National Health and Medical Research Council (NHMRC),
Australia.

P.-T. Yap et al. (Eds.): MBIA 2012, LNCS 7509, pp. 147–156, 2012.
© Springer-Verlag Berlin Heidelberg 2012

been extensively used for whole-brain tractography. Streamline methods follow the principal eigenvector in DT-MRI [2] or the dominant directions extracted from orientation distribution functions (ODF) [1] in HARDI to trace out a fibre trajectory in 3D.

Clustering methods can group the fibres from tractography, enabling large population studies of disease and genetic effects on tract shapes, or tract integrity. Various approaches have been proposed for automatically clustering fibres. One simple strategy selects anatomically well-known WM tracts that are "seeded" in regions of interest (ROI) [3]. One problem with this approach is that ROIs either have to be manually drawn on the scans, or must heavily rely on accurate registration of the scans to a previously labeled atlas. Image quality inevitably affects streamline tractography results, so many propagated streamlines fall short of reaching the ROIs and may be incorrectly excluded from the resulting tracts.

A typical framework for fibre clustering defines a pairwise similarity/distance between each pair of fibres in a large set of candidate fibres, to group them into separate and distinct tracts. The resulting similarity matrix (that compares all fibres with all others) can serve as the input for standard clustering algorithms [4]. It is difficult for a user to specify the number of clusters or a threshold to decide when to stop merging or splitting clusters. Clustering results vary drastically when different numbers of clusters are chosen. Without any anatomical information to guide the clustering, tracts may not correspond to any anatomically familiar subdivisions. Some recent work [5-6] has addressed this problem by adding atlas information into the framework. However, whole-brain tractography typically produces 10,000-100,000 fibres per subject. These "bottom-up" methods (clustering individual fibres into larger and larger groups until major tracts are aggregated) can fail to filter out the large number of erroneous fibres generated by streamline methods.

To group fibres into coherent tracts that are consistently labeled across a population, a labeled training dataset (atlas) can be used. In traditional image segmentation, a deformable atlas may be used, in which an expertly labeled atlas is non-rigidly registered to the image to be segmented. The resulting deformation can then be used to transfer the training labels onto the test image. Recently, *label fusion* became popular for registration-based image segmentation [7-8]. Multiple atlases and registrations are used to transfer multiple training labels to the test subject space. The final labeling is obtained by applying a weighting strategy to the labels transferred from different atlases. Label fusion has two advantages: (1) large individual variations in anatomy can be better accommodated if one does not need to rely on a single atlas; (2) multiple registrations improve robustness against occasional registration failures, and non-global minima of the registration cost function.

Here we introduce a *multi-atlas label fusion* framework to automatically extract anatomically meaningful WM tracts. By organizing the results of whole-brain tractography into familiar and recognizable tracts, we provide a robust clustering of fibres for population studies. Based on the ROIs from a publicly available parcellated WM atlas [9], we first manually construct a number of WM fibre tract atlases, each consisting of a set of several major WM tracts. In contrast to prior "bottom-up" methods, we use the WM tracts in multiple hand-labeled atlases as prior anatomical information. Our "top-down" approach transfers tract labels by selecting only fibres that are similar to the corresponding tracts in the atlases, based on a similarity measure. This eliminates many false positive fibres that may be otherwise hidden in the ~100,000 fibres per subject produced by streamline tractography. Multiple atlases help to adapt to the variability of tract shapes in new subjects, and further reduce the number of outliers arising from registering a single atlas to diffusion images or to whole-brain tractography from a new subject. Finally, we use a multi-stage fusion scheme to fuse the clustered results obtained from individual atlases. A workflow diagram is shown in Figure 1. To test the robustness of our algorithm, we applied it to a population study over 100 HARDI datasets.

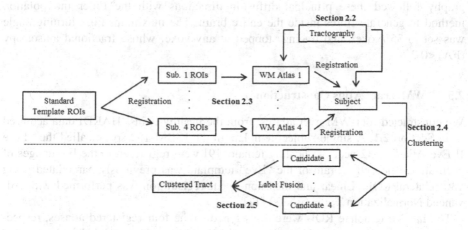

Fig. 1. A flow chart showing steps in our label fusion algorithm for clustering fibres

2   Label Fusion Clustering Framework

2.1   Data Acquisition

Our 100 subjects were selected from a much larger database of ~700 healthy young adult twins in their twenties from Australia. They were all right-handed. HARDI images were acquired with a 4-Tesla Bruker Medspec MRI scanner. Each 3D volume consisted of 55 2-mm axial slices and $1.79 \times 1.79 \text{mm}^2$ in-plane resolution with 128×128 acquisition matrix. 105 image volumes were acquired per subject: 11 with T2-weighted b0 images and 94 diffusion-weighted volumes (b = 1159 s/mm^2). We only used unrelated subjects in this analysis, leaving genetic analysis to future work.

2.2   Tractography

Raw HARDI images were corrected for eddy-current induced distortions with FSL (http://www.fmrib.ox.ac.uk/fsl/). We performed the whole-brain tractography with Camino (http://cmic.cs.ucl.ac.uk/camino/), an open source software package that uses both streamline and probabilistic algorithms to reconstruct fibre paths. The spherical harmonic (SH) representation provides faster ODF estimation, and is more robust to noise and arguably more accurate for detecting fibre crossings than the original numerical q-ball reconstruction method [10]. Explicitly, the SH basis may be expressed as follows: $Y_l^m(\theta, \varphi) = \sqrt{\frac{(2l+1)(l-m)!}{4\pi(l+m)!}} P_l^m(cos\theta)e^{im\varphi}$, where l denotes the order, m denotes the phase factor, $\theta \in [0, \pi]$, $\varphi \in [0, 2\pi]$, and P_l^m is an associated Legendre polynomial. Signal at each gradient direction may be approximated as a linear combination of a modified version of this SH basis. We used the 6th order (l=6) SH series to reconstruct ODFs for our HARDI data and a maximum of 3 local ODF maxima (where fibres mix or cross) were set to be detected at each voxel. Streamline tractography followed these principal diffusion directions with the Euler interpolation method to generate fibres inside the entire brain. The maximum fibre turning angle was set to 35°/voxel, and tracing stopped at any voxel whose fractional anisotropy (FA) <0.2.

2.3   WM Tract Atlas Construction

We constructed four WM tract atlases, from the healthy twins' HARDI data acquired as in **Section 2.1**. A single-subject template in the ICBM-152 space called the "Type II Eve Atlas" (a 32-year old healthy female) [9] were registered to the FA images of each atlas. The entire brain of the "Eve" template was previously parcellated using 130 bilateral ROIs. Linear and then non-linear registration was performed with Advanced Normalization Tools (ANTs) [11].

The labeled template ROIs were re-assigned to the four registered atlases, respectively, by warping them with the deformation fields generated by ANTs. Fibres that traversed the ROIs were extracted according to the lookup table in [12]. For example, the corticospinal tract was extracted from fibres passing between the precentral gyrus and the cerebral peduncle. Each tract was manually edited to remove visible outliers and to add any short fibres that incorrectly failed to reach the ROIs. Guevara *et al.* [13] used a single multi-subject atlas in their clustering algorithm. In principle, multiple atlases should be more robust to inaccuracies in registration.

Currently, each atlas is comprised of 13 major WM tracts: the left/right corticospinal tracts, left/right *cingulum*, left/right arcuate fasciculi (part of the superior longitudinal fasciculi), left/right inferior fronto-occipital/longitudinal fasciculi, and five segments of the corpus callosum – projecting to both frontal lobes, precentral gyri, postcentral gyri, superior parietal lobes, and the occipital lobes. We combined the inferior fronto-occipital fasciculus and inferior longitudinal fasciculus as one tract, as they had substantial overlap during manual atlas construction due to tractography and our image quality.

Figure 2 shows an example WM tract atlas that we created (*top, left side,* and *back* views).

2.4   Fibre Clustering

For each test subject (i.e., each new dataset to be labeled), whole-brain tractography was extracted using Camino as well. The same registration registered the subject's FA image to each of the four WM tract atlases' FA images, respectively. Each atlas's tracts were then warped to the subject space with the corresponding deformation fields generated from the FA registration. Ideally, an ODF-based registration method should be used to reorient the fibres between different spaces. However, such a registration scheme would have tremendous costs in terms of time (a few hours per registration) and computing resources if it were performed on a large-scale, as in the label fusion scheme. In contrast, FA registration only takes 5 minutes per registration on our datasets. Moreover, it has also been shown that fibre alignment is indeed improved significantly with that type of registration [14]. The use of multiple atlases also helps to reduce clustering errors due to imperfect registration.

We defined a fibre distance metric to decide the subject's fibres that should be included in any individual warped atlas tract, based on an empirical threshold obtained from our training data. For any pair of fibres γ_i and γ_j, we define the symmetric Hausdorff distance: $d_{\mathrm{H}}(\gamma_i,\gamma_j) = \max(d_{\mathrm{H'}}(\gamma_i,\gamma_j), d_{\mathrm{H'}}(\gamma_j,\gamma_i))$, where $d_{\mathrm{H'}}$ is the asymmetric Hausdorff distance. $d_{\mathrm{H'}}(\gamma_i,\gamma_j) = max_x\epsilon_{\gamma i}\, min_y\epsilon_{\gamma j}\, \|x - y\|$. $\|.\|$ is the Euclidean norm and the ordered pair (γ_i,γ_j) indicates an asymmetric distance from γ_i to γ_j. x's and y's are the coordinate points along fibres γ_i and γ_j, respectively [4].

For each fibre that belonged to a particular tract in an atlas, we computed the distance between this fibre and each fibre in the subjects' tractography that traversed within a neighborhood around the points along this atlas fibre. For a particular atlas, a group of the subject's fibres was identified as the clustering result for each atlas tract.

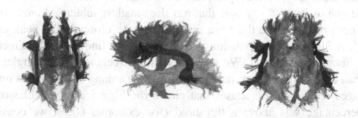

Fig. 2. A representative WM fibre atlas computed, and manually edited, from 4-Tesla 105-gradient HARDI data, showing major tracts. *Top*, *left side*, and *back* views are shown. Major tracts, distinguished in color, include the corticospinal tracts (*deep sky blue*), the cingulum on each side (*cyan*), arcuate fasciculi (*blue*), inferior fronto-occipital/longitudinal fasciculi (*green*), and multiple subdivisions of the corpus callosum (warm colors from *red* to *yellow*).

2.5   Multi-stage Label Fusion

To correctly fuse all the candidate fibres we obtained in **Section 2.4**, there are two pieces of information we need to consider: the position/geometric shape of the fibre, and the similarity between the atlases and the subject.

Majority Voting. We chose the Hausdorff distance metric in the fibre clustering phase because streamline tractography produces many false positives and this metric is relatively conservative in terms of including outliers. It will only pick streamlines with the similar geometric shapes that lie in the region where the particular atlas WM tract is located. However, due to the WM variability of individual atlases, they may nominate different candidates based on their own tract shapes. Majority voting, although it is probably the simplest label fusion method, has been proven to yield accurate segmentation results [15]. We decided that if a fibre appeared in at least 2 out of 4 individual clustering results, we considered it to be a true fibre that should be considered in the next step; otherwise, it was discarded.

Similarity of the Atlas to the Subject. The degree of correspondence between the atlas and the subject is another factor that should be taken into account. One way to measure it is to evaluate the registration quality locally along the candidate fibre. We first warped each candidate fibre that passed majority voting to the corresponding atlases (those who picked it out) with the inverse deformation fields generated by FA registration in Section 2.4. Then the angle between the fibre direction at each point on the warped fibre and the dominant direction of the ODF at the same point in the atlas was calculated. Camino uses the Euler method to interpolate fibre points. Therefore, the fibre direction is defined as: $(\vec{x}_{i+1}-\vec{x}_i)/\|\vec{x}_{i+1}-\vec{x}_i\|$, $i=1,\ldots,n-1$, where $\vec{x}_i$ is the point on the fibre, n is the number of points on the fibre, and $\|\cdot\|$ is the magnitude of the vector. The atlas ODF direction is the 3D linearly interpolated vector obtained through the closest ODF peak directions found in tractography at the 8 neighboring voxels. For each voxel, there may be multiple peak directions detected in tractography, so we picked the one or its 180° opposite that has the smallest subtended angle (that is, the largest inner product) from the fibre direction as the closest ODF peak direction at this voxel. A 3D linear interpolation was then used to find the ODF direction at the specified fibre point location. We calculated the percentage of the angles that were smaller than a threshold (for example, we used 25°) among all the points on that fibre and averaged it over all the atlases that chose the fibre for a particular tract. If the overall percentage was above a threshold (for example, 80%), we considered the overall registration quality to be good. The fibre picked out by those atlases was reliable and should be labeled as being part of that tract; otherwise, it was discarded. Figure 3 illustrates a good and a bad local registration based on our criterion.

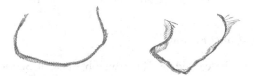

Fig. 3. This illustration shows the quality of the matching between the fibre direction of the subject and the local ODF principal direction of the atlas. A good match of a corpus callosum fibre is shown on the left and a poor match of another corpus callosum fibre is shown on the right (the fibre direction is in *red* and the ODF direction is in *green*).

3   Results

3.1   Automatic Clustering Results

Figure 4 shows how we obtain the left inferior fronto-occipital/longitudinal fasciculus (in *green*) in a test subject. The first row shows the four atlas versions of the tract. The second row shows the four different candidates for this tract in the same test subject, based on using each atlas to decide which fibres it should contain. We used the Hausdorff distance (see Section 2.4) with the threshold of 10mm to find potential fibre candidates. The final result for this tract was obtained by applying the label fusion scheme in Section 2.5. It is not hard to see that the label fusion process can help to eliminate outliers or add missing fibres in a single candidate. Figure 5 shows the label fusion results for the right cingulum (in *cyan*) in four *different* subjects. Despite individual variations, the overall tract shapes are consistent across the population. Figure 6 shows automatic WM fibre clustering results for two representative test subjects. Top, left side, and back views are shown. The types of tracts and their colors are as in Figure 1. The average fibre number in our clustering results is ~10,000 per subject, a 1 in 10 data reduction relative to the initial tractography.

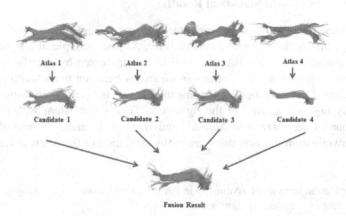

Fig. 4. Label fusion result for the left inferior fronto-occipital/longitudinal fasciculus (in *green*) in a test subject (viewed from the *left*)

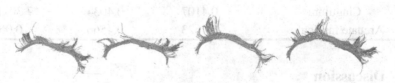

Fig. 5. Label fusion result for the right cingulum (in *cyan*) in four *different* subjects (viewed from the *left*)

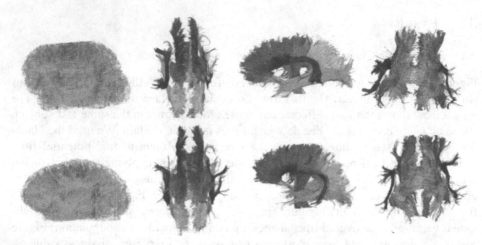

Fig. 6. Results of automatic fibre clustering, for two subjects. For the tract names and colors used to distinguish them, please see Fig. 1 (view from *top*, *left side*, and *back*, respectively). The leftmost column is the original whole-brain tractography, for comparison.

3.2   Population-Based Statistical Results

Many analyses are possible on these clustered tracts, for example, genetic analysis of fibre tract geometry, integrity, and connectivity. As one example of a typical application, we calculated the mean FA across all voxels traversed by specific tracts in 100 subjects, and tested for any differences in mean FA between the left and right hemispheres (Table 1). Interestingly, the mean FA of the left corticospinal tract is significantly higher than that of the right one. This is consistent with prior studies since all our subjects are right-handed, and there is a tendency towards a higher degree of myelination in tracts that control the right side of the body, at least in right-handers.

Table 1. Population analysis of asymmetry in FA for various tracts, in 100 subjects. * indicates that the difference is statistically significant.

Tract Name	Mean FA (Left/Right)		p-value
Corticospinal	0.4644	0.4528	$*1.15 \times 10^{-12}$
Inferior fronto-occipital	0.4501	0.4544	$*0.01$
Cingulum	0.4107	0.4034	$*7.30 \times 10^{-5}$
Arcuate fasciculus	0.4623	0.4566	0.06

4   Discussion

Multiple atlases were used in our framework to capture the individual variability of tract shapes. However, optimal selection of the number of atlases in label fusion is still an open question; for our application we will perform convergence tests once we have sufficient ground truth data. The focus of this paper is to show the benefit of using multi-atlases (Fig. 4). Based on our data, four atlases already offer a reasonable number of tracts to account for the WM shape variability in our sample, relative to the time needed to build atlases by hand.

We empirically decided on the Hausdorff threshold (Section 2.4), and the angle and the percentage (Section 2.5) as similarity metrics, to help recover similar numbers of fibres in the test subjects versus atlases, based on our training data. Quantitative analysis would be more convincing, but without having ground truth at the moment, a meaningful comparison is not easily achieved; currently, we are working on creating many hand labelled datasets to serve as ground truth.

Validation of any particular clustering of real fibre tract data is difficult, as there is no agreed ground truth on what fundamental elements the connectivity pattern contains. It is very difficult to validate clustering quantitatively except by careful visual inspection, as it is often clearer which fibres are false positives than true positives [4][6]. Clustering relies on fibres obtained from tractography, which is already tough to validate, except on phantoms, and phantoms may not be realistically complex. Comparing Dice coefficients between different approaches and hand-labeled tracts might be feasible and will be part of our future work, but is very time consuming. Instead, we show preliminary illustrations to indicate how label fusion can add missing fibres or delete obvious false positives, compared to a single atlas, in **Fig. 4**. We also used the FA statistics on the corticospinal tracts in **Section 3.2** to show that our method can pick up subtle known effects.

5   Conclusion

Here we presented an automatic fibre clustering pipeline that uses anatomical information from multiple manually made atlases. It can robustly segment the brain WM fibres into major tracts; we showed an illustrative example where we applied it to segment and cluster tracts in 100 subjects. The contribution of our work is to extend the well-established label fusion technique in atlas-based image segmentation to fibre clustering. This results in a powerful approach to large population studies in various neurological and psychiatric research fields, as well as in imaging genetics, where vast samples must be phenotyped to identify genes that affect brain integrity.

References

1. Tuch, D.S.: Q-Ball Imaging. Magn. Reson. Med. 52, 1358–1372 (2004)
2. Mori, S., Crain, B.J., Chacko, V.P., van Zijl, P.C.: Three-dimensional Tracking of Axonal Projections in the Brain by Magnetic Resonance Imaging. Ann. Neurol. 45, 265–269 (1999)
3. Wakana, S., Caprihan, A., Panzenboeck, M.M., Fallon, J.H., Perry, M., Gollub, R.L., Hua, K., Zhang, J., Jiang, H., Dubey, P., Blitz, A., van Zijl, P., Mori, S.: Reproducibility of Quantitative Tractography Methods Applied to Cerebral White Matter. NeuroImage 36, 630–644 (2007)

4. O'Donnell, L.J., Westin, C.F.: Automatic Tractography Segmentation using a High-dimensional White Matter Atlas. IEEE Trans. Med. Imag. 26, 1562–1575 (2007)
5. Maddah, M., Zöllei, L., Grimson, W.E., Westin, C.F., Wells, W.M.: A Mathematical Framework for Incorporating Anatomical Knowledge in DT-MRI Analysis. In: 5th IEEE ISBI, pp. 105–108 (2008)
6. Wassermann, D., Bloy, L., Kanterakis, E., Verma, R., Deriche, R.: Unsupervised White Matter Fibre Clustering and Tract Probability Map Generation. NeuroImage 51, 228–241 (2010)
7. Artaechevarria, X., Munoz-Barrutia, A., Ortiz-de-Solorzano, C.: Combination Strategies in Multi-Atlas Image Segmentation: Application to Brain MR Data. IEEE Trans. Med. Imag. 28, 1266–1277 (2009)
8. Sabuncu, M., Yeo, B.T., Van Leemput, K., Fischl, B., Golland, P.: A Generative Model for Image Segmentation Based on Label Fusion. IEEE Trans. Med. Imag. 29, 1714–1729 (2010)
9. Oishi, K., et al.: Atlas-based Whole Brain White Matter Analysis using Large Deformation Diffeomorphic Metric Mapping. NeuroImage 46, 486–499 (2009)
10. Descoteaux, M., Faria, A., Jiang, H., Li, X., Akhter, K., Zhang, J., Hsu, J.T., Miller, M.I., van Zijl, P.C., Albert, M., Lyketsos, C.G., Woods, R., Toga, A.W., Pike, G.B., Rosa-Neto, P., Evans, A., Mazziotta, J., Mori, S.: Regularized, Fast and Robust Analytical Q-ball Imaging. Magn. Reson. Med. 58, 497–510 (2007)
11. Avants, B.B., Tustison, N.J., Song, G., Cook, P.A., Klein, A., Gee, J.C.: A Repro-ducible Evaluation of ANTs Similarity Metric Performance in Brain Image Registration. NeuroImage 54, 2033–2044 (2011)
12. Zhang, Y., Zhang, J., Oishi, K., Faria, A.V., Jiang, H., Li, X., Akhter, K., Rosa-Neto, P., Pike, G.B., Evans, A., Toga, A.W., Woods, R., Mazziotta, J.C., Miller, M.I., van Zijl, P.C., Mori, S.: Atlas-Guided Tract Reconstruction for Automated and Comprehensive Examination of the White Matter Anatomy. NeuroImage 52, 1289–1301 (2010)
13. Guevara, P., Duclap, D., Poupon, C., Marrakchi-Kacem, L., Fillard, P., Le Bihan, D., Leboyer, M., Houenou, J., Mangin, J.F.: Automatic Fibre Bundle Segmentation in Massive Tractography Datasets using a Multi-subject Bundle Atlas. In: 14th MICCAI Workshop on CDMRI (2011)
14. Jin, Y., Shi, Y., Jahanshad, N., Aganj, I., Sapiro, G., Toga, A.W., Thompson, P.M.: 3D Elastic Registration Improves HARDI-derived Fibre Alignment and Automated Tract Clustering. In: 8th IEEE ISBI, pp. 822–826 (2011)
15. Rohlfing, T., Brandt, R., Menzel, R., Maurer Jr., C.R.: Evaluation of Atlas Selection Strate-gies for Atlas-based Imaging Segmentation with Application to Confocal Microsco-py Images of Bee Brains. NeuroImage 21, 1428–1442 (2004)

Comparative Characterisation of Susceptibility Weighted MRI for Brain White Matter Lesions in MS*

Maddalena Strumia[1], Constantin Anastasopoulos[2], Irina Mader[2],
Jürgen Henning[3], Li Bai[1], and Stathis Hadjidemetriou[3]

[1] School of Computer Science, University of Nottingham, UK
maddalena.strumia@nottingham.ac.uk
[2] Dep. of Neuroradiology, University Medical Centre Freiburg, Germany
[3] Dep. of Radiology, University Medical Centre Freiburg, Germany

Abstract. MR Images of the brain in Multiple Sclerosis (MS) show regions of signal abnormalities that can provide information for the diagnosis and for the pathogenesis of the disease. Two very commonly used MRI contrasts in this context are the T_1 weighted (T_1-w) and the FLAIR. This study shows that additional information can be extracted from the Susceptibility Weighted MRI (SWI) contrast. In particular, the signal and the contrast of white matter lesions in SWI are examined and compared to T_1-w and FLAIR contrasts. The lesions are analysed into hypo- and hyper-intense. Additionally, the spatial distributions for the two lesion types are computed and summarised with their expected distance from the ventricles. The data from 19 MS patients and 23 controls have been acquired and examined. The results show the presence of two lesion classes in SWI for MS patients, while T_1-w and FLAIR contrast mechanisms present only a single class each. The hypo-intense SWI lesions appear closer to the ventricles and are more correlated to the T_1-w signal rather than the FLAIR signal.

Keywords: Multiple Sclerosis, white matter lesions, brain MRI, Susceptibility Weighted MRI.

1 Introduction

Multiple Sclerosis (MS) is an inflammatory demyelinating disease of the central nervous system and its main hallmarks are demyelination plaques, inflammation, axonal damage, edema, and atrophy [10]. The pathogenesis of the lesions is still unclear and one of the most challenging aspects of the disease remains the understanding of the nature and mechanisms of tissue injury. MS pathology shows a typical spatial pattern of abnormalities in the MR signal of the White

---

* We acknowledge the funding support of the European Commission through the MIBISOC project (Marie Curie Initial Training Network, FP7 PEOPLE-ITN-2008, GA n. 238819).

P.-T. Yap et al. (Eds.): MBIA 2012, LNCS 7509, pp. 157–166, 2012.

Matter (WM), which is routinely used for disease diagnosis and to monitor the evolution of the lesions along time.

The T_2 weighted (T_2-w) MRI contrast is highly sensitive and the appearance of the hyper-intensities in the WM can correspond to a wide spectrum of pathologies ranging from edema and mild demyelination to necrosis. The FLAIR (Fluid Attenuated Inversion Recovery) sequence that is based on the T_2-w contrast together with water suppression is extensively used for imaging of brain lesions especially those surrounding the ventricles and proximal to the cortex. The T_1 weighted (T_1-w) contrast is less sensitive to the presence of lesions compared to the T_2-w contrast, but it is more specific to their clinical severity [9]. The SWI contrast is very sensitive to the presence of paramagnetic iron components. Thus, it can be used for lesion characterisation in relation to the vasculature. This information can help to better understand the connection between the pathogenesis of the disease and microvasculature abnormalities.

The role of vascular pathology in MS has been examined in various studies [1,5,6,8,11]. In [5] the authors have visually compared and classified the appearance of the lesions in different MRI contrasts acquired at different field strengths. Lesions are classified based on the MR sequence in which they appear, their contrast, and their spatial pattern. Similarly the WM lesions have been classified by visual observation in terms of their contrast with the surrounding normal appearing WM and with the rim around them [11]. That study also includes a postmortem analysis on a patient to correlate myelin in histological findings with the SWI signal.

This work considers a statistical investigation of the intensity and the contrast information of WM lesions in SWI alone as well as in comparison with the more commonly used T_1-w and FLAIR. The joint statistics of SWI and FLAIR as well as of SWI and T_1-w are computed to analyse the dependency between different contrasts. Also, an internal and a centre-surround contrast measure is defined, and the latter distinguishes the lesions into two classes. Atlases of different lesion types for the case of SWI are computed and their relation to the ventricles is examined.

2   Method

2.1   Patient Description and MR Imaging Protocol

In this study 19 chronic MS patients (11 women and 8 men; mean age 37.2 years; age range 28-55) and 23 controls (14 women and 9 men; mean age 27.2 years; age range 23-32) were included. The study was approved by the local review board and both patients and volunteers provided informed consent. The images were acquired with a 3T Siemens Trio MRI system equipped with head coils. The acquisition protocol consisted of a 3D T_1-w, FLAIR and SWI sequences. The T_1-w sequence gives a matrix of size $512 \times 512 \times 160$ with a voxel of size $0.5 \times 0.5 \times 1mm^3$ to provide an image $I_{T1} : \mathbf{x} \to [0...N\text{-}1]$, where $\mathbf{x} = (x, y, z)$ defines a voxel location in 3D space, and N is the number of intensity levels. The FLAIR sequence gives a matrix of size $512 \times 512 \times 176$ with a voxel of size $0.49 \times 0.49 \times 1mm^3$ to provide an image $I_{FLAIR} : \mathbf{x} \rightarrow [0...N\text{-}1]$. Finally, the SWI sequence gives a matrix of size $240 \times 320 \times 72$ with a voxel of size $0.72 \times 0.72 \times 1.2mm^3$ to provide an image $I_{SWI} : \mathbf{x} \rightarrow [0...N\text{-}1]$.

2.2   Image Pre-processing

The intensity inhomogeneity resulting from the use of the head coils has been restored jointly for the I_{T_1} and I_{FLAIR} with the intensity co-occurrence method [7]. This is followed by an intra-patient rigid co-registration performed with SPM8 [4]. The images of each patient $p = 0, ..., P\text{-}1$, where P is the number of patients, are rigidly registered within the subject by estimating the transformation $\mathcal{T}_{R,1}$ between I_{T_1} and I_{FLAIR} and $\mathcal{T}_{R,2}$ between I_{T_1} and I_{SWI}. The I_{T1} image is the reference, the nearest neighbour interpolation is used and the distance metric is the normalised mutual information. Then, an inter-patient spatial normalisation with reference the space of the I_{T1} in MNI [2] is performed with an affine registration $\mathcal{T}_{A,p}$:

$$I_p' = \mathcal{T}_{A,p}^{-1} \cdot \mathcal{T}_{R,i,p}^{-1} I_p,$$

where $I \in \{I_{T1}, I_{FLAIR}, I_{SWI}\}$, $i = 1$ for I_{FLAIR}, $i = 2$ for I_{SWI}, and $\mathcal{T}_{R,0,p}^{-1}$ is the identity transformation for I_{T1}. The spatially normalised images are used to analyse the WM lesion signal and WM lesion contrast within an image, within all subject data, and across all subjects.

Finally, tissue segmentation into Grey Matter (GM), White Matter (WM), and Cerebrospinal Fluid (CSF) is estimated based on I_{T1} with SPM8. This tool is not directly able to identify WM lesions and classifies them as GM due to the intensity range they occupy. However, the WM region provided can be assumed to be a reference for the normal appearing WM (NAWM) region in the I_{T1} image.

2.3   Joint Distribution between Images of Different Contrasts

The 2D joint statistics of the I_{SWI} with the I_{FLAIR} as well as of the I_{SWI} with the I_{T1} are computed over the regions of the lesions. The joint statistics are assumed to be a density and their covariance matrix is estimated. The eccentricity of the resulting ellipse is calculated as the ratio of the distance between the foci and the major axis length.

2.4   Definition of Lesion Contrast Measures in MR Images

In all patients and controls the WM lesions are manually annotated in I_{FLAIR} by an expert physician providing a binary lesion map $I_{LM,FLAIR}$. The $I_{LM,FLAIR}$ is projected to the I_{T1} and all the voxels that lie on NAWM I_{T1} tissue are removed from the binary lesion map to give rise to a second binary lesion map over I_{T1}, $I_{LM,T1}$.

The lesions are characterised in terms of their statistics. The histogram of the intensities over the domain of lesion l, $\forall l$, appearing in an image I is formulated as: $h_l(i) = \int_{I^{-1}(i) \cap l} d\mathbf{x}$ where $i \in [0...N\text{-}1]$. The mean value of the lesion intensities is computed as:

$$\mu_l = \frac{\int i h_l(i) di}{\int h_l(i) di},$$

and similarly for the standard deviation σ_l. The cumulative histogram of h_i is:

$$\mathcal{H}_l(i) = \int_0^i h_l(i') di'.$$

The dynamic range of the intensities in $\mathcal{H}_l$ is considered normalised to the range [0...1].

An internal and a centre-surround contrast measures are defined. The domain of the lesions can be $I_{LM,T1}$ or $I_{LM,FLAIR}$. The first measure is the *internal lesion contrast*, C_{Int}, to represent the variation of the intensities within a lesion. The 5% and 95% percentile of $\mathcal{H}_l$ are selected for noise robustness and to provide the internal lesion contrast as:

$$C_{Int} = \frac{\mathcal{H}_l(0.95) - \mathcal{H}_l(0.05)}{\sigma_s},$$

where σ_s is the standard deviation of the intensities in the region surrounding the lesion. The surrounding region is computed as a rim adjoining the lesion with volume equal to half of the lesion volume. The second measure is the *centre-surround lesion contrast*, C_{CS}, that compares the intensities within lesions with the intensities of the NAWM surrounding it. The cumulative histogram over the surrounding NAWM, $\mathcal{H}_s$, is also computed. The C_{CS} measure is represented by:

$$C_{CS} = \frac{\mathcal{H}_l(0.5) - \mathcal{H}_s(0.5)}{0.5 \times (\sigma_l + \sigma_s)},$$

where σ_l is the standard deviation of the intensities over the lesion, and $\mathcal{H}(0.5)$ is the median of the intensities. The C_{CS} measure is used to classify the lesions as hypo-intense when $C_{CS} \leq 0$ and as hyper-intense when $C_{CS} > 0$.

Typical examples of the appearance of lesions in two axial slices of I_{SWI}, I_{T1}, and I_{FLAIR} with both a hyper-intense (enclosed in a red circle) and a hypo-intense (enclosed in a blue circle) lesion is shown in figure 1. In this figure both lesions are hyper-intense in I_{FLAIR}, both are hypo-intense in I_{T1}, and in I_{SWI} they belong to different classes. In the following we will investigate the classification in images of all contrasts.

2.5   Atlases of Hypo- and Hyper-Intense WM Lesions

The hypo- and hyper-intense WM lesions are identified and their atlases are computed showing their individual spatial distributions. The atlases are the average of the registered lesion maps of all patients, the hypo-intense lesions

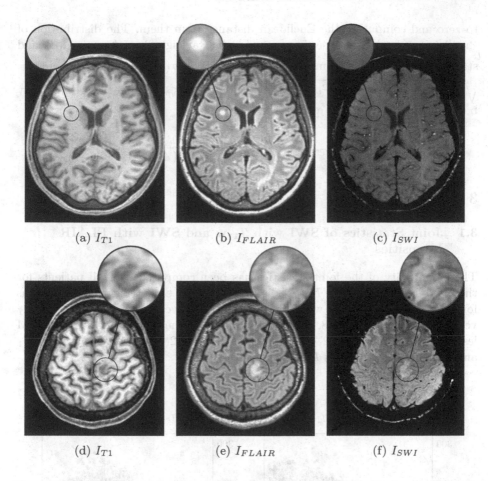

(a) I_{T1} (b) I_{FLAIR} (c) I_{SWI}

(d) I_{T1} (e) I_{FLAIR} (f) I_{SWI}

Fig. 1. Two axial slices of the same subject of I_{T1} in (a) and (d), of I_{FLAIR} in (b) and (e), and of I_{SWI} in (c) and (f). The red circle encloses a lesion that is hyper-intense in I_{SWI} (c) and the blue one encloses a lesion that is hypo-intense in I_{SWI} (f).

provide the hypo-intense atlas A_{hypo} and the hyper-intense lesions provide the hyper-intense atlas A_{hyper}. The intra- and inter-subject registration computed as described previously are used to place the WM lesion maps in the same anatomic space:

$$A = \frac{1}{P} \sum_{p=1}^{P} I'_{LM,p} = \frac{1}{P} \sum_{p=1}^{P} \mathcal{T}_{A,p}^{-1} \cdot \mathcal{T}_{R,i,p}^{-1} \cdot I_{LM,p},$$

where $A \in \{A_{hypo}, A_{hyper}\}$ and I_{LM} represents the domain of either the hypo- or the hyper-intense lesion maps in I_{SWI} respectively.

The two atlases are summarised with the expected distance of hyper- and hypo-intense lesions from the ventricles. The distance map $d(\mathbf{x})$ is computed over the brain region provided by MNI by fixing the regions occupied by the ventricles to zero and computing the Euclidean distance from them. The distribution of the distances for both atlases is assumed to be Rayleigh [3] with mean $\mu(d)$, and standard deviation $\sigma(d)$ computed as: $\mu(d) = \bar{\sigma}\sqrt{\frac{\pi}{2}}$, $\sigma(d) = \sqrt{\frac{4-\pi}{2}\bar{\sigma}^2}$, where $\bar{\sigma} = \sqrt{\frac{1}{2\int A(\mathbf{x})d\mathbf{x}}} \int (d(\mathbf{x}) \cdot A(\mathbf{x}))^2 d\mathbf{x}$ and $A \in \{A_{hypo}, A_{hyper}\}$. The discriminability between the two atlases is quantified as:

$$D_{hypo,hyper} = \frac{\mu(A_{hyper}) - \mu(A_{hypo})}{0.5 \cdot (\sigma(A_{hyper}) + \sigma(A_{hypo}))}.$$

3   Results

3.1   Joint Statistics of SWI with T_1-w and SWI with FLAIR Intensities

The eccentricity of the joint statistics has been computed over all patients for the hypo-intense lesions in I_{SWI}. The average of the eccentricity over all lesions for I_{SWI} versus I_{T1} is 0.81 which is larger than the average eccentricity for I_{SWI} versus I_{FLAIR} that is 0.78. A typical example of the joint statistics of a WM lesion are shown in figure 2, where the plot in figure 2(a) shows I_{SWI} versus I_{T1} and in figure 2(b) it shows I_{SWI} versus I_{FLAIR}.

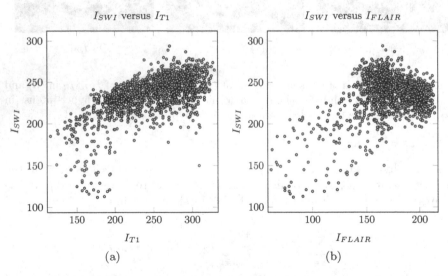

Fig. 2. The joint statistics for a typical hypo-intense I_{SWI} lesion over $I_{LM,T1}$ with I_{SWI} versus I_{T1} in (a), and I_{SWI} versus I_{FLAIR} in (b)

3.2 Statistical Analysis of Lesion Contrasts in SWI, T_1-w, and FLAIR

The C_{Int} and C_{CS} measures are computed for all the lesions in the patient data in the study both over $I_{LM,T1}$ and over $I_{LM,FLAIR}$. The graphs in figure 3 summarise the values of the two measures for different contrast images. The mean and the standard deviation over the subjects are computed for each lesion map $I_{LM} \in \{I_{LM,T1}, I_{LM,FLAIR}\}$ and for the image of every contrast $I \in \{I_{T1}, I_{FLAIR}, I_{SWI}\}$. The contrast measure $C \in \{C_{Int}, C_{CS}\}$ is defined as a function of both I_{LM} and I, the computation of the mean is given by $\mu_C = \frac{1}{P} \sum_{p=1}^{P} C(I_{LM,p}, I_p)$. The σ_C is computed similarly.

The C_{Int} measure assumes similar values over both lesion maps for all the contrast images. The C_{CS} measure presents some differences. The I_{T1} assumes a larger negative value when using its own lesion map. The contrast of I_{SWI} is greater over the $I_{LM,T1}$ map, $C_{CS}(I_{LM,T1}, I_{SWI})$, rather than over the $I_{LM,FLAIR}$ map, $C_{CS}(I_{LM,FLAIR}, I_{SWI})$. In the following, the statistical analysis is performed for contrasts defined over $I_{LM,T1}$.

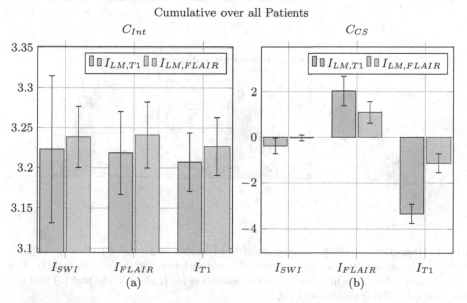

Fig. 3. In (a) are the comparative statistics for the C_{Int} measure and in (b) for the C_{CS} measure. In blue the results using $I_{LM,T1}$ and in red for $I_{LM,FLAIR}$. The bars represent the mean values while the error bars represent the standard deviation. To be noticed the larger negative value of the C_{CS} measure in I_{SWI} when calculated over $I_{LM,T1}$.

In figure 4 the histograms of the C_{CS} measures are presented in more detail highlighting a typical patient in figure 4(a-c) and for the cumulative histograms over all patient data in figure 4(d-f). The computation of C_{CS} for the images of all three contrasts shows the presence of both hypo- and hyper-intense lesions in I_{SWI}, only hypo-intense lesions in I_{T1}, and only hyper-intense lesions in I_{FLAIR}.

The normal control data investigated in this work have a small number of lesions in $I_{LM,FLAIR}$ and the majority of these lesions are NAWM in $I_{LM,T1}$. The C_{Int} and C_{CS} measures have been computed for I_{SWI}, I_{FLAIR} and I_{T1} for both lesions maps. A notable outcome is that the computation of the C_{CS} measure in normals over I_{SWI} results in only hyper-intense WM lesions.

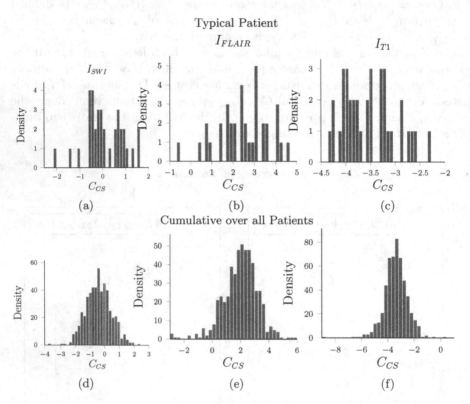

Fig. 4. Histograms of the C_{CS} measure of WM lesions of a typical patient in (a),(b), and (c). The cumulative histograms over all patients lesions are in (d),(e), and (f). The first column is for I_{SWI} in (a) and (d), the second is for I_{FLAIR} in (b) and (e) and the last column is for I_{T1} in (c) and (f).

3.3 Atlases of Hypo-Intense and Hyper-Intense WM Lesions in SWI

An atlas is computed for each of the hyper- and the hypo-intense lesions in I_{SWI}. In figure 5 a 3D surface rendering of both atlases is presented with an I_{T1} mid-sagittal slice in figure 5(a) and an I_{T1} mid-axial slice in figure 5(b). The results show that the hypo-intense lesions are on average closer to the ventricles compared to the hyper-intense lesions. The presence of intralesional-traversing veins could partially explain this periventricular accumulation of the dark appearing lesions in I_{SWI}. This is also shown by the lower range of distances occupied by the hypo-intense lesions, $16.2 \pm 8.4mm$, compared to the range occupied by the hyper-intense lesions, $19.7 \pm 10.2mm$. The results show that the hyper-intense lesions extend to regions farther from the ventricles compared to the hypo-intense lesions. The $D_{hypo,hyper}$ assumes a value of 0.36 since for the chronic patients considered in this study the hypo-intense periventricular lesions are more developed and thus cover a more extensive area.

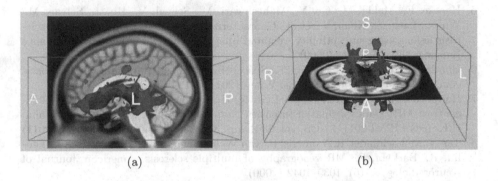

(a)   (b)

Fig. 5. A 3D surface rendering of the ventricles in gray, surrounded by A_{hypo} in blue and A_{hyper} in red with the mid-sagittal I_{T1} slice in (a) and the mid-axial I_{T1} slice in (b)

4   Discussion and Conclusion

This study analyses the brain WM lesions based on their appearance in an I_{SWI} image as hypo-intense and as hyper-intense. A higher eccentricity for hypo-intense lesion intensities has been found for I_{SWI} versus I_{T1} compared to I_{SWI} versus I_{FLAIR}, suggesting a relation closer to linear between the SWI and the T_1-w imaging contrasts. The centre-surround contrast measure C_{CS} provides more information about the lesions compared to C_{Int}. The statistical properties and the spatial distribution of the hypo- and hyper-intense groups have been elaborated. The hypo-intense lesions tend to surround the ventricles compared to the hyper-intense ones which can extend even farther closer to the cortex. This may also be related to the staging of the disease.

Initial results over control data show that in I_{SWI} there are only hyper-intense lesions suggesting that they are less severe [5]. The classification of the lesions can be improved by generalising the definition of the measures and by including possible iso-intensities. Statistical measures for the co-localization between venous vasculature and lesion type can also improve the understanding of the role of vascular abnormalities in the pathogenesis of the disease.

References

1. Dawson, J.: The histology of disseminated sclerosis. Trans. Roy. Soc. Edinb. 50, 517 (1916)
2. Evans, A., Collins, D., Mills, S., Brown, E., Kelly, R., Peters, T.: 3D statistical neuroanatomical models from 305 MRI volumes. In: Conference Record of Nuclear Science Symposium and Medical Imaging Conference, pp. 1813–1817. IEEE (1993)
3. Forbes, C., Evans, M., Hastings, N., Peacock, B.: Statistical distributions. Wiley Online Library (2011)
4. Friston, K.: Statistical parametric mapping: the analysis of functional brain images. Academic Press (2007)
5. Haacke, E., Makki, M., Ge, Y., Maheshwari, M., Sehgal, V., Hu, J., Selvan, M., Wu, Z., Latif, Z., Xuan, Y., et al.: Characterizing iron deposition in multiple sclerosis lesions using susceptibility weighted imaging. Journal of Magnetic Resonance Imaging 29(3), 537–544 (2009)
6. Haacke, E., Reichenbach, J., Xu, Y.: Susceptibility weighted imaging in MRI: basic concepts and clinical applications. Wiley (2011)
7. Hadjidemetriou, S., Buechert, M., Ludwig, U., Hennig, J.: Joint Restoration of Bi-contrast MRI Data for Spatial Intensity Non-uniformities. In: Székely, G., Hahn, H.K. (eds.) IPMI 2011. LNCS, vol. 6801, pp. 346–358. Springer, Heidelberg (2011)
8. Tan, I., van Schijndel, R., Pouwels, P., van Waldervenn, M., Reichenbach, J., Manoliu, R., Barkhof, F.: MR venography of multiple sclerosis. American Journal of Neuroradiology 21(6), 1039–1042 (2000)
9. Walderveen, M., Kamphorst, W., Scheltens, P.: Histopathologic correlate of hypo intense lesions in T1-weighted spin-echo MRI in multiple sclerosis. Neurology 50, 1282–1288 (1998)
10. Weinshenker, B., Bass, B., Rice, G., Noseworthy, J., Carriere, W., Baskerville, J., Ebers, G.: The natural history of multiple sclerosis: a geographically based study. Brain 112(1), 133–146 (1989)
11. Yao, B., Bagnato, F., Matsuura, E., Merkle, H., van Gelderen, P., Cantor, F., Duyn, J.: Chronic multiple sclerosis lesions: Characterization with high-field-strength MR imaging. Radiology 262(1), 206–215 (2012)

Constructing Fiber Atlases for Functional ROIs
via fMRI-Guided DTI Image Registration

Tuo Zhang[1,2], Lei Guo[1], Hanbo Chen[2], Xintao Hu[1], Kaiming Li[3], and Tianming Liu[2]

[1] School of Automation, Northwestern Polytechnical University, Xi'an, China
[2] Department of Computer Science and Bioimaging Research Center,
The University of Georgia, Athens, GA
[3] Department of Biomedical Engineering, Emory, GA

Abstract. Quantitative mapping of the relationship between brain structure and function has emerged as an active research field in order to answer the question of whether brain structure can predict its function. In the literature, it is widely believed that a brain region's structural connectivity pattern largely determines the function it performs. Based on this premise, we used multimodal diffusion tensor imaging (DTI) and task-based fMRI data to perform fMRI-guided DTI image registration and built structural fiber atlases for functional brain Regions of Interests (ROIs). First, we used working memory task-based fMRI-derived ROIs as the functional constraint to register DTI images into a template via an energy minimization procedure. Then, the regularity and variability of the warped white matter fibers for each ROI was quantitatively assessed, and it turns out that structural connection patterns for corresponding functional ROIs across different subjects are quite consistent. Therefore, we constructed the white matter fiber atlases for these functional ROIs, which can be used as intrinsic attributes of those ROIs for quantitative representation of cortical architecture. Our results provided evidence that there is deep-rooted regularity of the common human brain architecture and that structural connectivity is strongly correlated with brain function.

Keywords: DTI registration, functional constraint, fiber atlas.

1   Introduction

It is widely accepted that structural connection is a good predictor of a brain region's function [1, 2]. The basic premise is that each brain's cytoarchitectonic area has a unique set of extrinsic inputs and outputs called the 'connectional fingerprint' [1], and this unique set of brain connectivity patterns can be identified across subjects although certain degree of variability exists. In this paper, we attempt to construct a structural connectivity atlas for a functionally defined brain regions of interest (ROI) by using multimodal task-based fMRI and DTI data, the former of which provides benchmark functional ROIs and the latter of which provides structural connection information. In general, there are two critical requirements for building such an atlas. First, the atlas should reflect the regularity of the structural connectivity across

P.-T. Yap et al. (Eds.): MBIA 2012, LNCS 7509, pp. 167–174, 2012.

subjects; second, the atlas should be specifically labeled by brain function. To meet these two requirements, we propose a novel framework to apply functional constraints for deformable registration of DTI images. Specifically, task-based fMRI data was acquired to generate the functionally-defined ROIs. Then, they are integrated into the DTI registration process as functional constraint. The constrained registration is formulated and solved as an energy minimization procedure. Finally, consistent fiber bundles emanating from those ROIs are extracted to build the atlases.

Growing literature reports have shown that functionally-defined brain regions are not necessarily consistently located in relation to morphological landmarks on the cortex [3, 4, 5]. This issue has been recognized and several published studies have investigated the idea of incorporating functional information into anatomical alignment between subjects [6, 7, 8]. Closely related literature to this work includes DTI brain image registration [9, 10, 11] and cortical alignment based on functional constraints [6, 7]. The major contribution of this paper is that we used fMRI data to guide DTI image registration for the purpose of white matter fiber atlas construction, and achieved promising results.

2   Materials and Methods

The algorithmic pipeline is composed of three major steps (Fig. 1a). In the first step (green dashed box), we pre-processed individual subject's data including detection of functional ROIs from working memory task-based fMRI data and registration of fMRI and DTI data via the FSL FLIRT tool. DTI data was used as the standard space onto which functional ROIs were warped. In the second step (purple dashed box), we formulated the inter-subject DTI registration procedure as an energy minimization problem, in which the distance between tensor features and the distance between corresponding functional ROIs are defined as the similarity metrics. In the third step (red dashed box), the white matter fibers were extracted for the functional ROIs. After the assessment of regularity and variability of fiber tracts was performed, a probabilistic fiber atlas for each functional ROI was built.

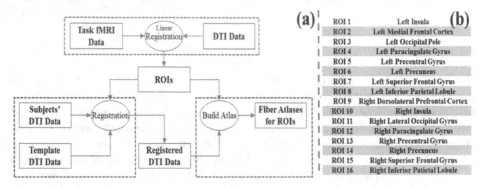

Fig. 1. (a) The flowchart of the algorithmic pipeline. The green, purple, and red boxes will be detailed in section 2.1, section 2.2, and section 2.3, respectively; (b) 16 working memory ROIs.

2.1   Data Acquisition and Pre-processing

Seventeen university students voluntarily participated in this study, and none of them were reported to have mental or physical disease. Each volunteer performed a modified version of the OSPAN task (3 blocks: OSPAN, Arithmetic and Baseline) while fMRI data was acquired [12]. DTI scans were also obtained for each volunteer. Both fMRI and DTI scans were acquired on a 3T GE Signa scanner with acquisition parameters as follows: fMRI: 64×64 matrix, 4mm slice thickness, 220mm FOV, 30 slices, TR = 1.5s, TE = 25ms, ASSET = 2; DTI: 128×128 matrix, 2mm slice thickness, 256mm FOV, 60 slices, TR = 15100ms, ASSET = 2, 3 B0 images, 30 optimized gradient directions, b-value = 1000.

Inputs to the individual subject preprocessing steps are task-based fMRI data and DTI data. Each volunteer's fMRI data of the OSPAN task was analyzed using the FSL FEAT. Individual activation map reflecting the OSPAN (complex span) contrast was identified. 16 highest activated ROIs were identified (Fig. 1b). The pre-processing of the DTI data is composed of brain skull removal and motion correction. Afterwards, the diffusion tensor is computed via the DTI Studio [14]. For each subject, the DTI space is used as the standard space [13], in which the gray matter (GM)/white matter (WM) surface is generated via a similar approach in [15] for visualization purpose. Co-registration between DTI and fMRI data is performed using the FSL FLIRT and the resulting global transform matrix is consequently applied to the activated ROIs to map them to the DTI space. In all of the experiments, one subject from the 17 candidates was randomly selected as the template, to which the other ones were registered using the following method.

2.2   DTI Registration with Functional Constraint

Let I_1 and I_2 be a pair of images to be registered, and U be the deformation field that warps voxel v in I_1 to I_2, and the warped location is denoted as $U(v)$. The goal of registration is to deform the DTI images of an individual subject to the template using an attribute matching method similar to that in [10], and meanwhile to ensure the locations of corresponding functional landmarks are close. Mathematically, the registration procedure is formulated as a problem of minimizing an energy function defined as:

$$E(U) = w_{ten}E_{ten}(U) + w_{func}E_{func}(U) \tag{1}$$

where $E_{ten}(U)$ and $E_{func}(U)$ are tensor distance term and functional constraint term respectively, and w_{ten} and w_{func} are weights of the two energy terms. $E_{ten}(U)$ requires that the features extracted from voxel v in the subject should be similar to that of its deformed counterpart $U(v)$ in the template. It can be mathematically defined as:

$$E_{ten}(U) = \sum_{v \in D} dist_1(f(v), f(U(v))) \tag{2}$$

where $f(\cdot)$ denotes the attribute vector of a voxel. $dist_1(\cdot, \cdot)$ measures the distance of two features. D denotes the entire set of voxels in the subject. In this paper, $f(\cdot)$ is defined as the geometry and orientation of diffusion tensors similar to that in [10].

E_{func} is designed to prevent the corresponding functional ROIs in the subject and template from being deformed far away from each other. For each of the 16 ROIs identified in section 2.1, we had a unique label to identify it across subjects. Currently, for each ROI, only the highest activated voxel was adopted. Let R denote the set of ROI voxels in the subjects and $C(\cdot)$ be the corresponding set of ROI voxels in the template. We defined $dist_2(\cdot,\cdot)$ to measure the Euclidean distance between the corresponding ROI voxels. The mathematical expression of the term is as follow:

$$E_{func}(U) = \sum_{v \in R} dist_2(C(v), U(v))$$

(3)

The functional constraint term in Eq. (3) was modeled according to the elastic deformation transformation (EDT) [16] to propagate the correspondences in Eq. (3) from functional ROIs to the whole image volume.

The energy function in Eq. (1) is minimized via a similar hierarchical scheme in HAMMER [17]. The resulted deformation field U is applied on the DTI image and the functional ROIs of subject to re-locate their positions. The white matter fibers are re-oriented via the approach in [10]. Moreover, because ROIs are relatively sparse voxels and the propagation of reliable correspondence of ROIs to the whole volume via EDT will benefit the framework by reducing the chance of being trapped in local minima.

2.3   Probabilistic Fiber Atlas Construction

The construction of fiber atlas, e.g., by the means of clustering [18] or by shape warping [19], might be affected by the variability of fiber bundles across individuals. Moreover, the regularity of the atlas can hardly be quantitatively measured by existing methods. In this section, we developed a simple and effective method to construct a probabilistic white matter fiber atlas for each ROI as illustrated in Fig. 2. Specifically, fiber tracts emanating from ROIs were firstly tracked and uniformly sampled using the constant-speed parameterization (Fig. 2a and Fig. 2b). Then, taking ROI j for example, fibers from all subjects were gathered in one set. As all the fibers were resampled into m points and the starting points were all located in the ROI regions, the atlas was defined as the one with m sequential probabilistic volume images. For each voxel in the $k^{th} \epsilon\ m$ volume image, the number of kth points of all the fibers passing through it was computed, and the accumulated number was normalized by

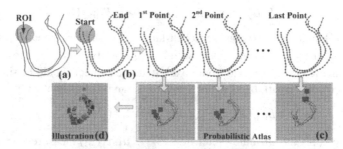

Fig. 2. Probabilistic fiber atlas construction. (a) Fiber tracking; (b) Fiber resampling; (c) Atlas construction; (d) Atlas for visualization.

dividing the total number of fibers (Fig. 2c). To measure how close a fiber bundle is to the atlas, we simply resampled each fiber tract into m points and map the kth points of all fiber tracts onto the kth sequential probabilistic volume atlas. The accumulated the value of all m points of all the fiber tracts is used as the measurement. For the purpose of visualization of the atlas, the m sequential probabilistic volume images were overlapped together as shown in Fig. 2d.

3   Experimental Results

3.1   DTI Registration with Functional Constraint

In order to verify the effects of the functional constraint for DTI registration, the final deformation field U generated by our method is applied on the ROIs to warp them into the template cortical surface. They are compared with results of linear (FSL FLIRT performed on FA images) and nonlinear (method in [10]) registration without functional constraint. A shown in Fig. 3a, by visual inspection, our method performs the best in terms of concentration of corresponding ROIs. Quantitatively, for each ROI, we computed the mean of distances between individual to the group center. The average distance by our method is 3.18 mm for all ROIs, which confirms that we achieved the objective in Eq. (3). In comparison, the average distance is much higher for the other two methods: 5.50 mm for FSL FLIRT and 4.72 mm for method in [10], suggesting the needs of using functional constraints in DTI image registration for atlas construction.

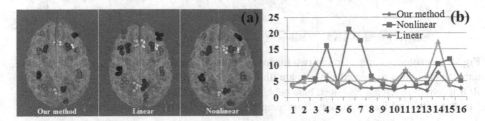

Fig. 3. (a) The 16 ROIs of 17 subjects warped in the template surface via three methods: our method (left), FSL FLIRT linear registration (middle) and nonlinear registration in [10] (right). The same ROIs are coded with the same color; (b) Mean Hausdorff metrics of each ROI for the three methods. ROIs are indexed on horizontal axis. The vertical axis is labeled with Hausdorff metric in mm unit.

3.2   Assessment of Fiber Bundle Regularity and Variability

We extracted fiber bundles from 16 ROIs and used the Hausdorff metric to measure the fiber bundle regularity and variability among subjects. Our rational is that the less variable of the fiber bundles are, the more suitable they can be used to construct atlases. The Hausdorff metric between two fiber bundles F_1 and F_2 is defined as:

$$Dist_H(F_1, F_2) = \max \left\{ sup_{f_i^1 \in F_1} \, inf_{f_i^2 \in F_2} \, d(f_i^1, f_i^2), sup_{f_i^2 \in F_1} \, inf_{f_i^1 \in F_2} \, d(f_i^1, f_i^2) \right\} \quad (4)$$

where $f_i^1 \in F_1(f_i^2 \in F_2)$ is a single fiber tract, sup represents the supremum, inf is the infimum, and $d(\cdot,\cdot)$ denotes the distance between two fiber curves, defined to be the minimum distance. The Hausdorff metric was computed between any two fiber bundles from the same ROI across subjects and the mean values for each ROI are shown in Fig. 3b, together with the ones via FSL FLIRT and nonlinear registration method in [10]. The average Hausdorff distance is 3.62 mm for our method, which is significantly better than the other two methods: 6.75 mm for FSL FLIRT and 8.21 mm for the method in [10]. This demonstrates that the fibers bundles are much more consistent across subjects by our method. The conclusion is more intuitively supported by visualizing the fiber bundles for two ROIs from three randomly selected subjects in Fig. 4.

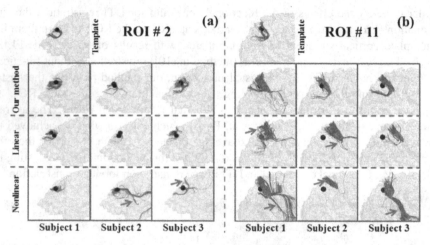

Fig. 4. Consistency comparison of two randomly selected bundles amongst three methods. The template and three registered subjects are illustrated. (a) ROI #2; (b) ROI #11. Black bubbles: ROI locations in template subject; blue bubbles: registered ROI locations by the three methods. Bundles with significant variations from templates are highlighted by green arrows.

3.3   Evaluation of Probabilistic Atlas

In section 3.2, the superiority of the method proposed in this paper is demonstrated both visually and numerically. The result suggests that the registered fiber bundles via our method are quite consistent with each other. Then, these fiber bundles are used to construct a fiber bundle atlas for each ROI via the approaches in section 2.3. The probabilistic atlases are visualized in Fig. 5a the same way as Fig. 2d. By visual inspection, the atlases are quite reasonable. To further prove the validity of the atlas, we adopted the leave-one-out strategy for cross-validation. Taking ROI j for example, the atlas is constructed on the corresponding fiber bundles from all subjects except subject i. Then, the atlas was mapped onto the entire fiber tracts of subject i, and only 5% of the fiber tracts with the highest probabilistic value were preserved. Finally, the Hausdorff metric is computed between the preserved fiber tracts and those extracted from ROI j of subject i.

We randomly selected seven subjects to conduct the leave-one-out test on all the 16 ROI fiber bundle atlases. Again, the FSL FLIRT linear registration and the method in [10] were used for comparisons. Fig. 5b shows the Hausdorff metric matrices, in which the element (i, j) denotes the Hausdorff metric for ROI j on the leave-one-out test of subject i. The mean values in the matrices are 5.05 *mm* (our method), 8.42 *mm* (FSL FLIRT linear registration), and 8.48 *mm* (nonlinear registration in [10]), respectively. It is evident that the method in this paper performs significantly better than the other two methods.

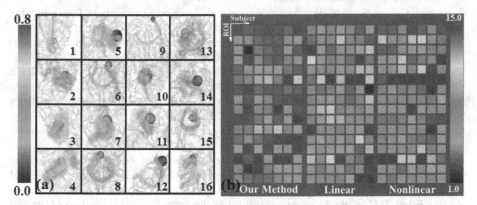

Fig. 5. (a) Probabilistic atlases of fiber bundles for 16 ROIs. To better visualize them, the probability is scaled in (0, 0.8). ROI bubbles are color coded the same way as that in Fig. 3a; (b) Comparison of the Hausdorff metric matrices in the leave-one-out test amongst the three methods.

4   Conclusion

In this paper, we presented a functionally-constrained DTI registration method, in which both functional correspondence and anatomical alignment are incorporated into an energy minimization framework. Also, we constructed probabilistic fiber bundle atlas for each of the aligned functional ROIs. Validation experiments were performed on both the registration result and the atlas construction result, and superiority of our method with functional constraint to others demonstrates the importance of applying functional principles for brain image registration and for statistical fiber atlas construction. Importantly, our results demonstrated that structural connection patterns of the corresponding functional ROIs are quite similar across different subjects, providing direct evidence to support the 'connectional fingerprint' hypothesis in [1]. Our results further suggest the close relationship between structural connectivity and brain function, which has deep-rooted regularity across different subjects despite the considerable variability.

Our future work will apply the developed fiber atlases of functional ROIs as prior knowledge for quantitative prediction of the corresponding ROIs in other subjects without fMRI data. This capability could facilitate numerous applications in quantitative assessment of brain connectivity in brain diseases that are associated with disruption of structural and functional connectivity.

Acknowledgement. Tuo Zhang is supported by Doctorate Foundation of Northwestern Polytechnic University and Chinese Government Scholarship and the China Government Scholarship.

References

1. Passingham, R.E., et al.: The anatomical basis of functional localization in the cortex. Nat. Rev. Neurosci. 3(8), 606–616 (2002)
2. Honey, C.J., et al.: Predicting human resting-state functional connectivity from structural connectivity. Proc. Natl. Acad. Sci. U S A 106(6), 2035–2040 (2009)
3. Rademacher, J., et al.: Topographical variation of the human primary cortices: implications for neuroimaging, brain mapping and neurobiology. Cereb Cortex 3(4), 313–329 (1993)
4. Dougherty, R.F., et al.: Visual field representations and locations of visual areas V1/2/3 in human visual cortex. J. Vis. 3(10), 586–598 (2003)
5. Li, K., et al.: Individualized ROI optimization via maximization of group-wise consistency of structural and functional profiles. In: NIPS (2010)
6. Sabuncu, M.R., et al.: Function-based intersubject alignment of human cortical anatomy. Cereb. Cortex 20(1), 130–140 (2010)
7. Yeo, B.T., et al.: Learning Task-Optimal Registration Cost Functions for Localizing Cytoarchitecture and Function in the Cerebral Cortex. In: IEEE TMI, pp. 1424–1441 (2010)
8. Van Essen, D.C., et al.: An integrated software suite for surface-based analyses of cerebral cortex. J. Am Med. Inform. Assoc. 8(5), 443–459 (2001)
9. Park, H.J., et al.: Spatial normalization of diffusion tensor MRI using multiple channels. Neuroimage 20(4), 1995–2009 (2003)
10. Yang, J.: Diffusion tensor image registration using tensor geometry and orientation features. Med. Image Comput. Comput. Assist. Interv. 11(Pt 2), 905–913 (2008)
11. Yap, P.T., et al.: TIMER: Tensor Image Morphing for Elastic Registration. Neuroimage 47(2), 549–563 (2009)
12. Anonymous
13. Li, K., et al.: Cortical surface based identification of brain networks using high spatial resolution resting state fMRI data. In: ISBI, pp. 656–659 (2010)
14. Jiang, H., et al.: DtiStudio: resource program for diffusion tensor computation and fiber bundle tracking. Comput Methods Programs Biomed. 81(2), 106–116 (2006)
15. Liu, T., et al.: Brain tissue segmentation based on DTI data. Neuroimage 38(1), 114–123 (2007)
16. Davatzikos, C., et al.: Image registration based on boundary mapping. IEEE Trans. Med. Imaging 15(1), 112–115 (1996)
17. Shen, D.: Image registration by local histogram matching. Pattern Recognition 40(4), 1161–1172 (2007)
18. O'Donnell, L., et al.: A high-dimensional fiber tract atlas. In: Proceedings of the ISMRM Annual Meeting (ISMRM 2006) (2006)
19. Corouge, I., Gouttard, S., Gerig, G.: A Statistical Shape Model of Individual Fiber Tracts Extracted from Diffusion Tensor MRI. In: Barillot, C., Haynor, D.R., Hellier, P. (eds.) MICCAI 2004. LNCS, vol. 3217, pp. 671–679. Springer, Heidelberg (2004)

Structural Feature Selection for Connectivity Network-Based MCI Diagnosis

Biao Jie[1,2], Daoqiang Zhang[1,2], Chong-Yaw Wee[2], and Dinggang Shen[2]

[1] Dept. of Computer Science and Engineering, Nanjing University of Aeronautics
and Astronautics, Nanjing 210016, China
[2] Dept. of Radiology and BRIC, University of North Carolina at Chapel Hill, NC 27599
{jbiao,dqzhang}@nuaa.edu.cn, dgshen@med.unc.edu

Abstract. Connectivity networks have been recently used for classification of neurodegenerative diseases, e.g., mild cognitive impairment (MCI). In typical connectivity network-based classification, features are often extracted from (multiple) connectivity networks and concatenated into a long vector for subsequent feature selection and classification. However, some useful network topological information may be lost in this type of approach. In this paper, we propose a new structural feature selection method which embeds the topological information of connectivity networks through graph kernel and then uses recursive feature elimination with graph kernel (RFE-GK) to select the most discriminative features. Furthermore, multiple kernel learning (MKL) is also adopted to combine multiple graph kernels for joint structural feature selection from multiple connectivity networks. The experimental results show the efficacy of our proposed method with comparison to the state-of-the-art method in MCI classification, based on the connectivity networks.

1 Introduction

Many methods have been developed for classification of Alzheimer's disease (AD) or its prodromal stage, i.e., mild cognitive impairment (MCI), based on either single or multiple modalities of biomarkers. Recently, connectivity networks have been used for diagnosis and classification of neurodegenerative diseases, e.g., schizophrenia and MCI [1, 2]. For example, Wee et al. proposed an effective network-based classification method to accurately identify MCI patients by using a collection of measures derived from white matter (WM) connectivity networks [1]. In their method, six types of connectivity networks as shown in Fig. 1 were first constructed from each subject by using six different physiological parameters, i.e., fiber count (FC), fractional anisotropy (FA), mean diffusivity (MD), and principal diffusivities (λ_1, λ_2, and λ_3), based on the parcellated 90 regions-of-interest (ROIs) of the brain, and then the clustering coefficient of each ROI in relation to the remaining ROIs is extracted from these connectivity networks as features for subsequent feature selection and classification.

In the conventional feature selection and classification methods, which solely rely on the feature vector obtained from previous feature extraction step (e.g., in [1]),

P.-T. Yap et al. (Eds.): MBIA 2012, LNCS 7509, pp. 175–184, 2012.

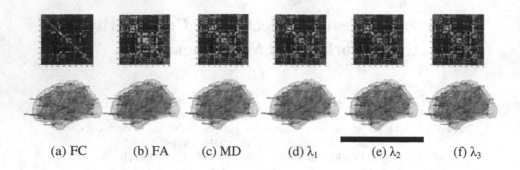

   (a) FC   (b) FA   (c) MD   (d) λ_1 (e) λ_2 (f) λ_3

Fig. 1. Six different connectivity matrices (networks) used in our structural feature selection method

some useful network topological information may be lost and thus the performance may be affected. In this paper, we address this problem by proposing a new structural feature selection method that preserves the network topological information to guide the feature selection. Specifically, graph kernel [3-5] is adopted to measure the topological similarity between a pair of graphs (i.e., connectivity networks) of individual subjects, and then support vector machine (SVM) with graph kernel is used to select the most discriminative features based on similar technique as recursive feature elimination (RFE) [6]. Moreover, to deal with multiple connectivity networks of each subject, we use multiple kernel learning (MKL) [7] to combine the graph kernels of each connectivity network for joint structural feature selection. The proposed method is evaluated on 10 MCI patients and 17 healthy controls, and promising experimental results are obtained.

2   Materials and Method

2.1   Materials

In this study, 10 MCI patients and 17 socio-demographically matched healthy controls were recruited. Informed consent was obtained from all participants, and the experimental protocols were approved by the institutional ethics board. All the recruited subjects were diagnosed by expert consensus panels.

Data acquisition was performed using a 3.0-Tesla GE Signa EXCITE scanner. Diffusion-weighted images of each participant were acquired axially parallel to the anterior and posterior commissures (AC-PC) line with twenty-five-direction diffusion-weighted whole-brain volumes using diffusion weighting values: b=0 and 1000s/mm^2, flip angle=90°, TR/TE=17000/78ms. The imaging matrix=128×128 and FOV=256×256 mm^2 were used, leading to a voxel size of 2×2×2 mm^3. A total of 72 contiguous slices were acquired.

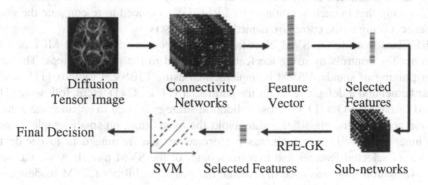

Fig. 2. Flowchart of the proposed method

2.2   Overview of Methodology

Fig. 2 shows the flowchart of the proposed method for connectivity network-based feature selection and classification, which contains three main steps:

i) Connectivity Network Construction and Feature Extraction. We followed the same procedure as in [1]. Specifically, each brain image was first parcellated into 90 ROIs by propagating the Automated Anatomical Labeling (AAL) ROIs [8] to each image using a deformable DTI registration algorithm called F-TIMER [9] with tensor orientation corrected using the method described in [10], and then six connectivity networks were constructed according to these ROIs and six physiological parameters, i.e., FC, FA, MD, and principal diffusivities ($\lambda1$, $\lambda2$, and $\lambda3$). Note that each connectivity network is a 90×90 symmetric matrix. After we obtained the connectivity networks, we computed the clustering coefficient [1] of each ROI in relation to the remaining ROIs from connectivity networks as features for subsequent feature selection and classification. It is worth noting that each ROI in each connectivity network corresponds to one feature, and thus there are totally 540 features (90 ROIs × 6 connectivity networks) for each subject.

ii) Feature Selection. We adopted a two-stage feature selection strategy. Specifically, a standard t-test was first performed to screen out those features that are not significant for discrimination between MCI patients and healthy controls, i.e., those features with p-value larger than a given threshold (0.05 in this paper) will be omitted. Since each feature corresponds to a ROI or node in each of six different connectivity networks, six sub-networks can be constructed for each selected ROI or network node in each subject, after eliminating those non-significant features (ROIs or nodes) from all six original connectivity networks. Then, we measured the topological similarity by computing graph kernel between pair of sub-networks from same network type across different subjects. Furthermore, to deal with multiple connectivity networks available in each subject, we used MKL technique to combine the graph kernels from different connectivity networks. Finally, we used the RFE with the above learned graph kernel, denoted as RFE-GK, to select the most discriminative features. It is worth noting that in each iteration step of RFE-GK, we need to re-compute the graph kernel according to the current remained feature subsets.

iii) Classification. A SVM classifier was adopted to identify the MCI patients from healthy controls by using the features selected in the previous steps. The classifier training of standard SVM is implemented using LIBSVM toolbox [11], with a linear kernel and a default value for the parameter C (i.e., C=1). Here, following [1], a nested Leave-One-Out (LOO) cross-validation strategy is used to enhance the generalization power of the classifier and to avoid the over-fitting on small sample dataset. The inner cross-validation loop was performed on the training data to decide the number of selected features and hyperparameter of the SVM models while the outer cross-validation loop was used to evaluate the generalizability of SVM models using unseen subjects.

2.3   Topology-Based Graph Kernel

Kernel-based learning methods work by first embedding the data into a higher dimensional feature space, and then searching for linear relations among the embedding data points. Given two subjects (vectors) x and x', the kernel can be defined as $k(x, x') = \langle \emptyset(x), \emptyset(x') \rangle$, where $\emptyset$ is a mapping function that maps data from original subject data space to feature space. Examples of common kernel function are linear function and Gaussian radial basis functions (RBF). Besides using feature vector, kernel can also be defined on more complex data types, e.g., graph, and the corresponding kernel is called graph kernel, which captures the semantics inherent in the graph structure. A number of methods have been proposed to define graph kernel [3-5], and have been successfully applied to a variety of problems such as image classification [3] and protein function prediction [5].

To define the graph kernel, some basic terms are first introduced. Here, a labeled graph G is defined as a triple (V, E, ℓ), where V is the set of vertices, E is the set of undirected edges, and $\ell: V \rightarrow L$ is a function that assigns labels from an alphabet L to nodes. A walk is a finite sequence of neighboring vertices, while a path is a walk such that all its vertices are distinct. A subtree is a subgraph of a graph, which has no cycles (i.e., any two vertices are connected by exactly one simple path). Subtree pattern extends the notion of subtree by allowing repetitions of nodes and edges. However, these same nodes (edges) are treated as distinct nodes (edges). Fig. 3 illustrates an example for subtree pattern. Comparing with path and walk, subtree pattern has better discriminative power to measure the similarity between graphs [3], thus it is used in this paper.

Given a pair of graph G and H, a graph kernel can be defined as $k(G, H) = \langle \emptyset(G), \emptyset(H) \rangle$, which takes into account the topology of the graph G and H. Generally, the computational complexity of graph kernel is very high. In order to improve the computational efficiency, Shervashidze and Borgwardt [4] proposed a new method to construct the subtree kernel based on the Weisfeiler-Lehman test of isomorphism. The basic process of the 1-dimensional Weisfeiler-Lehman test is as follows: First, every vertex of a graph is labeled with the number of edges connected to that vertex. Then,

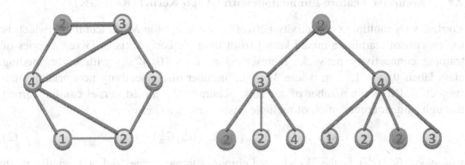

Fig. 3. A subtree pattern of height 2 rooted at the node 2

at each subsequent step (or iteration), the label of each vertex is updated based on its previous label and the label of its neighbors, i.e., parallelly augment the label of each vertex in graph by the sorted set of node labels of neighboring nodes, and compress these augmented labels into new, short labels. This process proceeds iteratively until the node label sets of two graphs differ, or the number of iteration reaches the maximum h. If the sets of new created labels are identical after h iteration, we cannot determine whether these two graphs are isomorphic or not.

Let G_0 and H_0 represent the initial two labeled graphs respectively, G_i and H_i be the corresponding labeled graphs at i-th iteration $(i = 1, ..., h)$, and $L_i = \{s_{i1}, s_{i2}, ..., s_{i|L_i|}\}$ be the set of letters that occur as node labels in G_i or H_i. Assume all L_i are pairwise disjointed. Without loss of generality, assume every L_i is ordered, then the Weisfeiler-Lehman subtree kernel on two graphs is defined as:

$$k(G, H) = \langle \emptyset_{WL}^{(h)}(G), \emptyset_{WL}^{(h)}(H)\rangle, \tag{1}$$

where

$$\emptyset_{WL}^{(h)}(G) = (\sigma_0(G, s_{01}), ..., \sigma_0(G, s_{0|L_0|}), ..., \sigma_h(G, s_{h1}), ..., \sigma_h(G, s_{h|L_h|}))$$

and

$$\emptyset_{WL}^{(h)}(H) = (\sigma_0(H, s_{01}), ..., \sigma_0(H, s_{0|L_0|}), ..., \sigma_h(H, s_{h1}), ..., \sigma_h(H, s_{h|L_h|})),$$

with $\sigma_i(G, s_{ij})$ and $\sigma_i(H, s_{ij})$ are the number of occurrences of the letter s_{ij} in G and H, respectively. Intuitively, the Weisfeiler-Lehman subtree kernel counts the common original and compressed labels in two graphs. It can be proved that this kind of kernel is positive definite and the computational complexity for N graphs is $O(Nhm + N^2hn)$, where n and m are the numbers of nodes and edges of graphs, respectively [4]. In our method, we compute the graph kernel based on the above algorithm on a pair of same type sub-networks across different subjects, as shown in Fig. 2.

2.4   Recursive Feature Elimination with Graph Kernel (RFE-GK)

To deal with multiple connectivity networks, we adopt the MKL technique which is the process of learning a mixed kernel from multiple basis kernels. Given a series of training connectivity networks represented as $G^i = \{G_m^i\}_{m=1}^M$, with corresponding class labels $y^i, i = 1, \dots, n$, where M is the number of connectivity networks of each subject, and n is the number of subjects, generally the mixed kernel can be learned through a linear combination of multiple basis kernels as below:

$$k(G^i, G^j) = \sum_{m=1}^M \mu_m k_m(G_m^i, G_m^j), \tag{2}$$

where $k_m(G_m^i, G_m^j)$ is the Weisfeiler-Lehman subtree kernel defined on the m-th connectivity network using Eq. 1, and μ_m is a nonnegative weight parameter with $\sum_{m=1}^M \mu_m = 1$. We adopt the simple MKL algorithm proposed in [7] to solve Eq. 2. Finally, we will perform structural feature selection using RFE based on graph kernel, which we call as RFE-GK, as shown in Algorithm 1.

It is worth noting that our RFE-GK method is different from the standard RFE framework. In the standard RFE-SVM, it eliminates features through ranking based on weight vector of a linear SVM, while in our method features are eliminated based on classification accuracy in a wrapper-like way. Moreover, there are two other key differences between the proposed feature selection method and the standard RFE-SVM, i.e., 1) the former uses graph kernel that preserves the topological (structural) information of data while the latter uses standard kernel on vector-type data without considering the structural information, and 2) the former uses MKL to combine multiple kernels from multiple connectivity networks to select features while the latter uses single kernel.

3   Experimental Results

3.1   Evaluating Classification Performance

A LOO cross-validation strategy was used to evaluate the classification performance. The performance of a classifier could be quantified by using accuracy, area under receiver operating characteristic curve (AUC), sensitivity and specificity, where the sensitivity represents the proportion of patients that are correctly predicted, and the specificity denotes the proportion of health controls that are correctly predicted. We compared our method with Wee's method and their classification performances are summarized in Table 1. Fig. 4 shows the ROC curves of compared methods. It is worth noting that in Table 1, 'All' denotes using all six connectivity networks, while FC, FA, MD, λ_1, λ_2 and λ_3 denote only using the individual connectivity network, respectively. Also, in Fig. 4 the proposed method and Wee's method [1] use all six connectivity networks, while the others using only single connectivity network.

As can be seen from Table 1 and Fig. 4, our method performs the best in terms of classification accuracy and AUC values. Specifically, our method achieves a classification accuracy of 92.59% and a AUC of 0.965, which are higher than the state-of-the-art connectivity networks-based MCI classification method [1], which achieves

---

Algorithm 1. Recursive Feature Elimination with Graph Kernel (RFE-GK)
Input: Training connectivity networks represented as $G_i = \{G_m^i\}_{m=1}^M, i = 1, ..., n$, and corresponding class labels $y^i, i = 1, ..., n$.
Output: Ranked feature (ROI) list F
Initialize: Subset of surviving features (ROIs) $S = [1,2,...,d]$, and ranked feature list $F = [\ ]$, where d is the number of surviving features in previous feature selection step.
Repeat until $S = [\ ]$
    For each $s \in S$
        For each pair of G^i and G^j, $i \neq j$, compute the combined graph kernel using Eq. 2 on sub-networks excluding feature (or ROI) s;
        Train Leave-One-Out SVM and get the accuracy
    End for
    Find s^* with corresponding maximum accuracy;
    Update ranked feature list $F = [s^*, F]$;
    Eliminate s^* from S
End repeat

---

the best classification accuracy of 88.89% and AUC of 0.929. Our proposed method successfully classified all the MCI patients while only misclassified 2 healthy controls. Table 1 also indicates that combining multiple connectivity networks will achieve much better performance than using single connectivity network alone.

Table 1. Comparison of classification performance of different methods using different connectivity networks

	Accuracy (%)		AUC		Sensitivity (%)		Specificity (%)	
	Wee's	Ours	Wee's	Ours	Wee's	Ours	Wee's	Ours
FC	70.37	70.37	0.653	0.565	-	60	-	76.47
FA	74.07	66.67	0.859	0.565	-	40	-	82.35
MD	59.26	74.07	0.647	0.641	-	40	-	94.12
λ_1	59.26	66.67	0.629	0.729	-	70	-	64.71
λ_2	55.56	62.96	0.594	0.582	-	30	-	82.35
λ_3	59.26	55.56	0.612	0.471	-	40	-	64.71
All	88.89	92.59	0.929	0.965	-	100	-	88.24

3.2   Evaluating Discriminative Power of Features

In this subsection, we evaluate the discriminative power of the selected features using the locality-preserving projection (LPP) approach [12]. Specifically, we used LPP to project the selected features by our method and Wee's method [1] into a 2-D space for visualization. For comparison, we also project the original features (i.e., 540 features) using LPP. Fig. 5 shows the 2-D visualization results of different methods. As can be

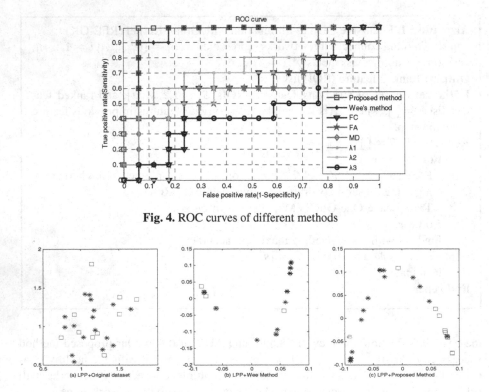

Fig. 4. ROC curves of different methods

Fig. 5. The 2-D visualization results of different methods. Each point represents a subject, and different shapes (or colors) indicate different class labels.

seen from Fig. 5, both feature selection methods (including ours and Wee's) can enhance the discrimination ability of features compared with the original features, with the selected features by our method being more discriminative than those by Wee's method.

3.3   The Most Discriminative Regions

To determine the most discriminative regions, we counted the frequency of features selected at different LOO folds, and ranked them according to their frequencies. The experimental results show that the most frequently selected ROIs include right rectus gyrus, right insuta, right superior temporal gyrus, and left Inferior frontal gyrus (triangular), which are in agreement with the previously reported brain regions related to MCI [1, 13, 14].

Furthermore, the "exclude-one" strategy was adopted to estimate the contribution of each selected ROI. That is, each time one ROI was excluded from the selected ROIs, and the classification performance was investigated using the remaining ROIs; the experiment was repeated for all 4 most frequently selected ROIs. The classification accuracies and AUC values are summarized in Table 2. As can be seen from Table 2, right rectus gyrus and right insula have the most discriminative power, because excluding either of them will cause the most apparent decline in both classification accuracy and AUC.

Table 2. The classification performance under the "exclude-one" strategy

Excluded ROI	Accuracy (%)	AUC
Right rectus gyrus	66.67	0.670
Right insula	70.37	0.759
Right superior temporal gyrus	81.48	0.865
Left Inferior frontal gyrus (triangular)	81.48	0.894

4   Conclusion

In this paper, we have proposed a novel structural feature selection method based on graph kernel, for enhancing the connectivity networks-based classification. Specifically, graph kernel was used to measure the topological similarity between two sub-networks of subjects. Furthermore, multiple kernel learning was used to combine multiple graph kernels obtained from multiple connectivity networks. Experimental results on MCI classification show not only significant improvement of classification performance in terms of accuracy and AUC value, but also show great potential of our method in detecting sensitive ROI regions for MCI. In the future, we will investigate combining the graph kernel used in the current study with the existing linear or Gaussian kernels for further improving performance.

Reference

1. Wee, C.Y., Yap, P.T., Li, W., Denny, K., Browndyke, J.N., Potter, G.G., Welsh-Bohmer, K.A., Wang, L., Shen, D.: Enriched white matter connectivity networks for accurate identification of MCI patients. Neuroimage 54, 1812–1822 (2011)
2. Shen, H., Wang, L.B., Liu, Y.D., Hu, D.W.: Discriminative analysis of resting-state functional connectivity patterns of schizophrenia using low dimensional embedding of fMRI. Neuroimage 49, 3110–3121 (2010)
3. Harchaoui, Z., Bach, F.: Image classification with segmentation graph kernels. In: 2007 IEEE Conference on Computer Vision and Pattern Recognition, Vols. 1-8, pp. 612–619 (2007)
4. Shervashidze, N., Borgwardt, K.M.: Fast subtree kernels on graphs. In: Advances in Neural Information Processing Systems 22, pp. 1660–1668 (2009)
5. Borgwardt, K.M., Kriegel, H.-P.: Shortest-path kernels on graphs. In: Fifth IEEE International Conference on Data Mining, pp. 74–81 (2005)
6. Rakotomamonjy, A.: Variable selection using SVM based criteria. Journal of Machine Learning Research 3, 1357–1370 (2003) (special issue on special feature)
7. Rakotomamonjy, A., Bach, F.R., Canu, S., Grandvalet, Y.: MKLsimple. Journal of Machine Learning Research 9, 2491–2521 (2008)

8. Tzourio-Mazoyer, N., Landeau, B., Papathanassiou, D., Crivello, F., Etard, O., Delcroix, N., Mazoyer, B., Joliot, M.: Automated anatomical labeling of activations in SPM using a macroscopic anatomical parcellation of the MNI MRI single-subject brain. Neuroimage 15, 273–289 (2002)
9. Yap, P.T., Wu, G., Zhu, H., Lin, W., Shen, D.: F-TIMER: fast tensor image morphing for elastic registration. IEEE Trans. Med. Imaging 29, 1192–1203 (2010)
10. Xu, D., Mori, S., Shen, D., van Zijl, P.C., Davatzikos, C.: Spatial normalization of diffusion tensor fields. Magn. Reson. Med. 50, 175–182 (2003)
11. Chang, C.C., Lin, C.J.: LIBSVM: a library for support vector machines (2001)
12. Belkin, M., Niyogi, P.: Laplacian eigenmaps and spectral techniques for embedding and clustering. Adv. Neur. In. 14, 585–591 (2002)
13. Lenzi, D., Serra, L., Perri, R., Pantano, P., Lenzi, G.L., Paulesu, E., Caltagirone, C., Bozzali, M., Macaluso, E.: Single domain amnestic MCI: a multiple cognitive domains fMRI investigation. Neurobiol. Aging 32, 1542–1557 (2011)
14. Schroeter, M.L., Stein, T., Maslowski, N., Neumann, J.: Neural correlates of Alzheimer's disease and mild cognitive impairment: A systematic and quantitative meta-analysis involving 1351 patients. Neuroimage 47, 1196–1206 (2009)

Groupwise Segmentation Improves Neuroimaging Classification Accuracy

Yaping Wang[1,2], Hongjun Jia[2], Pew-Thian Yap[2], Bo Cheng[2],
Chong-Yaw Wee[2], Lei Guo[1], and Dinggang Shen[2,*]

[1] School of Automation, Northwestern Polytechnical University,
Xi'an, Shaanxi Province, China
[2] Department of Radiology and BRIC, University of North Carolina at Chapel Hill, USA
dgshen@med.unc.edu

Abstract. Accurate diagnosis of Alzheimer's disease (AD), especially mild cognitive impairment (MCI), is critical for treatment of the disease. Many algorithms have been proposed to improve classification performance. While most existing methods focus on exploring different feature extraction and selection techniques, in this paper, we show that the pre-processing steps for MRI scans, i.e., registration and segmentation, significantly affect the classification performance. Specifically, we evaluate the classification performance given by a multi-atlas based multi-image segmentation (MABMIS) method, with respect to more conventional segmentation methods. By incorporating tree-based groupwise registration and iterative groupwise segmentation strategies, MABMIS attains more accurate and consistent segmentation results compared with the conventional methods that do not take into account the inherent distribution of images under segmentation. This increased segmentation accuracy will benefit classification by minimizing errors that are propagated to the subsequent analysis steps. Experimental results indicate that MABMIS achieves better performance when compared with the conventional methods in the following classification tasks using the ADNI dataset: AD vs. MCI (accuracy: 71.8%), AD vs. healthy control (HC) (89.1%), progressive MCI vs. HC (84.4%), and progressive MCI vs. stable MCI (70.0%). These results show that pre-processing the images accurately is critical for neuroimaging classification.

1   Introduction

Alzheimer's disease (AD) is the most common cause of dementia in the worldwide elderly population. It has been reported that the number of affected people is expected to rise above 100 million by 2050 [1] - 1 in 85 people will be affected. Thus, accurate diagnosis of AD and its prodrome, mild cognitive impairment (MCI), is important, particularly for the pre-symptomatic patients: patients with amnestic mild cognitive impairment (MCI) and those at increasing risk for developing AD. Many neuroimaging-based algorithms have been proposed for the classification of AD and MCI. Most

---

* Corresponding author.

P.-T. Yap et al. (Eds.): MBIA 2012, LNCS 7509, pp. 185–193, 2012.

of the proposed methods focus on applying different machine learning techniques in feature extraction and selection for improving classification accuracy [2]; less emphasis is placed on how the images are pre-processed. In this paper, we show that accurate and consistent image registration and labeling [3, 4] can help improve AD/MCI classification.

The recently proposed iterative multi-atlas based multi-image segmentation (MABMIS) [3] method has been demonstrated to be more accurate and consistent in labeling different brain tissues (or ROIs). Traditional pairwise methods propagate segmentation information from one or multiple atlases to a target image for segmentation. MABMIS is a multi-atlas based approach that gives significant improvement over pairwise methods by employing the following novel strategies: 1) a novel tree-based groupwise registration method for simultaneous registration of both atlases and target images to improve the registration performance; 2) an iterative groupwise segmentation strategy for simultaneous segmentation of multiple target images to correct inconsistent labeling of the same anatomical structure among different target images. MABMIS can attain more accurate and consistent segmentation results when compared with conventional methods. These approaches benefit the classification by minimizing outliers and inter-subject variability. As the first and fundamental step in the procedure of feature extraction, its accuracy will substantially affect the performance of the following steps and eventually affect the final classification accuracy. This is because the errors introduced in this step might propagate throughout the subsequent analysis steps. We hypothesize that by using advanced data pre-processing, such as groupwise registration and segmentation in MABMIS, the classification performance can be improved.

In this paper, we compare the classification performance between the MABMIS-based and the conventional data pre-processing methods using the ADNI dataset. The significantly better classification performance given by MABMIS indicates that the advanced data pre-processing techniques are crucial for the classification tasks associated with neurodegenerative disorders, e.g., AD and MCI.

2   Method

In this section, we first describe the image registration and segmentation procedures involved in MABMIS, followed by a detailed description of the experimental settings, including the feature selection method and classifiers used in this paper.

2.1   MABMIS

When ROI volumes are used as features for classification, an accurate and consistent delineation of different anatomical structures becomes a critical prerequisite [3]. Compared with the time-consuming manual segmentation executed by human experts, automatic atlas-based segmentation methods are highly efficient and are capable of yielding reproducible results with accuracy comparable to manual segmentation [5]. The basic assumption of atlas-based segmentation methods is that the knowledge regarding the atlas can be carried forward to the target image, modulated by some form of structural similarity measures that reflects anatomical resemblance [6]. However, this is true only if the atlas can match the target image sufficiently well. Instead of using a single "optimal" atlas, some approaches resort to using multiple atlases and requires that all the atlases to be registered to the target image, followed by the fusion of multiple segmentations into a final segmentation result [7]. The potential bias introduced by using only a single atlas can thus be compensated to some extent by combining information from multiple resources. The atlases can be either weighted globally with a constant weight for all voxels within a particular atlas [7], or locally with different weights assigned to different local patches [8]. Further studies show that the selection of a specific subset of atlases for each target image [9] may achieve more accurate segmentation results than using all atlases or a randomly selected subset. For further improvement, an iterative strategies [6] is also proposed for refining the atlas selection.

Nonetheless, the current multi-atlas-based segmentation methods are limited by the several factors as indicated in [3]: 1) The commonly used pairwise registration is problematic when a pair of images under registration have large shape difference; 2) The registration between atlases and target images is usually carried out independently, instead in a groupwise manner, which is more effective in achieving better and more consistent registration result; 3) Segmentation is performed one image at a time, which may lead to inconsistent segmentation across different target images; and 4) Many current implementations lack a feed-back loop among multiple target images for further segmentation refinement.

The MABMIS algorithm is designed for concurrent and consistent segmentation of a group of target images. The overall framework of MABMIS is summarized as follows [3]: First, a group of simulated atlases are generated for better coverage of the atlas space, and then all atlases, including the original and the simulated ones, are registered towards a common space, facilitated by a combinative tree structure. The atlases are represented as nodes on the tree, and the deformation fields related to the connected nodes are computed and stored for further use. By introducing simulated images in the tree, an expanded training set can be obtained, providing a better coverage of the image space. All the atlases are connected in the tree according to their similarity. Note that the differences between the neighboring images on the tree are relatively small, so the deformation between them can be estimated easily with higher accuracy. For each target image that needs to be segmented, an image on the tree that is most similar to it is located so that all atlases can be warped to the target image space by following the respective path on the tree based on the stored deformation fields. An initial segmentation result of the target image is obtained via label fusion. Since the target image and its best-matching atlas are relatively similar, the risk of being trapped by local minima is significantly reduced, good initialization is thus achieved, and the registration accuracy can be improved. Each target image is attached to the tree after being segmented. The atlas set is hence augmented and more information is included for the alignment of new target images, improving the accuracy of registration. On the other hand, we also account for the relationship among target images by performing registration between all atlases and the target image concurrently to improve the consistency.

The segmentation results of all target images are further refined with an iterative groupwise labeling strategy until the results converge. In each iteration, to update the segmentation result of each target image, MABMIS takes advantages of useful information from not only the warped atlases, but also the newly segmented target images. For the labeling of each voxel, the intensity similarity on local patch is used as weight to perform weighted label fusion. All other target segmentations and warped atlases contribute to the labeling of the current target image. Iterative updating will be terminated either when maximum number of iterations is reached, or when the average difference of the overlap ratio between two consecutive iterations is below a predefined threshold. This guarantees consistent labeling of anatomical structures across different target images.

The superiority of MABMIS has been demonstrated by the overlap ratio (Dice ratio) averaged over all ROIs between the estimated labels and the corresponding ground-truth on the LPBA40 dataset [10], with the best segmentation accuracy (82.8%), compared with 77.4% given by the conventional pairwise method. For segmentation accuracy evaluated as the average tissue overlap rate on white matter, gray matter and CSF, MABMIS achieves an accuracy of 83.1% on the ADNI dataset, compared with 80.5% given by the conventional pairwise method. Experimental results show that the groupwise registration framework proposed in MABMIS can significantly improve registration accuracy, especially for target images that have large anatomical differences compared with the atlases; and the iterative groupwise segmentation framework can dramatically improve segmentation consistency over a group of target images [3].

2.2   Experimental Settings

Details on experimental settings, including data pre-processing, feature extraction and selection, and classifier used, are provided as follows.

Data Pre-Processing: All subjects were pre-processed using the same pipeline: 1) anterior commissure (AC)-posterior commissure (PC) alignment correction was performed on all images; 2) nonparametric non-uniform intensity normalization (N3) algorithm [11] was applied to correct the intensity inhomogeneity; 3) skull stripping [12] was performed, and the skull stripping results were further manually reviewed to ensure clean skull and dura removal; 4) removal of the cerebellum; 5) segmentation of the brain into 3 different tissue types: grey matter (GM), white matter (WM), and cerebrospinal fluid (CSF) using the FAST algorithm [13] in the FSL package [14]; 6) histogram matching was performed on all images for overall intensity normalization; and 7) affine registration with default parameters (e.g., 12 degrees of freedom) was performed using FLIRT [15]. For consistency, all images were resampled to dimensions $256{\times}256{\times}256$ and resolution $1{\times}1{\times}1$ mm^3.

Feature extraction: Forty brain images from the LONI LPBA40 dataset [10] were manually labeled with a total of 54 ROIs on different cortical and sub-cortical regions. We utilized these 40 subjects together with the ground-truth labels as atlases in segmenting the ADNI dataset. For each ROI, the volume of GM, WM, and CSF were calculated from the segmented images, before they were collected into a feature vector with 162 (=54 × 3) elements.

Feature Selection: A simple *t*-test was utilized to select the most discriminative features from the training set. The optimal *p*-value was determined via grid search over the range of $(0.001 \leq p \leq 0.9)$.

Classification: Support vector machine (SVM) implemented in LibSVM [16], with a linear kernel and a default value for the parameter C (i.e., C=1), was adopted for classification. To evaluate the performance of different methods, 10-fold cross-validation strategy was used to compute the classification accuracy and the area under receiver operating characteristic curve (AUC). Specifically, the whole dataset was randomly partitioned into 10 subsets, with one subset was used as the testing sample and the remaining subsets were used for training SVM classifier. For each feature d_i in the training samples, a common feature normalization scheme was adopted, i.e., $d_i' = (d_i - \mu_i)/\sigma_i$, where μ_i and σ_i are the mean and standard deviation of the i-th feature across all training samples, respectively. The values of μ_i and σ_i will be used to normalize the corresponding feature of the test samples.

3   Experimental Results

A total of 832 subjects from the ADNI dataset (with age range 55~90 years), consisting of 229 HC, 404 MCI (including 168 progressive MCI (pMCI) and 236 stable MCI (sMCI)), and 199 AD, were considered in this study. Only the baseline scans were used in the experiments. MABMIS was compared with the conventional pairwise methods using 40, 20, 10, 5, and 1 atlas(es), which were randomly selected from the LPBA40 dataset [10]. For the conventional pairwise method, all images from the ADNI dataset were registered to each of these atlases. The images were then segmented by fusing segmentation labels from multiple atlases, based on local-patch similarity [3]. The results with 40, 20, 10, 5, and 1 atlas(es) are denoted as "pairwise", "S20", "S10", "S5", and "S1", respectively. Note that diffeomorphic demons [17] was applied for pairwise registration in this paper.

3.1   Results

Tables 1 - 4 provide the 10-fold cross-validation classification performance results given by all compared methods on different classification tasks. As can be seen from Tables 1 - 4, MABMIS consistently yields better classification performance in terms of accuracy, sensitivity, and specificity compared with the pairwise method. This indicates that accurate segmentation is conducive to improved classification accuracy. Specifically, MABMIS achieves a better classification accuracy of 71.8% compared with the pairwise method with 40 atlases (69.0%) for AD vs. MCI classification. The improvements in terms of accuracy are approximately 2.6%, 3.6%, and 2.3% for AD vs. HC, pMCI vs. HC, and pMCI vs. sMCI classification, respectively. It can be observed that the classification accuracy generally increases as the number of atlases

Table 1. Comparison between MABMIS and the pairwise methods for AD vs. MCI classification task. (ACC=Accuracy, SEN=Sensitivity, SPE=Specificity, AUC=Area under ROC).

Methods	ACC %	SEN %	SPE %	AUC
MABMIS	**71.8**	**40.3**	**87.0**	**0.745**
pairwise	69.0	35.2	85.4	0.717
S20	68.4	34.8	84.7	0.717
S10	68.4	36.7	83.7	0.713
S5	68.1	29.7	86.7	0.690
S1	66.6	30.0	84.2	0.701

Table 2. Comparison between MABMIS and the pairwise-based methods for AD vs. HC classification task. (ACC=Accuracy, SEN=Sensitivity, SPE=Specificity, AUC=Area under ROC).

Methods	ACC %	SEN %	SPE %	AUC
MABMIS	**89.1**	**86.1**	**91.8**	**0.928**
pairwise	86.5	85.2	87.6	0.923
S20	86.6	84.3	88.6	0.920
S10	87.4	86.4	88.3	0.924
S5	87.3	85.7	88.6	0.921
S1	87.1	84.5	89.4	0.922

Table 3. Comparison between MABMIS and the pairwise methods for pMCI vs. HC classification task. (ACC=Accuracy, SEN=Sensitivity, SPE=Specificity, AUC=Area under ROC).

Methods	ACC %	SEN %	SPE %	AUC
MABMIS	**84.4**	**79.4**	**88.1**	**0.905**
pairwise	80.8	75.8	84.5	0.884
S20	81.0	72.7	87.2	0.889
S10	80.8	73.5	86.3	0.891
S5	80.4	74.5	84.7	0.894
S1	79.6	74.5	83.4	0.896

Table 4. Comparison between MABMIS and the pairwise methods for pMCI vs. sMCI classification task. (ACC=Accuracy, SEN=Sensitivity, SPE=Specificity, AUC=Area under ROC).

Methods	ACC %	SEN %	SPE %	AUC
MABMIS	**70.0**	**66.7**	**72.3**	**0.726**
pairwise	67.7	66.4	68.6	0.719
S20	67.7	65.8	69.0	0.718
S10	65.8	63.7	67.3	0.709
S5	67.7	65.8	69.1	0.713
S1	64.2	61.0	66.4	0.695

used increases for the pairwise method, similar observation as in the previous studies [7, 8]. Note that the sensitivity value of the AD vs. MCI classification task is significantly lower than the specificity value due to imbalanced number of subjects between the two groups, i.e., the number of MCI subjects is two times that of AD subjects. Nevertheless, MABMIS still outperforms the pairwise method in terms of sensitivity value. As can be seen from the other experiments (AD vs. HC, pMCI vs. HC, and pMCI vs. sMCI), with matched subject ratio, the sensitivity and specificity values of MABMIS are relatively high and balanced.

The ROC curves of MABMIS and the pairwise method (with 40 atlases) for different classification tasks are provided in Fig. 1. It can be observed that MABMIS performed better than the pairwise method, particularly for AD vs. MCI and pMCI vs. HC classification tasks. The AUC values for MABMIS and the pairwise method are 0.745 and 0.717, respectively, for AD vs MCI classification; and 0.905 and 0.884, respectively, for pMCI vs. HC classification.

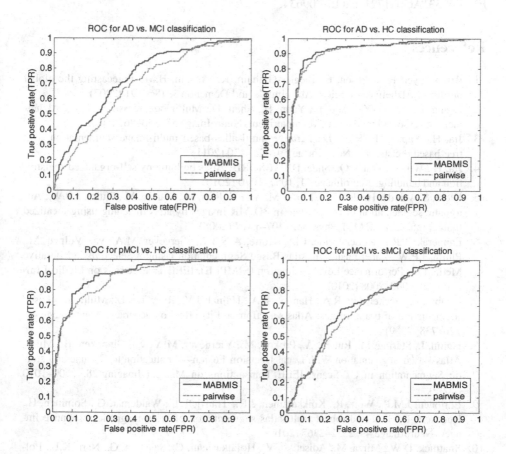

Fig. 1. ROC curves for different classification tasks given by MABMIS and the pairwise method

4   Conclusion

This paper shows the importance of image pre-processing steps in neuroimaging classification. Specifically, the classification results for AD vs. MCI, AD vs. HC, pMCI vs. HC, and pMCI vs. sMCI from the ADNI dataset indicate that the groupwise data pre-processing methods, e.g., MABMIS, is superior to the pairwise methods. MABMIS integrates a novel tree-based groupwise registration method (which registers atlases and target images concurrently) and an iterative groupwise segmentation strategy (which accounts for the relationship of all target images simultaneously), for simultaneous registration and segmentation to improve accuracy and across-image consistency in segmentation. The improved segmentation helps increase classification accuracy by reducing inter-subject variability.

Acknowledgements. This work was supported in part by NIH grants EB008374, EB006733, AG041721 and EB009634.

References

1. Brookmeyer, R., Johnson, E., Ziegler-Graham, K., Arrighi, H.M.: Forecasting the global burden of Alzheimer's disease. Alzheimer's and Dementia 3, 186–191 (2007)
2. Zhang, D., Wang, Y., Zhou, L., Yuan, H., Shen, D.: Multimodal classification of Alzheimer's disease and mild cognitive impairment. NeuroImage 55, 856–867 (2011)
3. Jia, H., Yap, P.-T., Shen, D.: Iterative multi-atlas-based multi-image segmentation with tree-based registration. NeuroImage 59, 422–430 (2011)
4. Jia, H., Wu, G., Wang, Q., Shen, D.: ABSORB: Atlas building by self-organized registration and bundling. NeuroImage 51, 1057–1070 (2010)
5. Klein, S., van der Heide, U.A., Lips, I.M., van Vulpen, M., Staring, M., Pluim, J.P.W.: Automatic segmentation of the prostate in 3D MR images by atlas matching using localized mutual information. Med. Phys. 35, 1407–1417 (2008)
6. Langerak, T.R., van der Heide, U.A., Kotte, A.N.T.J., Viergever, M.A., van Vulpen, M., Pluim, J.P.W.: Label Fusion in Atlas-Based Segmentation Using a Selective and Iterative Method for Performance Level Estimation (SIMPLE). IEEE Transactions on Medical Imaging 29, 2000–2008 (2010)
7. Aljabar, P., Heckemann, R.A., Hammers, A., Hajnal, J.V., Rueckert, D.: Multi-atlas based segmentation of brain images: Atlas selection and its effect on accuracy. NeuroImage 46, 726–738 (2009)
8. Isgum, I., Staring, M., Rutten, A., Prokop, M., Viergever, M.A., van Ginneken, B.: Multi-Atlas-Based Segmentation With Local Decision Fusion—Application to Cardiac and Aortic Segmentation in CT Scans. IEEE Transactions on Medical Imaging 28, 1000–1010 (2009)
9. Lötjönen, J.M.P., Wolz, R., Koikkalainen, J.R., Thurfjell, L., Waldemar, G., Soininen, H., Rueckert, D.: Fast and robust multi-atlas segmentation of brain magnetic resonance images. NeuroImage 49, 2352–2365 (2010)
10. Shattuck, D.W., Mirza, M., Adisetiyo, V., Hojatkashani, C., Salamon, G., Narr, K.L., Poldrack, R.A., Bilder, R.M., Toga, A.W.: Construction of a 3D probabilistic atlas of human cortical structures. NeuroImage 39, 1064–1080 (2008)

11. Sled, J.G., Zijdenbos, A.P., Evans, A.C.: A nonparametric method for automatic correction of intensity nonuniformity in MRI data. IEEE Transactions on Medical Imaging 17, 87–97 (1998)
12. Wang, Y., Nie, J., Yap, P.-T., Shi, F., Guo, L., Shen, D.: Robust Deformable-Surface-Based Skull-Stripping for Large-Scale Studies. In: Fichtinger, G., Martel, A., Peters, T. (eds.) MICCAI 2011, Part III. LNCS, vol. 6893, pp. 635–642. Springer, Heidelberg (2011)
13. Zhang, Y., Brady, M., Smith, S.: Segmentation of brain MR images through a hidden Markov random field model and the expectation-maximization algorithm. IEEE Transactions on Medical Imaging 20, 45–57 (2001)
14. Smith, S.M., Jenkinson, M., Woolrich, M.W., Beckmann, C.F., Behrens, T.E.J., Johansen-Berg, H., Bannister, P.R., De Luca, M., Drobnjak, I., Flitney, D.E., Niazy, R.K., Saunders, J., Vickers, J., Zhang, Y., De Stefano, N., Brady, J.M., Matthews, P.M.: Advances in functional and structural MR image analysis and implementation as FSL. NeuroImage 23(Suppl. 1), S208–S219 (2004)
15. Jenkinson, M., Smith, S.: A global optimisation method for robust affine registration of brain images. Medical Image Analysis 5, 143–156 (2001)
16. Chang, C.-C., Lin, C.-J.: LIBSVM: a Library for Support Vector Machines (2001)
17. Vercauteren, T., Pennec, X., Perchant, A., Ayache, N.: Diffeomorphic demons: Efficient non-parametric image registration. NeuroImage 45, S61–S72 (2009)

DWI Denoising Using Spatial, Angular, and Radiometric Filtering

Pew-Thian Yap and Dinggang Shen

Department of Radiology and Biomedical Research Imaging Center (BRIC)
The University of North Carolina at Chapel Hill, U.S.A.
{ptyap,dgshen}@med.unc.edu

Abstract. In this paper, we study the effectiveness of the concurrent utilization of spatial, angular, and radiometric (SAR) information for denoising diffusion-weighted data. SAR filtering smooths diffusion-weighted images while at the same time preserves edges by means of nonlinear combination of nearby and similar signal values. The method is noniterative, local, and simple. It combines diffusion signals based on both their spatio-angular closeness and their radiometric similarity, with greater preference given to nearby and similar values. Our results suggest that SAR filtering reveals structures that are concealed by noise and produces anisotropy maps with markedly improved quality.

1 Introduction

Diffusion-weighted imaging (DWI) reveals microscopic tissue properties through measurements of local tissue water diffusion, and has been extensively utilized for *in vivo* investigation of micro-structural and connectivity changes related to brain diseases, development, and aging. A more recent form of DWI — high angular resolution diffusion imaging (HARDI) — applies magnetic field diffusion gradients to the brain, in up to hundreds of different directions, to precisely detail the directional structures of neuronal pathways. For better separation of different compartments within each voxel, increasing the diffusion-weighting (b-value) is often required for higher angular contrast. This, however, comes with the price of lowered signal-to-noise ratio (SNR) of the acquired images. Noise is severely detrimental to the analysis of diffusion-weighted data, potentially causing the inference of more than actual intra-voxel complexity, such as over-estimating the number of fiber populations.

To reduce noise, acquisitions are often performed in a number of repetitions and diffusion-weighted images corresponding to a particular diffusion gradient direction are averaged to produce diffusion data with greater SNR. This approach, however, prolongs scan time substantially. With the mounting demand for higher angular resolution and hence the need for scanning in a greater number of directions, repetition is often limited by practical time constraints that are associated with any expensive shared resources and invites complications such as artifacts caused by subject movement.

P.-T. Yap et al. (Eds.): MBIA 2012, LNCS 7509, pp. 194–202, 2012.

To mitigate the need for multiple DW measurements, we propose in this paper a filtering technique, which considers concurrently spatial, angular, and radiometric (SAR) information, to denoise DW images. The premise underlying SAR filtering is that *close* and *similar* signals, when averaged to produce the denoised signals, will have greater tendency to preserve image structures. This has in fact been demonstrated effective by bilateral filtering [1,2]. Closeness refers to vicinity in the spatio-angular domain, and similarity to vicinity in the radiometric range. Domain filtering often enforces closeness by weights that fall off with distance. Similarly, the weights in radiometric filtering decay with radiometric dissimilarity. These weights are used to combine signal values for estimation of noise-free signals. These two kinds of information are complementary in nature: domain filtering ensures that the local structural continuity is respected, whereas radiometric filtering encourages the preservation of edges; domain filtering alone blurs structures, whereas radiometric alone distorts structures. A combination of these pieces of information to boost complementary strengths and to dampen individual weaknesses is hence important for effective denoising.

In contrast to existing approaches, our method offers the following advantages:

1. **Angular Extension:** Distinct from scalar images, each voxel location in DWI is characterized by a spherical function of diffusion signals. This angular dimension has not been sufficiently explored in existing methods in the context of denoising. We note that many DWI statistical quantities, such as anisotropy, are very sensitive to the regularity of the spherical profile. Inaccuracy in the estimation of these quantities, on which clinical diagnosis often relies, will potentially result in diagnostic error. We will demonstrate that this angular dimension is crucial for DWI denoising.

2. **Rician Adaptation:** The magnitudes of a magnetic resonance (MR) image is Rician-distributed. Although this distribution can often be conveniently approximated as Gaussian when the SNR is sufficiently high, this approximation is often implausible in DWI due to the typically lower SNR. Our formulation takes explicit consideration of the Rician nature of the noise distribution in DWI for more effective denoising.

3. **Low Computation Cost:** With our formulation, empirical evidence indicates that it is sufficient to compute signal differences/similarities based on the individual values alone. Methods such as non-local means (NLM) filtering [3–6] compares contextual information surrounding a pair of voxel locations to evaluate the similarity of these voxels. The size of the voxel neighborhoods that provide this contextual information has to be sufficient large to ensure sufficient characterization of local structures for distance evaluation. From the point of view of DWI, which generates essentially 4D data, this is clearly computationally prohibitive. The relative simplicity of the algorithm discussed in this paper makes applications in real-world scenarios much more feasible.

Our evaluation based on software phantoms and *in vivo* data suggests that SAR filtering reveals structures that are concealed by noise and produces anisotropy maps with markedly improved quality.

2   Method

2.1   SAR Filtering

The SAR filter estimates the denoised signal $\hat{S}(\mathbf{x}_i, \hat{\mathbf{q}}_k)$ at voxel location $\mathbf{x}_i \in \mathbb{R}^3$ and at angular direction $\hat{\mathbf{q}}_k \in \mathbb{S}^2$ by nonlinear combination of the observed signal values of voxels in a spatial neighborhood $\mathcal{N}(\mathbf{x}_i)$, i.e., $S(\mathbf{x}_j, \hat{\mathbf{q}}_l)$, $\forall j : \mathbf{x}_j \in \mathcal{N}(\mathbf{x}_i)$ and $\forall l : \hat{\mathbf{q}}_l \in \mathbb{S}^2$. The weights w_{ijkl} are carefully formulated so that only values that are spatially close and radiometrically similar are combined to trade-off between the retention of image structures, such as edges and corners, and the removal of noise. The SAR filter is defined as

$$\hat{S}(\mathbf{x}_i, \hat{\mathbf{q}}_k) = \sqrt{\left[\frac{\sum_{j,l} w_{ijkl} S^2(\mathbf{x}_j, \hat{\mathbf{q}}_l)}{\sum_{j,l} w_{ijkl}} - 2\sigma_{\text{rician}}^2 \right]_+} \tag{1}$$

where

$$[a]_+ = \begin{cases} a, & a > 0; \\ 0, & \text{otherwise.} \end{cases} \tag{2}$$

The case $(j = i) \wedge (l = k)$ results in a very large weight due to self-similarity and can be skipped to avoid over-weighting [4]. Note that the squared signal values are used here so that the statistical bias $2\sigma_{\text{rician}}^2$ can be removed for unbiased estimation. This is derived from the fact the second order moment of a Rician distributed quantity is given as

$$E(\mathbf{S}^2) = S_{\text{true}}^2 + 2\sigma_{\text{rician}}^2, \tag{3}$$

where S_{true} is the true signal value. The noise variance σ_{rician}^2 associated with the Rician distribution [7] can be estimated from the background signal ($S_{\text{true}} = 0$) using $\sigma_{\text{rician}}^2 = \sqrt{\langle S_{\text{background}}^2 \rangle}/2$. The determination of weights w_{ijkl} is dependent on the spatial, angular, and radiometric relationship of each pair of voxels. We can hence decompose w_{ijkl} as

$$w_{ijkl} = w_{ij,\text{spatial}} \times w_{kl,\text{angular}} \times w_{ijkl,\text{radiometric}}. \tag{4}$$

Each component is discussed in the subsequent sections.

2.2   The Spatio-Angular Component

Spatial coherence arises naturally from the inherent regularity of images of natural objects and has long been exploited for denoising. The weight related to the spatial component of the formulation is defined as

$$w_{ij,\text{spatial}} = \exp\left(-\frac{d_{ij}^2}{2\sigma_{\text{spatial}}^2} \right). \tag{5}$$

where $d_{ij}^2 = ||\mathbf{x}_i - \mathbf{x}_j||^2$ is the distance between two voxel locations and $\sigma_{\text{spatial}}^2$ determines the rate of decay of the weight with respect to spatial extent. The angular component, defined as

$$w_{kl,\text{angular}} = \exp\left[\kappa K(\mathbf{x}_i, \hat{\mathbf{q}}_k)\left(\hat{\mathbf{q}}_k^{\mathrm{T}}\hat{\mathbf{q}}_l\right)^2\right], \tag{6}$$

acknowledges the fact that DWI data capture directional information and the directionality of the image structures should be respected when combining the signals. Function

$$K(\mathbf{x}_i, \hat{\mathbf{q}}_k) = \frac{||S(\mathbf{x}_i, \hat{\mathbf{q}}_k)||^2 - 2\sigma_{\text{rician}}^2}{\max_{i,k} ||S(\mathbf{x}_i, \hat{\mathbf{q}}_k)||^2 - 2\sigma_{\text{rician}}^2} \tag{7}$$

falls within $[0, 1]$ and encourages smoothing of background noise and prevents over-smoothing of high SNR signals. Equation (5) is in fact a modified form of the probability density function (PDF) of the Watson distribution [8, 9], which is a natural choice for characterizing angular distribution. The parameter κ determines the concentration of the distribution. A larger κ value will give a more pointed distribution, with a greater weight in the direction pointed by $\hat{\mathbf{q}}_k$. A smaller κ value will give a more uniform distribution, allowing signals in different directions to be treated more equally.

2.3   The Radiometric Component

Radiometric range information is totally absent in the spatio-angular component. Combining signal values from the whole range spectrum is detrimental to image structures, since boundaries of different anatomical entities are often manifested as steep differences in radiometric range. At a more fine-grained level, resolving the micro-architecture within each voxel requires a spherical profile of DWI signals that shows clear delineation between the distinct fiber population. For this to be possible, again, we need a clear separation in radiometric values. The appropriate solution to the denoising problem is hence to combine spatio-angular and radiometric filtering. In our case, the radiometric component is defined as:

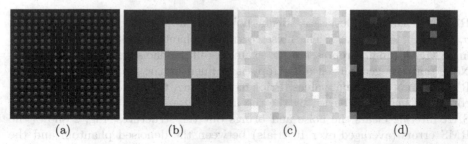

(a)   (b)   (c)   (d)

Fig. 1. Denoising the phantom. (a) The fiber orientation distribution functions (ODFs) of the DWI phantom; (b) The generalized anisotropy map of the phantom; (c) The noise corrupted phantom with $\sigma_{\text{rician}} = 5$; (d) Result from SAR filtering.

$$w_{ijkl,\text{radiometric}} = \exp\left(-\frac{|S^2(\mathbf{x}_j, \hat{\mathbf{q}}_l) - S^2(\mathbf{x}_i, \hat{\mathbf{q}}_k)|}{2\sigma_{\text{radiometric}}^2 K(\mathbf{x}_i, \hat{\mathbf{q}}_k)}\right). \tag{8}$$

Function $K(\mathbf{x}_i, \hat{\mathbf{q}}_k)$ is similarly defined as in the previous section. Note again that we have chosen to use the squared signal values for comparison in order to avoid signal-dependent bias due to the Rician-distributed nature of the magnitude signal.

3   Experiments

In this section, we validate the effectiveness of SAR filtering by using both a Rician noise corrupted software phantom and also a real image. For all cases, we set $\sigma_{\text{spatial}} = 1$, $\kappa = 0.5$, and $\sigma_{\text{radiometric}} = \sigma_{\text{rician}}$.

3.1   Synthetic Data

Phantom. We used a mixture of diffusion tensors to generate a DWI phantom for representing the crossing of two fiber populations (see Fig. 1(a)). Each fiber population was simulated by a tensor with $\lambda_1 = 1.5 \times 10^{-3}\,\text{mm}^2/\text{s}$, $\lambda_2 = \lambda_3 = 5 \times 10^{-4}\,\text{mm}^2/\text{s}$, and $b = 2000\,\text{s}/\text{mm}^2$. The (120) gradient directions were taken from the *in vivo* dataset. One group of tensors is oriented in the horizontal direction and the other in the vertical direction. The two fiber populations cross at the center of the image. Note that these diffusion parameters were carefully chosen to mimic the *in vivo* data.

Generation of Rician Noise. For the signal at each voxel location and gradient direction, we computed the Rician noise corrupted signal $\tilde{S}$ as:

$$\tilde{S} = \sqrt{(S + n_1)^2 + (n_2)^2} \tag{9}$$

where n_1 and n_2 are sampled from normal distributions with zero mean and variance σ_{rician}^2. The value $\tilde{S}$ is a realization of a random variable with a Rician PDF with parameters S and σ_{rician}.

Results. Different levels of Rician noise was applied to the phantom, i.e., $\sigma_{\text{rician}} = 5, 10, 15, 20, 25$. The noise-corrupted phantom was then denoised using SAR filtering. A representation example of the denoising is shown in Fig. 1. Note that the generalized anisotropy is defined as the standard deviation to RMS ratio of the signal values. Prior to denoising, the structures in the noise-corrupted image are buried by the the noise and are hence not readily visible. SAR filtering clears the noise and brings out the structures. Fig. 2 shows the RMS errors (averaged over 10 trials) between the denoised phantom and the original noise-free phantom. SAR filtering consistently reduces the RMS error for all levels of Rician noise. To demonstrate the importance of the angular component, we excluded it by setting $w_{kl,\text{angular}} = \delta_{kl}$, the Kronecker delta, and

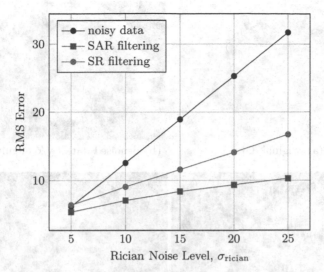

Fig. 2. RMS errors for different levels of Rician noise

tested the performance of the resulting spatioradiometric (SR) filtering. It is clear from Fig. 2 that excluding the angular component results in a significant decrease in denoising performance.

3.2   In Vivo Data

Data Acquisition. Diffusion-weighted images were acquired for 4 subjects using a Siemens 3T TIM Trio MR Scanner with an EPI sequence. Diffusion gradients were applied in 120 non-collinear directions with diffusion weighting $b = 2000\,\mathrm{s/mm^2}$, flip angle = $90°$, repetition time (TR) = $12{,}400\,\mathrm{ms}$ and echo time (TE) = $116\,\mathrm{ms}$. The imaging matrix was 128×128 with a rectangular FOV of $256 \times 256\,\mathrm{mm^2}$. 80 contiguous slices with a slice thickness of $2\,\mathrm{mm}$ covered the whole brain.

Qualitative Results. Denoising the raw DWI data can lead to greater robustness in subsequent fitting of various diffusion models [5,6,10]. Fig. 3 demonstrates that denoising the DWI data give significantly greater structural clarity. Note that in the figure we have included the results for filtering with the full spatial, angular, and radiometric information (Fig. 3(d)) as well as that without the spatial component (Fig. 3(c)). Although using the full information will generally give better structural smoothness as well as a cleaner background, filtering without the spatial component gives comparable results (despite with lesser structural smoothness) and, more important, a massive improvement in computation speed (see Section 4). We have also included the result given by denoising without the angular component (Fig. 3(b)); the resulting filter is conceptually equivalent to

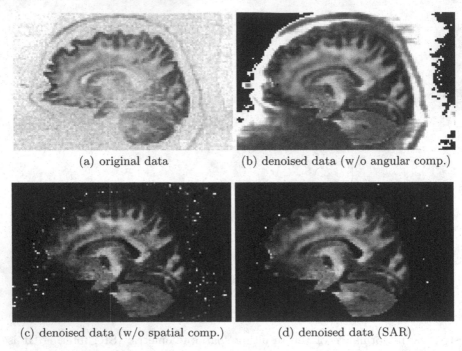

(a) original data   (b) denoised data (w/o angular comp.)

(c) denoised data (w/o spatial comp.)   (d) denoised data (SAR)

Fig. 3. Typical denoising results for *in vivo* data

the bilateral filter [1, 2]. It is clear from the the figure that, without considering the angular component, the result is far from satisfactory.

Quantitative Results. To quantify denoising performance, we evaluated and compared the contrast of the anisotropy maps before and after denoising. It is a well-accepted fact that on an anisotropy map the white matter (WM) voxels will show the brightest values owing to diffusion anisotropy resulting from restricted diffusion. This is followed by the gray matter (GM) voxels, which generally exhibit a lower degree of anisotropy, and then the cerebrospinal fluid (CSF) voxels, which captures isotropic diffusion. Therefore, on the anisotropy map, the brightness decreases from WM, GM, to CSF. Based on this observation, we used GM as the reference and evaluated how much brighter on average the WM voxels are and how much dimmer the CSF voxels are. A larger difference in the average brightness values implies greater contrast. Fig. 4 shows the results for the 4 subjects using different denoising schemes. The brightness differences were computed by subtracting the average GM brightness from the average WM brightness and the average CSF brightness. It can be observed from the figure that other than SAR and AR filtering, the WM−GM and CSF−GM contrast is not as expected in the sense that the CSF voxels are in average brighter than the GM voxels. The diffusion signal for CSF is typical low and a small amount of noise will cause a large anisotropy value. The original DWI data with no denoising are obviously effected by this. The SR and SA filters are not capable

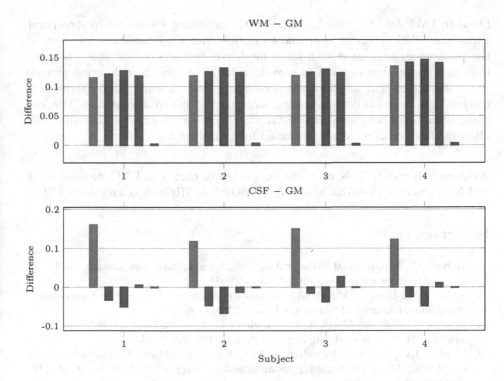

Fig. 4. Brightness differences for different denoising schemes: No (NIL, ■) filtering; spatial, angular, and radiometric (SAR, ■) filtering; angular and radiometric (AR, ■) filtering; spatial and radiometric (SR, ■) filtering; and spatial and angular (SA, ■) filtering. The brightness differences are computed by subtracting the average GM brightness from the average WM brightness and the average CSF brightness.

of denoising CSF voxels effectively. The results also indicate that, by not considering the radiometric component, the DWI data can be over-smoothed with significant loss in angular content, as evident in the marked loss of anisotropy.

4 Computation Time

On a machine with a quad-core 2.2GHz Intel processor, the SAR filter denoised each 3D DWI volume, corresponding to one gradient direction, in less than 1 minute. By not considering the spatial component and slightly compromising structural smoothness (i.e., the AR filter), each 3D volume can be denoised in less than 2 seconds. SAR filtering therefore requires a very modest time cost and can be easily adapted to clinical settings.

5 Conclusion

We have presented in this paper an effective and efficient denoising algorithm for raw DWI data. With the plethora of available diffusion models that can be fitted to DWI data for varied analysis with increasing sensitivity to structural variations, DWI denoising is crucial to ensure that the estimation accuracy of the parameters associated with these models is not affected by noise. Evaluation based on a phantom and *in vivo* data indicates that SAR filtering reveals image structures that are hidden in noise and produces white matter structural images, such as the anisotropy image, with markedly increased quality. The low computation cost associated with SAR filtering is an added advantage that will allow quality denoising to be performed in clinical settings.

Acknowledgment. This work was supported in part by a UNC start-up fund and NIH grants (EB006733, EB008374, EB009634, MH088520, and AG041721).

References

1. Tomasi, C., Manduchi, R.: Bilateral filtering for gray and color images. In: International Conference on Computer Vision (1998)
2. Smith, S.M., Brady, J.M.: SUSAN - a new approach to low level image processing. International Journal of Computer Vision 23(1) (1997)
3. Buades, A., Coll, B., Morel, J.M.: A review of image denoising algorithms, with a new one. Multiscale Modeling & Simulation 4, 490–530 (2005)
4. Manjón, J.V., Carbonell-Caballero, J., Lull, J.J., García-Martí, G., Martí-Bonmatí, L., Robles, M.: MRI denoising using non-local means. Medical Image Analysis 12(4), 514–523 (2008)
5. Descoteaux, M., Wiest-Daesslé, N., Prima, S., Barillot, C., Deriche, R.: Impact of Rician Adapted Non-Local Means Filtering on HARDI. In: Metaxas, D., Axel, L., Fichtinger, G., Székely, G. (eds.) MICCAI 2008, Part II. LNCS, vol. 5242, pp. 122–130. Springer, Heidelberg (2008)
6. Wiest-Daesslé, N., Prima, S., Coupé, P., Morrissey, S.P., Barillot, C.: Rician noise removal by non-local means filtering for low signal-to-noise ratio MRI: applications to DT-MRI. In: 11 (ed.) Medical Image Computing and Computer Assisted Intervention, Part 2, pp. 171–179 (2008)
7. Nowak, R.D.: Wavelet-based Rician noise removal for magnetic resonance imaging. IEEE Transactions on Image Processing 8(10), 1408–1419 (1999)
8. Watson, G.: Equatorial distributions on a sphere. Biometrika 52, 193–201 (1965)
9. Schwartzman, A., Dougherty, R.F., Taylor, J.E.: False discovery rate analysis of brain diffusion direction maps. Annals of Applied Statistics 2(1), 153–175 (2008)
10. Basu, S., Fletcher, T., Whitaker, R.T.: Rician Noise Removal in Diffusion Tensor MRI. In: Larsen, R., Nielsen, M., Sporring, J. (eds.) MICCAI 2006. LNCS, vol. 4190, pp. 117–125. Springer, Heidelberg (2006)

MRI Estimation of T_1 Relaxation Time Using a Constrained Optimization Algorithm

Fang Cao[1], Olivier Commowick[1], Elise Bannier[1], Jean-Christophe Ferré[2], Gilles Edan[2], and Christian Barillot[1]

[1] VisAGeS U746 INSERM/INRIA, IRISA UMR CNRS 6074, Rennes, France
[2] University hospital Pontchaillou, Rennes, France

Abstract. We propose a new method to improve T_1 mapping with respect to the popular *DESPOT1* algorithm. A distance function is defined to model the distance between the pure signal and the measurements in presence of noise. We use a constrained gradient descent optimization algorithm to iteratively find the optimal values of T_1 and M_0. The method is applied to MR images acquired with 2 gradient echo sequences and different flip angles. The performance of T_1 mapping is evaluated both on phantom and on in vivo experiments.

Keywords: T_1 relaxometry, *DESPOT1*, quantitative analysis, MRI.

1 Introduction

The longitudinal relaxation time, T_1, is tissue specific at a given field strength. It can be measured to identify and differentiate healthy or pathological tissues, and is particularly relevant for clinical studies involving quantitative MRI analysis. Hence, T_1 relaxometry is now progressively used in neurological studies to investigate the structural modifications occurring during brain development [13].

Conventionally, T_1 maps can be estimated using saturation-recovery (SR) sequences with multiple repetition times or on inversion recovery (IR) sequences with multiple inversion times. However, these conventional sequences require long acquisition times in order to measure the longitudinal magnetization at multiple time points. Moreover, long repetition times are needed for accurate T_1 measurements.

Several methods have been proposed to bring forth rapid and accurate T_1 relaxometry. The acquisition of high-resolution T_1 maps in a clinically acceptable time frame has been demonstrated with several approaches [5,14,16]. Currently, the most popular rapid and high-resolution T_1 estimation algorithm is Driven Equilibrium Single Pulse Observation of T_1 (*DESPOT1*) [10,1], originally introduced in [3] and further investigated by [15,6,7]. Deoni *et. al.* [6] first extracted the T_1 map from a pair of gradient echo images with optimal flip angles, and showed that, using *DESPOT1*, a 3D acquisition of $1 \times 1 \times 1 \text{mm}^3$ can be achieved in less than 8 minutes on a 1.5T scanner.

In practice, however, T_1 map estimation can be biased:

P.-T. Yap et al. (Eds.): MBIA 2012, LNCS 7509, pp. 203–214, 2012.

1. The explicit solution of T_1 is sensitive to noise, especially in the background and skull areas where the signal to noise ratio (SNR) is low.
2. Negative and extremely high T_1 values may appear in CSF and lesion areas due to the discontinuity and the locally high derivative of GRE equation.
3. Partial volume effects.
4. Flip angle inaccuracy related to B_1 inhomogeneity.
5. T_1 changes related to temperature drift.

In this work, we focus on noise sensitivity and on the negative and extremely high values of T_1 (item 1 and 2), and improve T_1 mapping with respect to the popular *DESPOT1* algorithm. We propose a constrained distance function and use a gradient descent optimization algorithm to iteratively estimate the optimal T_1 value. Evaluation on phantom and on in vivo studies indicates the improvement of the T_1 measurement.

2 Basic *DESPOT1* Theory

DESPOT1 uses a gradient echo sequence acquisition scheme [6]. The measured signal can be derived from the following equation:

$$S_\theta = \frac{M_0(1 - \exp(-TR/T_1)) \sin\theta}{(1 - \exp(-TR/T_1) \cos\theta)} \tag{1}$$

θ: flip angle (MR acquisition parameter)
TR: repetition time (MR acquisition parameter)
S_θ: gradient-echo sequence with flip angle θ (the acquired image)
T_1: longitudinal relaxation time (unknown parameter, tissue specific at a given magnetic field strength)
M_0: equilibrium magnetization (unknown parameter, related to tissue and MR setup)

S_θ can be corrupted by noise, and θ can be inaccurate due to the acquisition related limitations. As demonstrated in [15], holding TR constant and changing θ, equation (1) can be reformulated as a simple linear equation

$$Y = aX + b \tag{2}$$

in which X and Y are parameterized as $Y = S_\theta/\sin\theta$ and $X = S_\theta/\tan\theta$. The slope and intercept are

$$a = \exp(-TR/T_1), b = M_0(1 - \exp(-TR/T_1)) \tag{3}$$

Thus, we can extract T_1 and M_0 from a and b

$$T_1 = -\frac{TR}{\ln b}, M_0 = \frac{a}{1 - b} \tag{4}$$

From equation (2), we can find the explicit solution for T_1 and M_0 if we have 2 input signals ($S_{\theta 1}$ and $S_{\theta 2}$). Fig. 1 shows that acquiring 2 points $S_{\theta 1}$ and $S_{\theta 2}$, we can calculate the explicit solution of T_1 and M_0, and generate a solid curve with incrementally increasing θ. It should be noted that the factor M_0 only changes the absolute value of the signal intensity S_θ, not the shape of the curve.

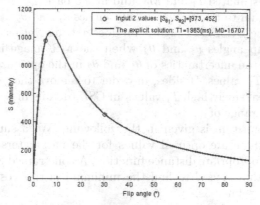

Fig. 1. The simulated plot of signal S from 2 acquisitions $(S_{\theta 1}, S_{\theta 2})$ with flip angles θ_1 and θ_2: $\theta_1 = 5°$, $\theta_2 = 30°$, TR = 15ms, acquired on a human brain

3   Optimized DESPOT1 Method

The basic *DESPOT1* algorithm provides an analytical solution for T_1 estimation. However, in the presence of noise, the analytical solution may not be the optimal value. For example, a background voxel (highly corrupted by noise) in a real brain image can get $S_{\theta 1}$ and $S_{\theta 2}$ equal to $S_{5°} = 7$ and $S_{30°} = 3$, leading to a T_1 value of 2245ms using *DESPOT1*. However, a calculated T_1 on a real gray matter voxel in the same image equals to 2493ms with $S_{5°} = 739$ and $S_{30°} = 298$. In this case, the T_1 values from the noise and from the signal are very close.

An intuitive method to suppress the influence of noise is to set thresholds to remove the background and skull signal before applying *DESPOT1*, and restrict T_1 estimation to a certain range [2]. However, choosing specific thresholds precludes the use of the method for multicenter studies, involving multiple MRI systems from different manufacturers with different image contrast and signal to noise ratio.

In this paper, we introduce an optimization algorithm to estimate the T_1 value without any prior knowledge on the images. In fact, if we consider the basic *DESPOT1* algorithm as an optimization process, the analytical solution of T_1 and M_0 from equation (2) is actually the solution of the following unconstraint cost function:

$$\underset{(\hat{T}_1, \hat{M}_0)}{\operatorname{argmin}} |\mathbf{S}_{\hat{\theta}} - \mathbf{S}_{\theta}|^2 \tag{5}$$

$$\mathbf{S}_{\hat{\theta}} = [S_{\hat{\theta}1}, S_{\hat{\theta}2}], \quad \mathbf{S}_{\theta} = [S_{\theta 1}, S_{\theta 2}]$$

$S_{\theta 1}$ and $S_{\theta 2}$ are the 2 input signals in Sect. 2. $S_{\hat{\theta}1}$ and $S_{\hat{\theta}2}$ are the 2 estimated signals following GRE equation

$$S_{\hat{\theta}} = \frac{\hat{M}_0(1 - \exp(-TR/\hat{T}_1))\sin\hat{\theta}}{(1 - \exp(-TR/\hat{T}_1)\cos\hat{\theta})} \tag{6}$$

$\hat{T}_1$ and $\hat{M}_0$ are the estimated T_1 and M_0, and in the basic *DESPOT1* algorithm, $\hat{\theta}_1$ and $\hat{\theta}_2$ are set equal to the prescribed flip angles θ_1 and θ_2.

However, the basic *DESPOT1* algorithm does not take into account the small variations of the flip angles θ_1 and θ_2 when the MR image is acquired. We propose to consider the uncertainties of $\hat{\theta}_1$ and $\hat{\theta}_2$ in the optimization algorithm to get the optimal T_1 values. Besides, in order to remove the possible negative T_1 values and the extremely high T_1 values in CSF (details in Sect. 4.1), we add a constraint for the range of $\hat{T}_1$.

The proposed algorithm is given in the following. We assume that, in the presence of noise, there are optimal values for the parameters $(\hat{T}_1, \hat{M}_0, \hat{\theta}_1, \hat{\theta}_2)$ with respect to an appropriate distance function. A constrained gradient descent optimization algorithm is used to find the minimum of this cost function. The distance function is defined as:

$$\underset{(\hat{\theta},\hat{T}_1,\hat{M}_0)}{\mathrm{argmin}} \left[\lambda|\hat{\theta} - \theta|^2 + (1 - \lambda)|\mathbf{S}_{\hat{\theta}} - \mathbf{S}_\theta|^2 \right] \tag{7}$$

with $\hat{\theta} = [\hat{\theta}_1, \hat{\theta}_2]$, $\theta = [\theta_1, \theta_2]$, $\mathbf{S}_{\hat{\theta}} = [S_{\hat{\theta}1}, S_{\hat{\theta}2}]$, $\mathbf{S}_\theta = [S_{\theta1}, S_{\theta2}]$

- $S_{\theta1}$ and $S_{\theta2}$ are the acquired MR images
- $S_{\hat{\theta}1}$ and $S_{\hat{\theta}2}$ are the estimated MR images
- θ_1 and θ_2 are the prescribed flip angles
- $\hat{\theta}_1$ and $\hat{\theta}_2$ are the estimated flip angles
- $\hat{T}_1$ and $\hat{M}_0$ are the estimated T_1 and M_0
- $\hat{\theta}$, $\hat{T}_1$, $\hat{M}_0$ and $S_{\hat{\theta}}$ follow the GRE equation (6)
- λ is a constant scale factor to balance the 2 terms in the distance function
- We constrain $\hat{T}_1$ in the range of $[1, 5000]$ based on prior knowledge on human body at 3T [9,4,12].

The algorithm starts from the initial values of $(\hat{T}_1 = 1, \hat{M}_0 = 0, \hat{\theta}_1 = \theta_1, \hat{\theta}_2 = \theta_2)$, and iteratively finds the first minimum. We allow the optimization to vary around nominal values of θ_1 and θ_2 because of the uncertainties on these parameters (modeled as noise here). We found that it is necessary to include the estimation of $\hat{\theta}_1$ and $\hat{\theta}_2$ in the distance function in order to get the optimal value of T_1.

4   Results

We tested our algorithm on in vivo MR acquisitions performed on a 3T Siemens Verio (VB17) scanner with a 32-ch head coil. T_1 relaxation was calculated based on two gradient echo sequences acquired with flip angles of 5° and 30° as well as a repetition time of 15ms [8]. The voxel size was $1.3 \times 1.3 \times 3.0\text{mm}^3$.

4.1   Synthetic Experimental Results on Sample Points

We found that our proposed algorithm is efficient to correct 3 typical types of errors in T_1 mapping.

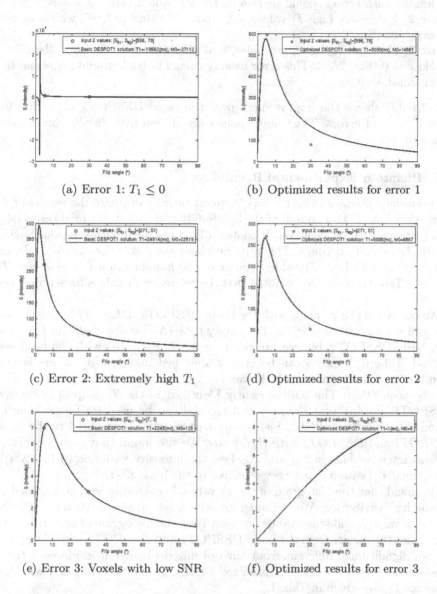

(a) Error 1: $T_1 \leq 0$

(b) Optimized results for error 1

(c) Error 2: Extremely high T_1

(d) Optimized results for error 2

(e) Error 3: Voxels with low SNR

(f) Optimized results for error 3

Fig. 2. Left column gives 3 different kinds of errors in the basic *DESPOT1* method. Right column gives the corresponding results of *optimized DESPOT1* algorithm. The $(S_{\theta 1}, S_{\theta 2})$ pairs are chosen from in vivo brain measurements.

Error 1: $T_1 \leq 0$ which is not possible (Fig. 2(a)). This error usually occurs in lesion and CSF areas. Since we are interested in the further study of these lesions, such errors should be removed before quantitative analysis.

Error 2: Extremely high T_1 values, e.g. above 20000ms in CSF, which are not expected (Fig. 2(c)).

Error 3: $S_{\theta 1}$ and $S_{\theta 2}$ are pure noise, and the estimated T_1 value should be close to 0 (Fig. 2(e)). This error usually occurs in background areas and the air-filled cavities in the skull.

Fig. 2(b,d,f) shows the improvement over the basic *DESPOT1* algorithm for these 3 types of errors. The sample points are chosen from in vivo brain measurements.

4.2   Phantom Experimental Results

We performed phantom experiments to quantitatively evaluate the results of T_1 estimation. The TO4 phantom of the SpinSafety test-objects[1] is made especially for T_1 accuracy assessment [11]. It contains 12 tubes filled with solutions having known T_1 relaxation times. The tube numbers are shown in Fig. 3(a). Tubes 1, 6, 9, 10 and 11 have T_1 values similar to the human brain (see reference T_1 values in Tab. 1). It should be noted that the reference T_1 values have a variance of 20%.

We compared the T_1 maps with the basic *DESPOT1*, *DESPOT1 with thresholds* and our algorithm (Fig. 3). The empty tube (Air) is not visible in Fig. 3(b) with basic *DESPOT1*, but we can see it clearly in Fig. 3(d) with the proposed method. Tube 6, 7 and 8 can be clearly identified in Fig. 3(d). There is also a bulb of the thermometer which was used to monitor the temperature during the acquisition. The bulb is clearly identified in the T_1 map of *optimized DESPOT1* showing that the proposed method can be used for target identification. *Optimized DESPOT1* yields improved results as compared to the basic *DESPOT1* and *DESPOT1 with thresholds*. We also found that even there is an obvious intensity bias in $S_{\theta 1}$ and $S_{\theta 2}$ (see the intensity variation in Fig. 3(a)), the estimated T_1 map is not very sensitive to the bias effect.

We found that the histogram of the T_1 values in each tube can be modeled as a Gaussian distribution. We utilize an iterative least squares method to estimate the mean value μ and standard deviation σ from the histogram of each tube. We found that the results from the basic *DESPOT1* and *DESPOT1 with thresholds* are not significantly different from our optimized algorithm inside each tube. The estimated μ and σ for the *optimized DESPOT1* method, together with the reference T_1, are given in Tab. 1.

The relative deviation (RD) is between 10% and 16% in all the cases. Given the fact that the reference T_1 value is known with 20% accuracy, we believe that the estimated μ falls well in the range of the reference value. The standard deviation is small (< 20) in most cases, except from tubes with high reference T_1

---

[1] The SpinSafety® test-objects (Spin Safety Ltd, Rennes, France) is a commercially available version of the Eurospin test-objects.

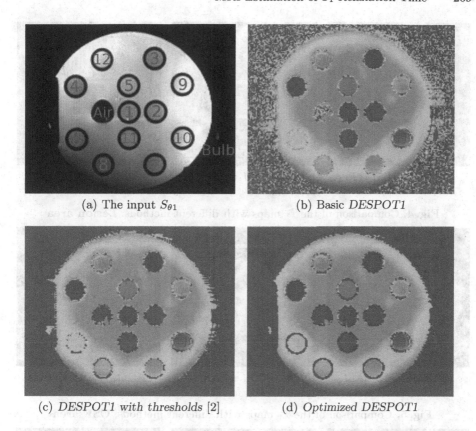

(a) The input $S_{\theta 1}$ (b) Basic *DESPOT1*

(c) *DESPOT1 with thresholds* [2]   (d) *Optimized DESPOT1*

Fig. 3. Comparison of the T_1 maps from the basic *DESPOT1*, *DESPOT1 with thresholds* and *optimized DESPOT1* on the TO4 SpinSafety phantom

Table 1. Quantitative analysis of the precision of T_1 map for the proposed method: R is the reference T_1 value (20% variance), μ the estimated mean value and δ the standard deviation for Gaussian modeling. RD is the relative deviation defined by $|\mu - R|/R$ (%)

Tube	R(ms)	Estimating T_1 (ms) μ	δ	RD (%)
1	107	94.6334	6.6591	11.5576
2	115	102.8524	3.4007	10.5631
3	98	86.4381	3.4564	11.7979
4	91	80.0732	3.6266	12.0075
5	162	143.2431	3.2002	11.5783
6	301	258.3710	6.6461	14.1624
7	360	309.7457	10.3142	13.9595
8	518	447.2865	18.0648	13.6513
9	703	599.4820	14.3356	14.7252
10	770	652.4993	24.4054	15.2598
11	1092	951.1581	40.9323	12.8976
12	719	607.3630	21.9891	15.5267

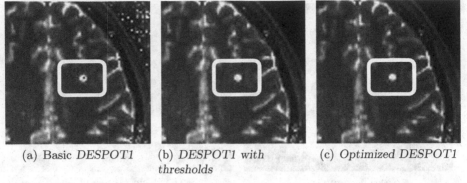

(a) Basic *DESPOT1*   (b) *DESPOT1 with*   (c) *Optimized DESPOT1*
                           thresholds

Fig. 4. Comparison of the T_1 maps with different methods: **Lesion area**

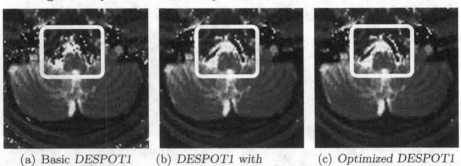

(a) Basic *DESPOT1*   (b) *DESPOT1 with*   (c) *Optimized DESPOT1*
                           thresholds

Fig. 5. Comparison of the T_1 maps with different methods: **CSF area**

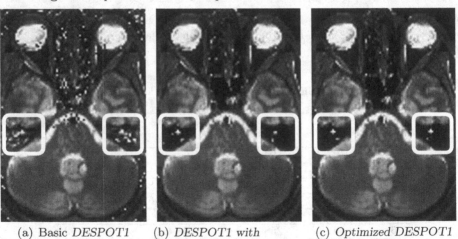

(a) Basic *DESPOT1*   (b) *DESPOT1 with*   (c) *Optimized DESPOT1*
                           thresholds

Fig. 6. Comparison of the T_1 maps with different methods: **Low SNR area**
DESPOT1 with thresholds and *optimized DESPOT1* remove the discontinuity effect
of black holes in lesions and CSF (near arteries). *Optimized DESPOT1* shows the best
performance to suppress noise in the lower part of the brain and preserve the tissue
signal with low SNR.

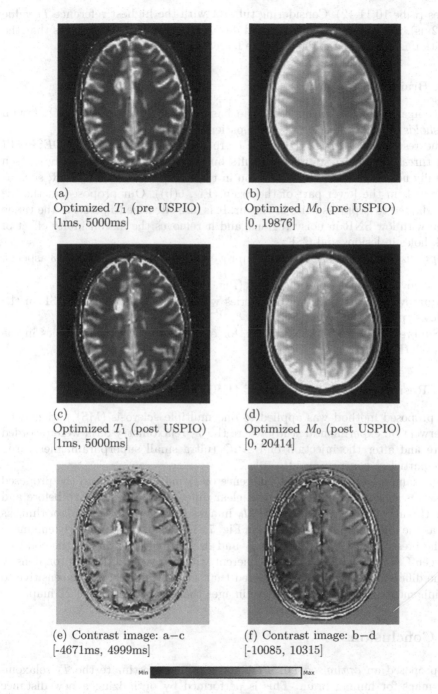

(a)
Optimized T_1 (pre USPIO)
[1ms, 5000ms]

(b)
Optimized M_0 (pre USPIO)
[0, 19876]

(c)
Optimized T_1 (post USPIO)
[1ms, 5000ms]

(d)
Optimized M_0 (post USPIO)
[0, 20414]

(e) Contrast image: a−c
[-4671ms, 4999ms]

(f) Contrast image: b−d
[-10085, 10315]

Min ▮▮▮▮▮▮▮▮▮▮ Max

Fig. 7. T_1 maps and M_0 images before and after the injection of USPIO. [min, max] gives the range of the colorbar for each image.

values (tube 10,11,12). Considering tube 11 with the highest reference T_1 value (1092ms), the corresponding standard deviation is over 40. This shows that the variation is increasing as the T_1 value increases.

4.3   Brain T_1 Mapping

We compared our algorithm with the basic *DESPOT1* and *DESPOT1 with thresholds* on multiple sclerosis (MS) patients.

The results of the basic *DESPOT1* are very sensitive to noise. *DESPOT1 with thresholds* shows improved results but the thresholds need to be chosen carefully not to preclude T_1 estimation in tissue regions with low SNR, such as the vessels in the lower part of the brain (Fig. 6(b)). Our proposed method is well adapted to suppress noise in the air. It is also effective to preserve the tissue signal with low SNR in noisy regions, and it removes the discontinuity effect of black holes in lesions and CSF.

Optimized DESPOT1 algorithm improves the brain T_1 mapping in 3 aspects.

1. Remove the black holes in lesions (Fig. 4).
2. Improve the identification of arteries which are surrounded by CSF in the lower part of the brain (Fig. 5).
3. Suppress noise in low SNR areas, for example the air filled cavities in the skull (Fig. 6).

4.4   Results on One MS Patient (USPIO)

The proposed method was applied to one multiple sclerosis (MS) patient who underwent on experimental study where the T_1 relaxometry data were recorded before and after the injection of USPIO (ultra small superparamagnetic iron oxide particles) contrast agent.

An example of the estimated difference of T_1 map according to the proposed method is shown in Fig. 7. We found clear difference in the T_1 map before and after the injection of USPIO. The M_0 images calculated by our algorithm, as well as the difference, are also given in Fig. 7. The lesion area is clearly enhanced by the presence of USPIO in both T_1 and M_0. On the M_0 image, the contrast between CSF and white matter is coherent with the variation of proton density in the different tissues. It can be noted that the M_0 image is more sensitive to the inhomogeneity bias in the native images than the quantitative T_1 map.

5   Conclusion

We proposed an *optimized DESPOT1* algorithm to estimate the T_1 relaxometry maps for human brain. This is performed by optimizing a new distance function to estimate the optimal values of T_1 and M_0 in presence of noise. A constraint gradient descent optimization algorithm is provided to give reliable T_1 estimation. Experimental results on phantom, synthetic relaxometry data and real brain measurements utilizing our algorithm show clear improvement over standard methods. Further work will focus on discussing the effect of initialization, the computation burden, extending the algorithm and assessing the method on a large database of MS patients. The framework will also be extended to T2 and T2* relaxometry mapping.

Acknowledgments. The study was supported by a grant from ARSEP and USPIO products were offered by BAYER-SCHERING. The authors would also like to thank the PRISM imaging platform for lending the test-objects.

References

1. Bagher-Ebadian, H., Jain, R., Paudyal, R., Nejad-Davarani, S.P., Narang, J., Jiang, Q., Mikkelsen, T., Ewing, J.R.: Magnetic resonance estimation of longitudinal relaxation time (T1) in spoiled gradient echo using an adaptive neural network. In: IJCNN, pp. 2557–2562 (2011)
2. Cao, F., Commowick, O., Bannier, E., Crimi, A., Barillot, C.: T1 and T2 mapping in patients with multiple sclerosis for project USPIO–6. In: ARSEP (June 2012)
3. Christensen, K.A., Grant, D.M., Schulman, E.M., Walling, C.: Optimal determination of relaxation times of fourier transform nuclear magnetic resonance. determination of spin-lattice relaxation times in chemically polarized species. J. Phys. Chem. 78(19), 1971–1977 (1974)
4. Dagia, C., Ditchfield, M.: 3t mri in paediatrics: challenges and clinical applications. Eur. J. Radiol. 68(2), 309–319 (2008)
5. Deichmann, R., Hahn, D., Haase, A.: Fast T1 mapping on a whole-body scanner. MRM 42(1), 206–209 (1999)
6. Deoni, S., Rutt, B., Peters, T.: Rapid combined T1 and T2 mapping using gradient recalled acquisition in the steady state. MRM 49(3), 515–526 (2003)
7. Deoni, S.C.L., Peters, T.M., Rutt, B.K.: Determination of optimal angles for variable nutation proton magnetic spin-lattice, T1, and spin-spin, T2, relaxation times measurement. MRM 51(1), 194–199 (2004)
8. Ferré, J.C., Tourbah, A., Berry, I., Barillot, C., Freeman, L., Galanaud, D., Maarouf, A., Pelletier, J., Portefaix, C., Ranjeva, J.P., Wiest-Daesslé, N., Edan, G.: MRI USPIO analysis in 35 clinically isolated syndrome patients. In: ECTRIMS 2011 vol. (5), pp. 399–416 (2011)
9. Gelman, N., Gorell, J., Barker, P., Savage, R., Spickler, E., Windham, J., Knight, R.: MR imaging of human brain at 3.0T: preliminary report on transverse relaxation rates and relation to estimated iron content. Radiology 210(3), 759–767 (1999)
10. Lee, C., Baker, E., Thomasson, D.: Normal Regional T1 and T2 Relaxation Times of the Brain at 3T, p. 959 (2006)
11. Ollivro, S., Eliat, P., Hitti, E., Tran, L., de Certaines, J., Saint-Jalmes, H.: Preliminary MRI quality assessment and device acceptance guidelines for a multicenter bioclinical study: The GO glioblastoma project. J. Neuroimaging (2011)
12. Stanisz, G., Odrobina, E., Pun, J., Escaravage, M., Graham, S., Bronskill, M., Henkelman, R.: T1, T2 relaxation and magnetization transfer in tissue at 3T. MRM 54(3), 507–512 (2005)

13. Tofts, P.: Quantitative MRI of the Brain: Measuring Changes Caused by Disease. John Wiley & Sons, Ltd. (2003)
14. Vaithianathar, L., Tench, C.R., Morgan, P.S., Constantinescu, C.S.: Magnetic resonance imaging of the cervical spinal cord in multiple sclerosis–a quantitative T1 relaxation time mapping approach. J. Neurology 250(3), 307–315 (2003)
15. Wang, H.Z., Riederer, S.J., Lee, J.N.: Optimizing the precision in T1 relaxation estimation using limited flip angles. MRM 5(5), 399–416 (1987)
16. Wang, J., Qiu, M., Kim, H., Constable, R.T.: T1 measurements incorporating flip angle calibration and correction in vivo. J. Magn. Reson. 182(2), 283–292 (2006)

Robust Cerebral Blood Flow Map Estimation in Arterial Spin Labeling

Camille Maumet[1,2,3,4], Pierre Maurel[1,2,3,4], Jean-Christophe Ferré[1,2,3,4,5], and Christian Barillot[1,2,3,4]

[1] University of Rennes 1, Faculty of medicine, F-35043 Rennes, France
[2] INSERM, U746, F-35042 Rennes, France
[3] CNRS, IRISA, UMR 6074, F-35042 Rennes, France
[4] Inria, VISAGES project-team, F-35042 Rennes, France
[5] CHU Rennes, Department of Neuroradiology, F-35033 Rennes, France

Abstract. Non-invasive measurement of Cerebral Blood Flow (CBF) is now feasible thanks to the introduction of Arterial Spin Labeling (ASL) Magnetic Resonance Imaging (MRI) techniques. To date, the low signal-to-noise ratio of ASL gives us no option but to repeat the acquisition in order to accumulate enough data to get a reliable signal. Perfusion signal is usually extracted by averaging across the repetitions. However, due to its zero breakdown point, the sample mean is very sensitive to outliers. A single outlier can thus have strong detrimental effects on the sample mean estimate.

In this paper, we propose to estimate robust ASL CBF maps by means of M-estimators to overcome the deleterious effects of outliers. The behavior of this method is compared to z-score thresholding as recommended in [8]. Validation on simulated and real data is provided. Quantitative validation is undertaken by measuring the correlation with the most widespread technique to measure perfusion with MRI: Dynamic Susceptibility weighted Contrast (DSC).

1 Introduction

Arterial Spin Labeling (ASL), a Magnetic Resonance Imaging (MRI) technique introduced in the early 1990s, allows non-invasive quantification of Cerebral Blood Flow (CBF) [2]. Contrary to Dynamic Susceptibility weighted Contrast (DSC), the most widespread technique to measure perfusion with MRI, ASL does not rely on the injection of an exogenous contrast agent.

During the ASL acquisition, blood water, used as an endogenous tracer, is labeled with a radio-frequency pulse in the neck of the patient. After a delay of a few hundred of milliseconds, called inversion time, a labeled image of the brain is acquired. A control image is acquired without prior labeling and the difference between control and label image leads to a perfusion weighted image. A model is then applied to this image to obtain a quantification of CBF. Besides the absence of allergic reaction risk compared to DSC, ASL is particularly well suited for longitudinal studies or studies on patients with difficult venous access

P.-T. Yap et al. (Eds.): MBIA 2012, LNCS 7509, pp. 215–224, 2012.

such as children. However this comes at the cost of low signal to noise ratio (SNR) and lower spatial resolution than DSC.

Due to the low SNR of the ASL sequence, a single pair of control and label image is not sufficient to measure perfusion. The acquisition is usually repeated several times, leading to R pairs of images (usually R≥30). Perfusion information is then usually extracted by pair-wise subtracting the control and label images and averaging across the repetitions.

Though sample average, as an unbiased estimate of mean, ensures convergence as R grows, it has a zero breakdown point and is thus very sensitive to outliers. In particular, sudden subject motion may not be correctly corrected by registration and cause strong corolla-shaped artefacts. To avoid the detrimental effects that a few abnormal repetitions could have in the final perfusion map, it is often suggested to ignore the volumes corresponding to the motion peaks using an appropriate threshold [7]. However the choice of these thresholds is empirical and there is no common rule across studies nor automatic methods to tune these ad-hoc parameters. In [8], the authors proposed an automatic algorithm for outlier rejection in ASL perfusion series based on z-score thresholding at the volume (or slice) level. Their method produced satisfactory results on a qualitative validation based on ratings made by medical experts.

How to appropriately deal with outliers has been largely studied in the statistical literature and a large range of methods has emerged. Z-score is known to be sensitive upon sample size and is suffering from masking effects when more than one outliers is present in the serie [6]. Indeed, in a dataset containing more than one outlier, the standard deviation estimate will be artificially inflated which may prevent z-score based outlier detection. On the other hand, M-estimators are robust techniques to estimate location and scale in the presence of outliers [5]. We focus on Huber's M-estimator [3], as it is the most widely used.

In this paper, we propose to estimate robust ASL CBF maps by means of Huber's M-estimator. This method is compared to z-thresholding as proposed in [8]. Validation is undertaken by measuring the voxel-to-voxel correlation between ASL CBF maps and DSC CBF maps as an affine relationship is expected between these estimates of CBF [9].

Section 2 presents the statistical methods and the validation procedure. Section 3 presents the results on simulated data and on real datasets from patients diagnosed with brain tumors.

2 Material and Methods

2.1 Robust CBF Map Creation

Starting from a perfusion-weighted serie, namely a 4D volume made of the R repetitions obtained after pair-wise subtracting the control and label scans, the objective is to compute a single perfusion weighted volume. This section presents z-score thresholding and M-estimators as statistical method to compute robust CBF maps.

Z-Score Thresholding. In [8], an outlier rejection algorithm based on z-scores is proposed in order to remove outliers from the perfusion-weighted serie. The outlier rejection is performed both on a volume-by-volume and a slice-by-slice basis. For each volume (respectively slices) v, the mean μ_v and standard deviation σ_v of in-brain voxel intensities is computed. Assuming a gaussian distribution of μ_v and σ_v, a volume is then rejected if:

$$|\mu_v| > \text{avg}_{i=1}^R(\mu_i) + 2.5 \ \text{avg}_{i=1}^R(\mu_i),$$
$$\text{or} \ \ \sigma_v > \text{avg}_{i=1}^R(\sigma_i) + 1.5 \ \text{std}_{i=1}^R(\sigma_i) \tag{1}$$

where avg and std stand for the sample mean and sample standard deviation. The constants 1.5 and 2.5 were determined empirically. To avoid over-filtering, series verifying $\ln(\max_{i=1}^R(\sigma_i) - \min_{i=1}^R(\sigma_i)) < 1$ are not searched for outliers. Once the outliers are identified, the perfusion map is then computed by averaging the remaining repetitions.

M-Estimators. Another solution to deal with outliers is to employ robust statistics such as M-estimators, which will not be overly influenced by outliers. In [3], M-estimators are defined, given a function ρ, as solutions $\hat{\theta}$ of:

$$\hat{\theta} = \underset{\theta}{\text{argmin}}\left(\sum_{i=1}^n \rho(x_i, \theta)\right). \tag{2}$$

If ρ is differentiable, and ψ is its derivative then eq. (2) can be solved by finding the root of:

$$\sum_{i=1}^n \psi(x_i, \theta) = 0. \tag{3}$$

The sample average can be seen as an M-estimator with $\rho(x_i, \theta) = (x_i - \theta)^2$ and $\psi(x_i, \theta) = 2(x_i - \theta)$ leading to $\hat{\theta} = \frac{\sum_{i=1}^n x_i}{N}$.

The M-estimator of location proposed by Huber in [3] is defined by:

$$\psi(x_i, \theta) = \gamma\left(\frac{x_i - \theta}{\sigma}\right) \quad \text{where } \gamma(x) = \begin{cases} -k, & x < -k \\ x, & -k < x < k \\ k, & x > k \end{cases} \tag{4}$$

k will be set to 1.345 throughout this paper corresponding to 95% efficiency in gaussian data [4]. Likewise, σ is estimated by a robust estimator: the median absolute deviation divided by 0.6745. Huber's M-estimator is applied voxel by voxel on the perfusion weighted serie to obtain the robust perfusion weighted map.

2.2   Validation

Simulated Data. In order to assess the efficiency of each technique, we generated simulated data with a known quantity of outliers based on two real datasets. Outliers were drawn from a uniform distribution with extrema (-100;100). These values were determined empirically. Indeed, in an uncorrupted perfusion-weighted map, the values usually range between -10 and +10 and voxel standard deviation can in fact be up to 50. Also, by looking at the values of identified outliers in a real dataset, we found values as big as 300 in absolute value.

As data corruption usually affects multiple voxels per volume [8], outlier simulation was undertaken by corrupting from 0% to 50% percent of the volumes. We will refer lately to these volumes as outlier volumes. Then, 2%, 20% or 50% of the voxels in each outlier volume were replaced by random outliers leading to low, medium and high level of volume corruption respectively. Each simulation was repeated 30 times in order to get estimates of the standard deviation. Simulated data were based on two real datasets as described below.

The first dataset was a perfusion-weighted serie with a large number of repetitions, R=250, from a healthy subject. The perfusion-weighted map obtained by averaging the 250 repetitions was considered as the ground truth. The 60 first volumes of the serie were extracted and used as dataset for robust CBF map estimation. The quality of the maps produced by each method was measured in term of sum of square difference (SSD) with the estimated ground truth.

The second dataset was built on the perfusion-weighted map of one patient diagnosed with a brain tumor. The original ASL CBF map of this subject presented few artefacts identified by visual inspection and a very low level of motion (<0.5mm and $<0.2°$ in all directions). As DSC is currently the reference method to estimate perfusion with MRI, the quality of the maps produced by each method was measured by computing the Pearson linear correlation coefficient with the DSC CBF map. This assumes an affine relationship between CBF maps produced by ASL and DSC [9].

Experiments on Real Clinical Data Sets. The efficiency of both algorithms was estimated on a dataset of 14 perfusion-weighted maps of patients diagnosed with brain tumors. The quality of the ASL CBF map was assessed by voxel-to-voxel correlation with the DSC CBF map.

2.3 Data

Data: 14 patients diagnosed with brain tumors were involved in this study. Data acquisition was performed on a 3T Siemens Verio MR scanner with a 32-channel head-coil. Patients were scanned in the context of clinical practice. The imaging protocol included a 3D T1-weighted anatomical sequence (TR: 1900ms, TE: 2.27ms, FOV: 256 x 256 x 176mm^3, flip angle: 9°, resolution: 1 x 1 x 1mm^3), a PICORE Q2TIPS sequence with crusher gradients (TR: 3000ms, TE: 18ms, FOV: 192 x 192mm^2, flip angle: 90°, in plane resolution: 3x3mm^2, slice thickness: 7mm, inter-slice gap: 0.7mm, TI: 1700ms, TI_{wd}: 700ms, R = 60), a DSC sequence (GRE EPI, TR: 1500ms, TE: 30ms, FOV: 230 x 230mm^2, flip angle: 90°, in plane resolution: 1.8 x 1.8mm^2, slice thickness: 4mm, inter-slice gap: 1.2mm) and 3D T1-weighted post gadolinium sequence (TR: 1900ms, TE: 2.27ms, flip angle: 9°, FOV: 250 x 250 x 176mm^3, resolution: 1 x 1 x 1mm^3).

1 healthy subject was involved in this study, the imaging protocol included a 3D T1-weighted anatomical sequence (same parameters as above) and a PICORE Q2TIPS sequence with crusher gradients (TR: 2500ms, TE: 19ms, flip angle: 90°, in plane resolution: 3x3mm^2, slice thickness: 7mm, inter-slice gap: 0.7mm, TI: 1800ms, TI_{wd}: 700ms, R = 250).

Pre-processing: Image pre-processing was performed using SPM8 (Wellcome Department of Imaging Neuroscience, University College, London) Matlab toolbox. A six-parameter rigid-body registration of the ASL volumes was carried out in order to reduce undesired effects due to subject motion. Coregistration on grey matter map was then performed based on normalised mutual information. The average of unlabeled volumes was used to estimate the geometrical transformation to apply to each volume.

The 60 unlabeled and labeled ASL volumes were pair-wise subtracted in order to obtain a perfusion weighted serie per subject. Robust ASL perfusion-weighted map was then carried out as described in section 2. A standard kinetic model [1] was then applied in order to obtain quantitative ASL CBF maps.

The DSC images were processed using MR manufacturer software by manually choosing an arterial input function to calculate CBF and mean transit time maps. Similarly to ASL, DSC CBF maps were coregistered on grey matter maps.

3 Results

3.1 Validation on Simulated Data

Dataset with 250 Repetitions: Figure 1 presents the simulation study based on a healthy subject data. The performances of sample average, z-score thresholding [8], and Huber's M-estimator are assessed by measuring the SSD of the ASL CBF map with the ground truth estimated by averaging a large number of repetitions.

As described in fig. 1, with a medium or a high level of corruption, z-score thresholding and Huber's M-estimator perform equally and better than averaging until 20% of volumes are corrupted. If more than 20% of the volumes are affected by outliers, then M-estimators provide better estimates than both z-score thresholding and averaging. The robust M-estimator CBF map is closer to the ground truth and less sensitive in an increase in the number of outliers. The same behavior is observed with a low number of corrupted voxels per volume except that the separation point is at 5% of corrupted volumes instead of 20%. The lower performances of z-thresholding when the number of corrupted volumes exceed 20% (or 5% with low corruption) is a consequence of the masking effect which penalize this estimator when several outliers are present in the serie. Moreover, the performance of Huber's M-estimator always depicts a smaller variance than z-thresholding.

Both Huber's M-estimator and z-score thresholding provide better estimate than the sample average. As the level of corruption per volume decreases, the separation point between Huber's M-estimator and z-score thresholding tends to become lower. This can probably be explained by the fact that the method proposed in [8] is based on a global mean and standard deviation estimate per volume (or slice) and is therefore less suited to detect lowly corrupted volumes.

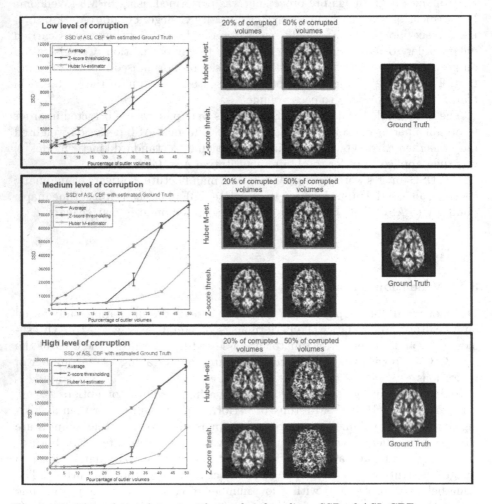

Fig. 1. Healthy subject dataset with simulated outliers: SSD of ASL CBF map, computed by M-estimator, z-score thresholding [8] and sample average, with the estimated ground truth. Low, medium and high level of volume corruption, from 0% to 50% of corrupted volumes. In all configuration Huber's M-estimators is either better or as good as z-thresholding to estimate robust CBF maps. In the presence of outliers, Huber's M-estimator is always more accurate than the sample average.

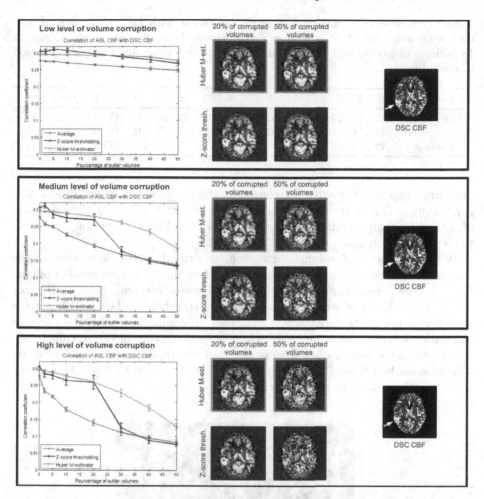

Fig. 2. Patient dataset with simulated outliers: correlation of ASL CBF map, computed by M-estimator, z-score thresholding [8] and sample average, with the DSC CBF map. Low, medium and high level of volume corruption, from 0% to 50% of corrupted volumes. The white arrow points the tumor site. A similar behavior as for healthy subject simulation (fig. 1) is observed outlining that correlation with DSC CBF is a valuable indicator to measure the quality of the ASL CBF estimates.

Simulation Based on Pathological Data: Figure 2 presents the simulation study based on pathological data of a subject suffering from a brain tumor. The performances of sample average, z-score thresholding [8], and Huber's M-estimator are assessed by measuring the correlation coefficient of ASL CBF with DSC CBF.

The simulation involving a high level of volume corruption leads to very similar results than the one obtained in the previous section on healthy subject data. Both Huber's M-estimator and z-thresholding perform better than averaging until 20% of corrupted volumes. After this threshold, z-thresholding performances

Table 1. Real clinical dataset: correlation coefficient with DSC CBF map of ASL CBF map computed by M-estimator, z-score thresholding [8] and sample average in 14 patients diagnosed with brain tumors. Last column: mean and standard deviation across subjects.

Patients	1	2	3	4	5	6	7	8	9	10	11	12	13	14	Mean ± std.
Huber M-est.	.45	.32	.29	.51	.52	.34	.28	.12	.14	.27	.35	.16	.17	.17	.29 ± .13
z-score thresh.	.45	.24	.27	.53	.51	.35	.28	.15	.14	.30	.35	.18	.16	.20	.29 ± .13
Average	.46	.25	.20	.42	.52	.31	.25	.12	.14	.25	.32	.13	.17	.12	.26 ± .13

drop until reaching the same correlation as the sample average for 30% of outlier volumes. This result suggests that correlation with DSC is a good measure of ASL CBF map quality. For medium level of volume corruption, the same tendency is observable.

With a low level of volume corruption, the trend is less clear. Overall the correlation coefficient seems much less affected by the increasing number of outliers. Z-score thresholding and Huber's M-estimator are both better estimator of the mean than the sample average. Z-score thresholding however displays a higher variance in its performance estimates. In comparison with the previous simulation study, there is probably a higher level of noise in the so-called "uncorrupted" pathological data than in the "uncorrupted" healthy subject data. The inherent higher level of noise in pathological data might prevent the correct detection of low level of volume corruption.

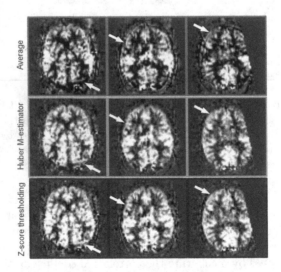

Fig. 3. Example of robust CBF map in one patient: three contiguous axial slices are depicted. White arrows outlines large artefacts presents in the averaged perfusion-weighted map and correctly corrected by both z-score thresholding and M-estimator.

3.2 Validation on Real Data

Table 1 presents the correlation coefficient obtained for 14 patients diagnosed with brain tumors. Overall, there is a significant improvement of both Huber's M-estimator (p=0.007) and z-score thresholding (p=0.010) over the sample average (paired two sample t-test). In this dataset, there was no significant difference between the two filtering methods (paired t-test p=0.84).

Fig. 3 presents an example of robust ASL CBF maps in which motion artefacts are significantly reduced by both Huber's M-estimator and z-thresholding.

4 Conclusion

We studied the ability of Huber's M-estimator to compute robust CBF maps in ASL. The behavior of this estimator was studied in both simulated and real clinical datasets and compared to an outlier removal technique based on z-thresholding previously introduced in the ASL literature [8].

Out of this study, it is confirmed that outlier filtering, either via outlier removal or M-estimation, provides more robust CBF maps than the sample average. Though, on real clinical datasets, both robust methods performed equally, the simulation study clearly stated the superior robustness of M-estimators over z-score thresholding. Overall Huber's M-estimates are either as good as or better than z-thresholding and are always less variable.

As M-estimators are able to deal with a broader range of outliers, we recommend the use of M-estimators as robust method to compute ASL CBF maps. This study focused on patients diagnosed with brain tumors, as DSC sequence is part of their routine clinical protocol. Other pathologies might be related with different outlier patterns and a larger validation study on real datasets is therefore needed in order to outline the cases in which M-estimator will have a significantly better behavior than z-thresholding. Future work will also investigate the effect of other types of M-estimators like Tukey's Biweight.

References

1. Buxton, R.B., Frank, L.R., Wong, E.C., Siewert, B., Warach, S., Edelman, R.R.: A general kinetic model for quantitative perfusion imaging with arterial spin labeling. Magnetic Resonance in Medicine 40(3), 383–396 (1998)
2. Detre, J.A., Leigh, J.S., Williams, D.S., Koretsky, A.P.: Perfusion imaging. Magnetic Resonance in Medicine 23, 37–45 (1992)
3. Huber, P.: Robust estimation of a location parameter. The Annals of Mathematical Statistics (1964)
4. Krasker, W.S., Welsch, R.E.: Efficient bounded-influence regression estimation. Journal of the American Statistical Association 77(379), 595–604 (1982)
5. Rousseeuw, P., LeRoy, A.: Robust Regression and Outlier Detection. Wiley series in probability and mathematical statistics. Probability and mathematical statistics. Wiley-Interscience (2003)
6. Shiffler, R.: Maximum Z scores and outliers. The American Statistician (1988)

7. Sidaros, K., Olofsson, K., Miranda, M.J., Paulson, O.B.: Arterial spin labeling in the presence of severe motion. Journal of Cerebral Blood Flow and Metabolism (2005)
8. Tan, H., Maldjian, J.A., Pollock, J.M., Burdette, J.H., Yang, L.Y., Deibler, A.R., Kraft, R.A.: A fast, effective filtering method for improving clinical pulsed arterial spin labeling MRI. Journal of Magnetic Resonance Imaging 29(5), 1134–1139 (2009)
9. Warmuth, C., Günther, M., Zimmer, C.: Quantification of Blood Flow in Brain Tumors: Comparison of Arterial Spin Labeling and Dynamic Susceptibility-weighted Contrast-enhanced MR Imaging. Radiology 228(4), 523–532 (2003)

Author Index